Current Concepts in Orthopaedic Surgery
Consulting Editor: P. Bedeschi

Volume 2

The Elbow

Traumatic Lesions

Editor: L. Celli
Translator: A. Warr

Springer-Verlag Wien GmbH

Luigi Celli, M.D.
Orthopaedic Surgeon, Head of the 2nd Orthopaedic Clinic, University of Modena, Italy
Paolo Bedeschi, M.D.
Director of the Institute of Clinical Orthopaedics, University of Modena, Italy
Amy Warr
Bachelor of Arts in History, Brown University, U.S.A.

Translation from the Italian edition
Il Gomito. Patologia traumatica
© by Aulo Gaggi Editore, Bologna

ISBN 978-3-7091-4129-8   ISBN 978-3-7091-4127-4 (eBook)
DOI 10.1007/978-3-7091-4127-4

Sole distribution rights: Springer-Verlag Wien-New York

With 476 Figures (170 single illustrations)

CONTENTS

Introduction

P. Bedeschi

This is the second volume in the monographic series *Current Concepts in Orthopaedic Surgery*, published with customary distinction by Aulo Gaggi, under the direction of the Institute of Clinical Orthopaedics and Traumatology of the University of Modena.

The subject of this text, "Traumatic lesions of the elbow", is very current and we believe it worthy of more attention than it has received in recent years.

The text begins with a chapter on the physiopathology of the elbow, which is important because of some interesting links between trauma and functional damage as well as between some traumatic lesions and consequent treatment.

Next are two important chapters on overwork syndromes of the elbow, which are mostly of microtraumatic origin and affect the periarticular musculotendinous, osteoarticular, and nerve structures.

A careful study of these two chapters will provide a clear understanding of the etiologic and pathogenetic stages, the clinical features, and the differential therapeutic indications.

Traumatic lesions of the elbow in children are dealt with separately, since the nature of the damage, the therapeutic approach, and the possible long-term complications are quite different in a growing child than in an adult.

The traumatic lesions in the adult are first classified and then analyzed in several chapters: distal humeral, proximal ulnar, and proximal radial fractures, dislocations, fracture-dislocations, and Monteggia lesions.

Each chapter is interesting because it reflects an important personal experience and contains an honest critical evaluation of the results.

The two following chapters give an updated analysis of the neural and vascular complications of elbow trauma from a pathogenetic, clinical, and therapeutic standpoint.

The next chapter is an update on nonunions of the elbow with special reference to therapeutic problems.

The difficulty of long-term evaluation of treatment of radial head fractures is examined in two interesting chapters that describe the long-term results of radial head resection and prosthetic replacement.

The next few chapters deal with a very current topic — treatment of postraumatic stiffness of the elbow. Problems related to arthroscopic and surgical arthrolysis, arthroplasty, and prosthetic replacement are discussed in detail.

The next chapter discusses the role of physical therapy in the treatment of postraumatic elbow stiffness, followed by a chapter of conclusions by Professor Lamberto Perugia.

I believe that a careful reading of this text will serve not only as an update for orthopaedic surgeons, but also as a stimulating, in-depth examination of as yet unresolved diagnostic and therapeutic problems in the field of traumatic lesions of the elbow.

Anatomophysiopathology of the elbow

A. Mingione - F. Barca

While the shoulder directs the spatial movement of the upper limb, the elbow, with its wide range of movements, steers the hand in desired directions, bringing food to the mouth, facilitating the grasp with adjustments in height and length, and guiding the hand to the most functional position.

These spatial abilities constitute a relatively recent acquisition for humans in the context of their evolution from stooping quadripeds to stooping bipeds and finally to upright bipeds.

Upright posture is achieved by the torsion of the distal humeral head on the axis of the proximal humeral epiphysis (Figs. 1,2); this explains the present anatomical status of the trochlea *and the pronation occurring in cases of obstetric paralysis due to lack of torsion of the distal head* (7).

From a strictly anatomical standpoint the elbow joint is unique, since it is encased in a single capsule (8,15); the joint cavity reaches its maximum capacity in moderate flexion, when neither the anterior nor the posterior portion is tense.

The capsule is reinforced by two collateral ligaments (8,15), whose function is to contain the joint and prevent lateral movement (Fig. 1).

The **ulnar collateral ligament**, the stronger of the two, arises from the medial epicondyle and divides into three bundles (Fig. 3):

a) the **anterior** bundle reinforces the orbicular ligament by means of its insertion on the anteromedial side of the coronoid process;

b) the **middle** bundle, or Poirier's ligament *de l'entorse*, is the most powerful and inserts on the medial side of the coronoid process;

c) the **posterior**, or Bardinet's, bundle is reinforced by the transverse fibers of Cooper's ligament, and moves toward the medial side of the olecranon.

Whatever the position of the joint, two of the three bundles are always tense.

The **radial collateral ligament** (Fig. 4) inserts centrally on the orbicular ligament, and the anterior and posterior faces insert on the edges of the radial surface of the ulna. It arises from the lateral epicondyle and divides into three bundles:

a) the **anterior** bundle reinforces the

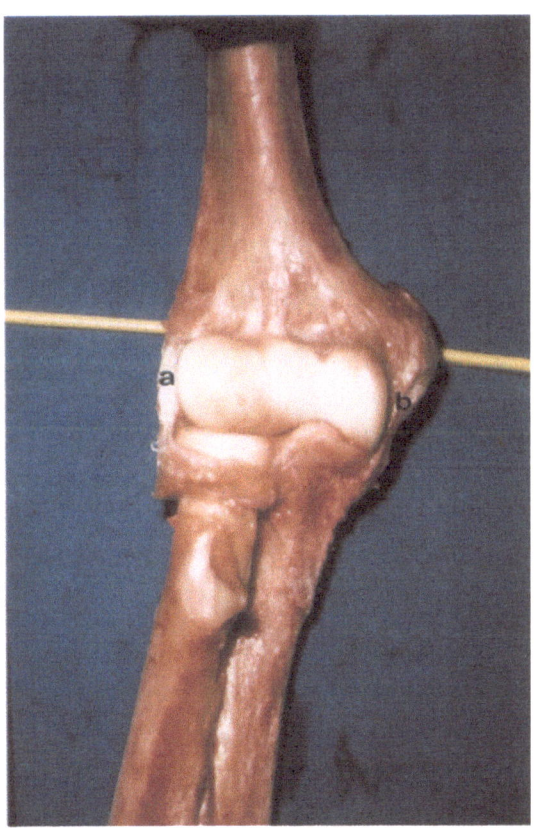

Fig. 1. - Anterior view of the elbow joint showing a) the radial collateral ligament and b) the ulnar collateral ligament.

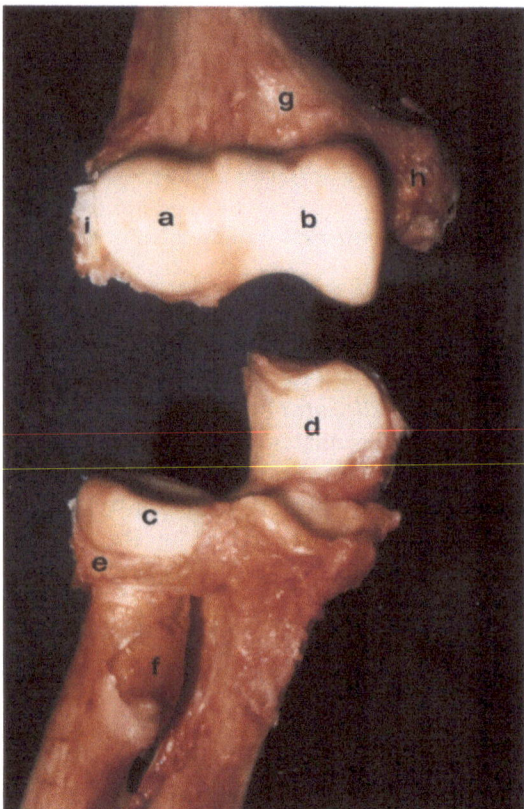

Fig. 2. - Anterior view of the individual joint components: a) capitulum, b) trochlea, c) radial head, d) semilunar notch, e) orbicular ligament, f) distal insertion of biceps, g) coronoid fossa, h) medial epicondyle, i) lateral epicondyle.

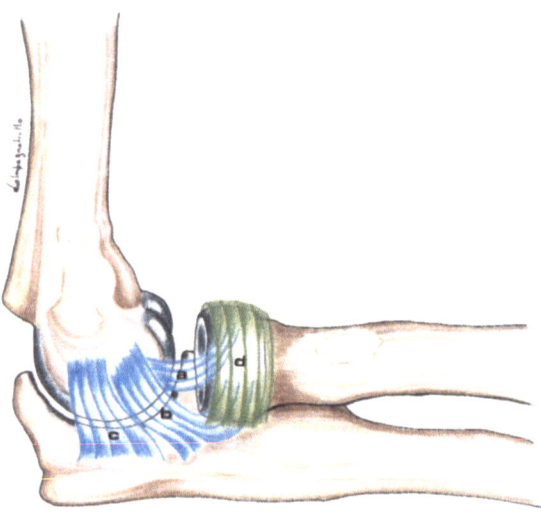

Fig. 4. - Radial collateral ligament: a) anterior bundle, b) middle bundle, c) posterior bundle, d) orbicular ligament.

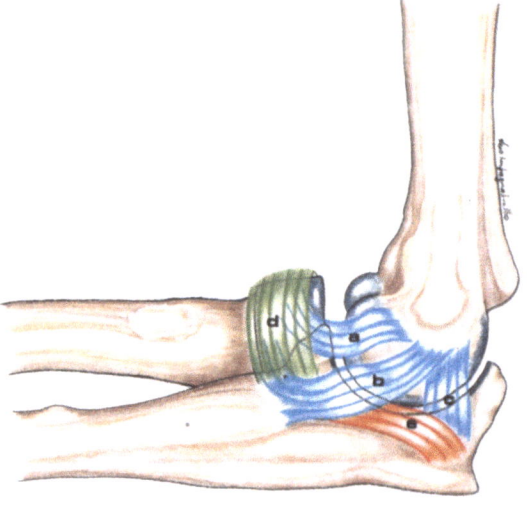

Fig. 3. - Ulnar collateral ligament: a) anterior bundle, b) middle bundle, c) posterior bundle, d) orbicular ligament, e) Cooper's ligament.

anterior portion of the orbicular ligament by inserting on the radial groove of the ulna;

b) the **middle** bundle posteriorly reinforces the orbicular ligament;

c) the **posterior** bundle covers the lateral side of the olecranon.

The radial collateral ligament tightens the orbicular ligament and helps regulate flexion and extension in the humeroulnar joint. *The anterior bundle of the ulnar collateral ligament and the anterior and middle bundles of the radial collateral ligament, which insert on the orbicular ligament may retract during trauma, impairing pronation- supination.*

The collateral ligaments also limit flexion and extension, *while their deficit can cause lateral instability of the elbow.* In particular, the collateral ligaments are especially tight in extension while the middle and posterior bundles are loose, and in flexion the contrary occurs.

Other capsular reinforcements also exist.

The ulnar collateral ligament is reinforced by the flexors of the forearm, which detach from the epitrochlea while several fibers of the supinator muscle join at the radial collateral ligament; the anterior portion of the capsule is covered by the brachialis muscle, whose deep fibers become a part of its framework, as if it were a true elbow joint muscle.

The epicondylar extensor carpi radialis muscles cover the radial head, with the extensor brevis especially adhering very closely to the capsule.

Finally, the posterior capsular wall is covered by the anconeus and more internally by the tendon of the triceps.

From a functional standpoint the elbow is a complex joint in which three main components must be considered (Figs 1,2):

1) the **humeroulnar component**, a hinge joint;

2) the **humeroradial** component, a gliding joint;

3) the **proximal radioulnar** component, a pivot joint

HUMEROULNAR JOINT

The flexion and extension of the elbow are made possible by the articulation of the semilunar notch of the ulna with the humeral trochlea (Figs. 1-2).

The latter is shaped like a section of a screw (6) (Fig. 6), anteriorly vertical (Fig. 2), oblique at the bottom and posteriorly bulging (Fig. 9A); therefore, in extension-supination (Fig. 7 A, B) the posterior portion, which juts obliquely outward, brings the forearm into a valgus angulation of about 20 degrees.

At maximum extension, the diaphyseal axes of the humerus and ulna (Fig. 7 A, B) form an obtuse angle facing outward, bisected by a line passing through the distal epiphysis of the humerus, which is responsible for flexion and extension.

The valgus angulation of the elbow helps to protect and unload the humeroradial joint; pressure along the longitudinal axis of the extended limb decreases as the limb is supinated. Thus the ulnar collateral ligament is, paradoxically, stressed in tension due to the "cubital angle".

While extended, the limb can exhibit an outward-facing valgus angulation of up to 158 degrees, which disappears in pronation (Fig. 8A) because after the radial shaft passes over the ulna, moving from a parallel to an oblique position, it comes into a medial position with respect to the ulna (Fig. 8B).

In flexion (Fig. 9 A, B), the anterior vertical portion of the trochlear groove (Figs. 1-2) guides the forearm, bringing it to be perfectly superimposed on the arm. The forearm rotates on its longitudinal anatomical axis during flexion and extension whatever the degree of pronation or supination; this explains how *a rotation or linear shift of a distal fragment of the humerus has no effect upon the humerus-forearm relationship in flexion and extension unless inclination is also involved.*

The singular anatomical structure of the trochlea produces an internal rotation of 5 degrees at the start of flexion, balanced by an external rotation of 5 degrees at maximum flexion.

Such rotatory mobility explains the frequency of prosthetic loosening.

Flexion is aided by the 45 degree angle formed anteriorly by the distal head and shaft of the humerus (Fig. 10), like the anterior-facing 45 degree angle formed by the semilunar

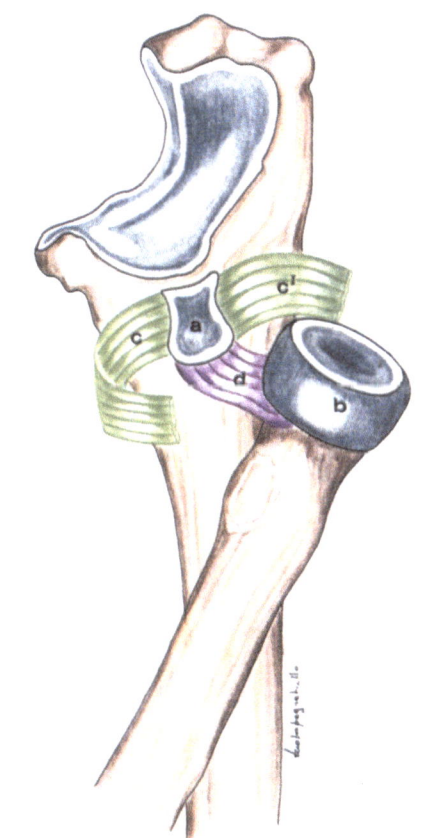

Fig. 5. - Proximal radioulnar joint: a) radial notch, b) radial head, c,c') open orbicular ligament, d) Denucé quadrate ligament.

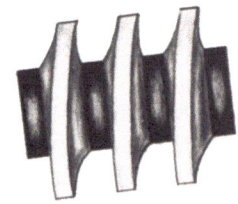

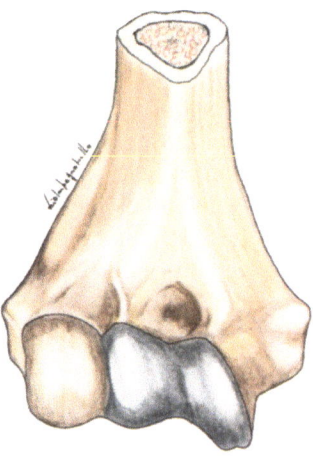

notch and the shaft of the ulna; thus the coronoid process slips into its fossa only when the arm and forearm are parallel.

In reality, the entrance of the coronoid process into the coronoid fossa never occurs because active movement is limited by muscular mass to 145 degrees; passive movement can reach 160 degrees, but is then limited by the impact of both the radial head upon the radial fossa and the coronoid process upon the coronoid fossa, the increasing tension of the posterior portion of the capsule, and the resistance of the marginal posterior fibers of the lateral ligaments.

Under normal conditions, elbow extension is limited by the impact of the olecranon fossa, the tension of the anterior portion of the capsule, the biceps, and the anterior portion of the brachialis muscle, whose strength

Fig. 6. - The drawing illustrates the comparison between the trochlea and a section of a screw (modified by Castaing [6]).

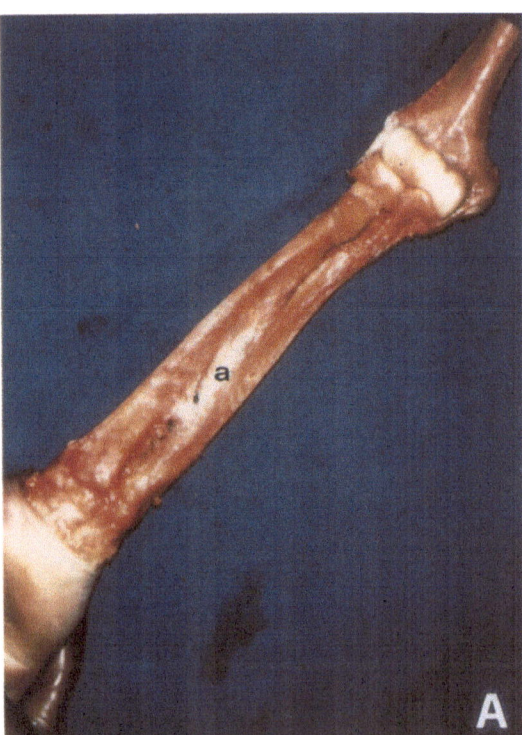

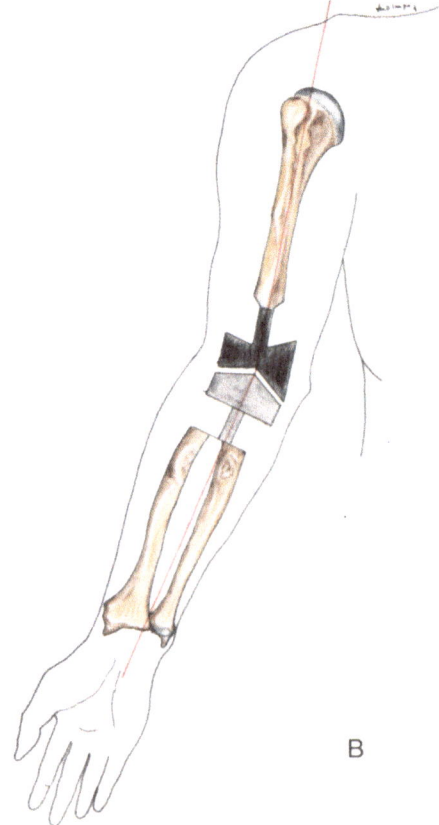

Fig. 7. - Anatomical specimen (A) and drawing (B) show the valgus angulation of the forearm compared to the arm in supination: a) anterior surface of the interosseous membrane.

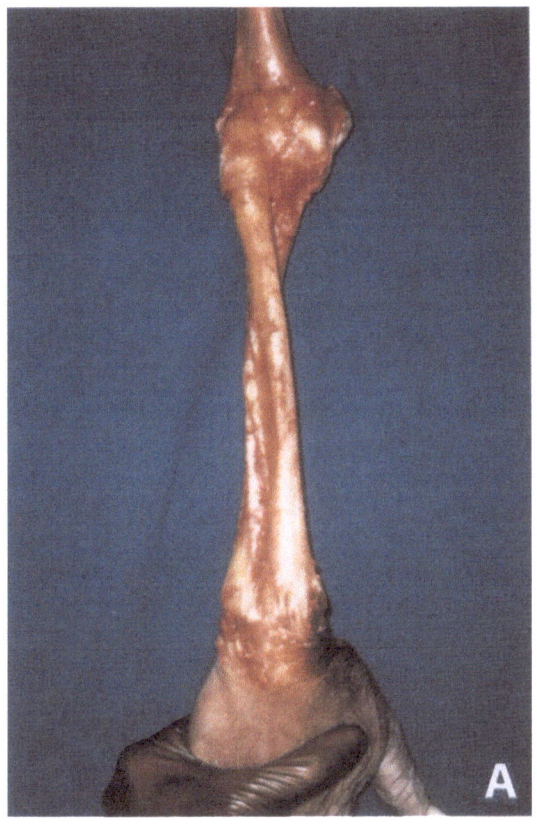
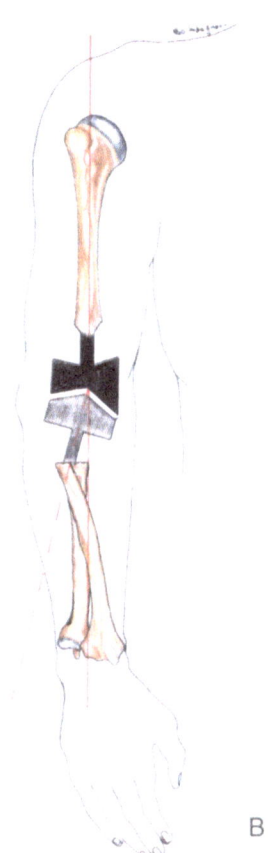

Fig. 8. - Anatomical specimen (A) and drawing (B) show the disappearance of the valgus deformity in pronation.

is sometimes overcome by *hyperextension trauma that cause supracondylar fractures of the humerus and can bring on paralysis of the median nerve.*

In 1% of elbows a supracondylar apophysis is present, from the apex of which a ligament originates (described by Struthers in 1849) that inserts on the epitrochlea, forming a tunnel that contains the median nerve, sometimes the brachial artery, and occasionally even the ulnar nerve. *Pathology of this ligament may cause compression of the structures occupying this tunnel.*

The ulnar nerve, together with the artery, runs through the olecrano-epitrochlear groove and is vascularized in this part of the elbow by an anastomotic arterial system which includes the supratrochlearis and the posterior ulnar recurrent arteries.

The proximal and distal portions of the nerve are protected by muscles, *while the portion of the nerve inside the tunnel is very vulnerable to compression.*

The floor of the tunnel is formed by the ulnar collateral ligament and, at its deepest point, by the internal lip of the trochlea.

The roof of the tunnel is the arcuate ligament, which originates at a fixed point on the epitrochlea and has a variable insertion on the olecranon, bridging the two ends of the anterior cubital muscle whose arch tightens, decreasing the volume of the tunnel.

The deep branch of the radial nerve also crosses the joint line, penetrating the semitendinous groove of the supinator muscle and innervating it. Before slipping in between the two muscle layers which form the so-called "supinator canal", this nerve branch coils around the radial head, *the fracture or luxation of which can injure the branch, resulting in motor paralysis without sensory deficit.*

HUMERORADIAL JOINT

The portion of the humerus which articulates with the radius consists of a condyle with a hemispheric surface in which the vertical diameter is greater than the anteroposterior diameter (Figs. 1-2). For this reason the radius moves distally as it goes from flexion to extension, thus contributing to the containment of the valgus (Fig. 1). Most of the articular surface of the condyle is anterior, only 1/3 being inferior (Fig. 2).

In maximum extension only the anterior half of the radial head articulates with the condyle, while in maximum flexion the edge of the radial head extends anterosuperiorly in the radial fossa.

The capitulum is oval-shaped (Figs. 2-5); during movement from supination to pronation, the position of the longer diameter varies with respect to the ulna, causing the radial head to move away from the ulna, which in turn allows the biceps tendon to pass over the biceps tuberosity.

At maximum supination the radial shaft is vertical, while in maximum pronation it is oblique and the plane of the radial head is inclined outward.

RADIOULNAR JOINT

The lateral edge of the capitulum articulates with the radial notch of the ulna (Fig. 5).

The proximal radioulnar joint is completed by the orbicular ligament, which together with the Denucé quadrate ligament prevents joint incongruity (Fig. 5).

The thickest fibers of the anterior portion of the Denucé quadrate ligament stabilize the radial head more forcefully in the proximal radiocubital joint, helping to minimize the lateral rotation of the radius and ensuring its vertical stability.

In children, the conical shape of the radial head is barely perceptible and the orbicular ligament is quite loose, *for which reason the radius can easily be moved in a longitudinal direction with respect to the ulna.*

PRONATION AND SUPINATION

Pronation and supination (Figs. 7-8) involve the contemporaneous action of the hu-

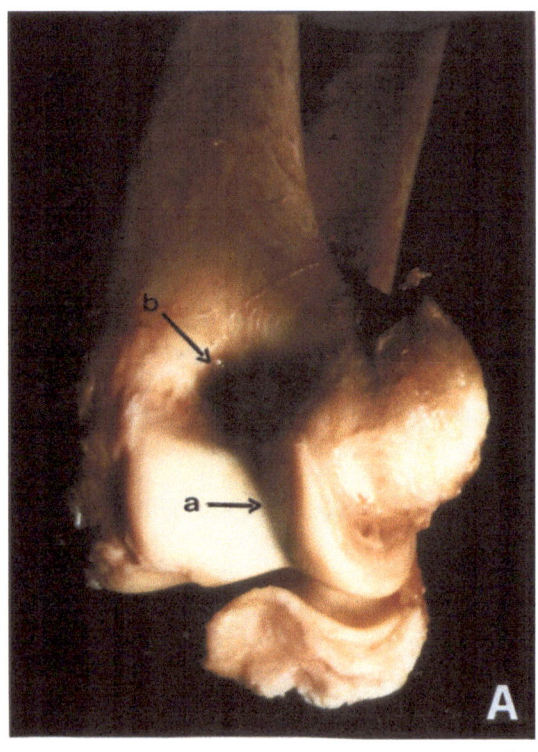
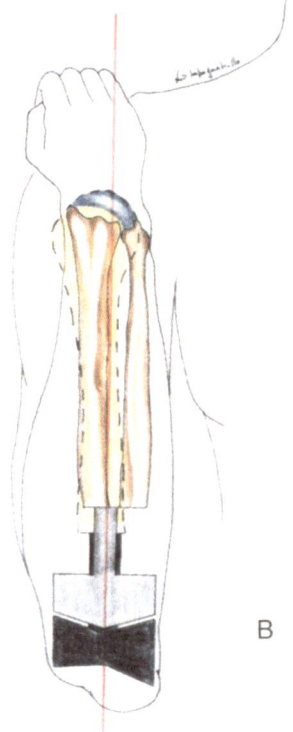

Fig. 9. - Anatomical specimen (A) and drawing (B) show the disappearance of the valgus deformity in maximum elbow flexion: a) Oblique posterior trochlear groove, b) olecranon fossa.

meroradial joint and the proximal and distal radioulnar joints, which can be considered a sole functional unit. These two movements are possible whatever the position of the elbow.

Together they have an overall range of 150 degrees, 80 degrees for supination and 70 degrees for pronation; this range can be increased by involving the shoulder. The extreme degrees of forearm rotation are limited by the respective ligaments, tendons, and muscles, but less by the interosseous membrane (Fig. 7), which is involved primarily in proximal and distal movements of the two bones. *If, however, the interosseous membrane is pathologically retracted, a proportionate reduction of the range of supination can occur.*

Rather than the anterior and posterior radioulnar ligaments, the anterior and posterior bundles of the triangular ligament are instrumental in limiting pronation and supination. In order to execute these movements three conditions must be met:

1) **the radioulnar joints must be free.**

2) **The two bones must have shapes which allow them to cross.** The radius has two curves: one anterior or supinator with its concave side facing forwards, and one medial or pronator with its concave side facing the ulna.

At the apex of the supinator curve is the insertion of the biceps, and at the apex of the pronator curve is the insertion of the pronator teres. *Retraction of one or both of these muscles limits the range of extension, pronation, and supination.*

The proximal portion of the ulna has an anteriorly concave curve.

If the two bones are shaped incorrectly or are not parallel, the range of pronation decreases proportionately.

3) **The two bones must be equal in length.**

INTEROSSEOUS MEMBRANE

While on the subject of rotation, it may be useful to mention the interosseous membrane, the extremely strong structure which holds together the radius and ulna. It consists of two layers:

— *the anterior layer* (Fig. 7A), the fibers of which are oblique both inferiorly and internally, is the more important of the two;

— *the posterior layer*, whose fibers are oblique both superiorly and externally, is associated with the *Weitbrecht oblique cord ligament* (Fig. 11).

The insertion of the superior edge of the interosseous membrane is 2.5 cm below the radial tuberosity, but inferiorly it becomes part of the distal radioulnar joint capsule.

The oblique cord ligament tightens distally from the ulnar tuberosity towards the radius at a point which is distal to the insertional tuberosity of the biceps, whose tendon (Fig. 11), during pronation, winds around the radial neck between the capsule and the Weitbrecht oblique cord ligament, transmitting to the ulna the traction stress which acts upon the radius.

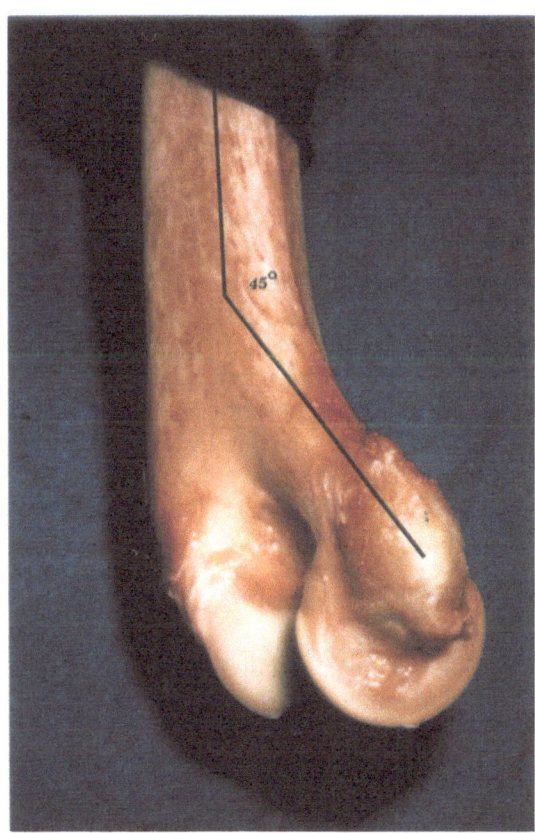

Fig. 10. - On the lateral aspect of the elbow is shown the 45-degree forward-facing angle made by the distal humeral head and the shaft.

The interosseous membrane has a three-fold biomechanical role:

1) It limits rotation and therefore supination, during which all components of the interosseous membrane are tightened with the help of the Denucé quadrate ligament, "**weak brake**", and the triangular ligament, "**strong brake**"; these structures loosen during pronation (10, 5).

2) It helps maintain the respective positions of the two bones preventing slippage of the radius with respect to the ulna. Proximal slippage of the radius is "braked" by the anterior fibers, while distal slippage is "braked" by the posterior fibers and the Weitbrecht oblique cord ligament.

3) It transmits axial pressure from the hand towards the humerus and vice versa.

The ulna transfers the forces of the body on the hand to the radius by means of the fibers of the interosseus membrane, and vice versa permits the radius to convey the forces of the hand on the body to the ulna. In supination the forces travel from the interosseous membrane to the middle portion of the ulna, which sends them directly to the humerus. In pronation the transmission of the forces is identical, even though the fibers of the interosseous membrane are loose. Various mechanisms explain this fact: on the one hand there is the accentuation of the bone curves under lateral pressure, and on the other the tightening of the interosseous membrane by the muscles inserted onto it.

The interosseous membrane is in maximum tension when the forearm is in zero position, that is when the distance between radius and ulna is the greatest; *therefore the immobilization of the forearm in this position helps insure against synostosis of complex fractures* (14).

The destabilizing forces acting on the elbow are:
— longitudinal traction
— longitudinal pressure
— laterality.

These forces are opposed by:
— in the case of longitudinal traction, the two collateral ligaments and the triceps, biceps, brachioradialis, epitrochlearis, and epicondylar muscles;
— in the case of longitudinal pressure, the bone contact of the radius, which can either fracture itself or the condyle, and of the coronoid process, which in breaking at impact causes posterior dislocation of the elbow;
— in the case of laterality, the two collateral ligaments. At 90 degrees the elbow is perfectly stable and only the radius, in case of orbicular ligament rupture, is pushed forward by the dislocating action of the biceps. The brachioradialis muscle opposes this destabilizing force.

The primary elbow flexors are the biceps and the anterior brachialis, innervated by the musculocutaneous nerve, and the brachioradialis, innervated by the radial nerve, which contributes, by means of several nerve branches, to the innervation of the anterior brachialis.

The biceps, starting from its two proximal superglenoid and coracoid insertion points,

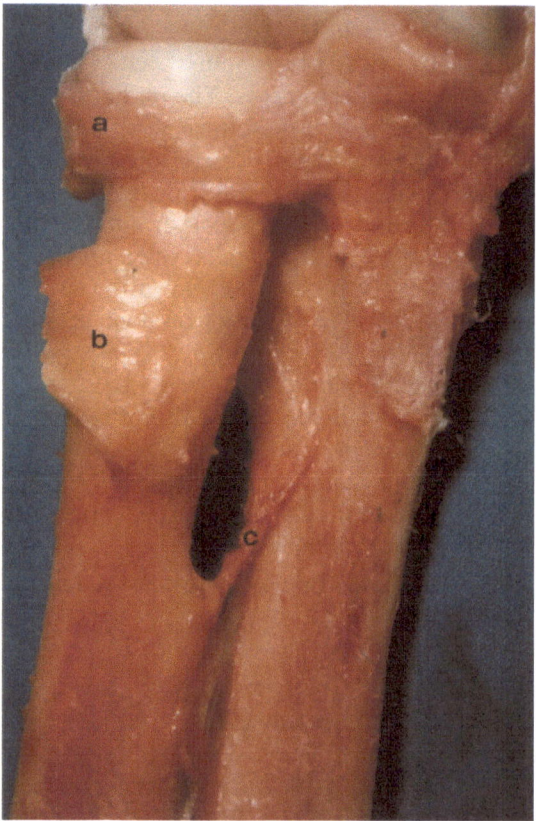

Fig. 11. - The proximal radioulnar joint: a) orbicular ligament, b) distal insertion of the biceps, c) Weitbrecht oblique cord ligament.

inserts on the posterior aspect of the radial tuberosity by means of a short, strong tendon (Figs. 2-11) which is separated from the anterior aspect of the tuberosity by a synovial bursa. The biceps is the primary flexor, yet it has a secondary role in supination and assists in the coaptation of the glenohumeral joint (11).

The anterior brachialis is active during slow flexion, while the brachioradialis enters into action as the load on the partially flexed forearm increases (17). The anterior brachialis, which does not modify its line of traction upon rotation of the arm, exerts considerable force in every position during both rapid and slow movements. The brachioradialis is inefficient as flexion begins because it acts only to compress the joint; its efficiency improves at 45 degrees and is maximized at 120 degrees; it functions therefore as a reserve, contributing during rapid movements or flexion of the pronated forearm when the biceps is less active.

The angle of maximum flexor efficiency is situated between 80 and 90 degrees, and the best position for lifting objects is with the forearm in zero position, while in maximum supination the maximum force by means of isometric contraction of the elbow is generated between 90 and 120 degrees of flexion.

The secondary flexors are the epitrochlearis muscles, all of which originate at the anterior portion of the epitrochlea and all of which, with the exception of the anterior cubitus, are innervated by the median nerve. Under normal conditions these muscles contribute little to forearm flexion, but their action increases if transplanted more proximally, acquiring a function similar to that of the supinator muscle (13, 4).

With the wrist in dorsiflexion, the epicondylar muscles together with the extensor carpi radialis longus and brevis produce elbow flexion (Steindler effect) (14).

The only true elbow extensor is the triceps, with its two heads that act only on this joint; even the long head contributes significantly to extension, especially if the arm is projected forward at shoulder-level, abducted, and rotated externally (1). At maximum flexion, the tendon is stretched from behind into the upper part of the trochlea that acts as a pulley, and is most efficient at 20-30 degrees of flexion (16). It is a two-joint muscle and its action on the arm depends on the efficiency of its long portion; it is most powerful when the limb is flexed and the elbow and the limb extend simultaneously from this position (3). It is less important in the combined movements of shoulder flexion and elbow extension.

The most important part of the triceps in elbow extension is the medial portion; the lateral and long portions are recruited only when more force is needed, while the anconeus, which splays out from the lateral epicondyle to a more spread out insertion on the lateral edge of the olecranon, acts as a stabilizer in both pronation and supination.

Further contributing to the extension of the elbow are the extensor carpi radialis brevis, the extensor digitorum, the extensor of the little finger, and the articularis cubiti, all of which are innervated by the posterior interosseous nerve.

The primary muscles in pronation are the pronator teres and the pronator quadratus, both innervated by the median nerve.

The first has an ulnar belly with two origins, one at the medial edge of the coronoid process and one at the internal supratrochlear ridge; its distal insertion point is at the apex of the pronator curve of the radius.

The pronator quadratus, flat and quadrilateral, covers the distal 1/4 of the radius and ulna and inserts on their volar sides.

During pronation this muscle is contracted, while the pronator teres is most active in elbow flexion and against resistance.

The palmaris longus, which originates together with the palmaris brevis at the epitrochlea, is a weak pronator. The brachioradialis also contributes to pronation, but acts only in maximum supination.

The anconeus is an accessory muscle during pronation; Ray and Johnson (12) as well as Basmajian (2) have verified its pronatory action with the elbow flexed. Pronation increases the lever potential in the arm and therefore the extent of flexion contracture of all the flexors except the anterior brachialis, whose contracture potential remains the same in all positions, and the biceps, whose potential decreases. For the same reasons, the overall flexor force increases up to just past the right angle and then decreases.

Supination is initiated by the elastic return of pronation; the contraction of the brachioradialis is continued by the supinator, supplemented by the biceps as resistance increases.

The supinator muscle, which extends up to the radial neck, is instrumental in forearm supination. It is assisted by the abductor pollicis and the extensor pollicis longus, all innervated by the posterior interosseous nerve.

The biceps intervenes with maximum force when the elbow is flexed and against resistance, while its action is minimal when the forearm is pronated and extended.

Familiarity with both the insertions and the actions of the individual muscles is especially important in reduction of forearm fractures at different levels (9) (Fig. 12).

Fracture displacement occurs at the insertion of the pronator teres in proximal fractures due to the action of the biceps, which forces the proximal fragment into supination, and the pronator teres, which forces the distal fragment into pronation (Fig. 12A).

Reduction and cast immobilization must be performed with the limb in supination.

At the insertion of the pronator teres in distal fractures, the proximal fragment is held in an intermediate position by the balance of the biceps and the pronator teres, while the distal fragment is forced into pronation by the pronator quadratus (Fig. 12B).

In this case, reduction and cast immobilization must be performed with the forearm in zero position.

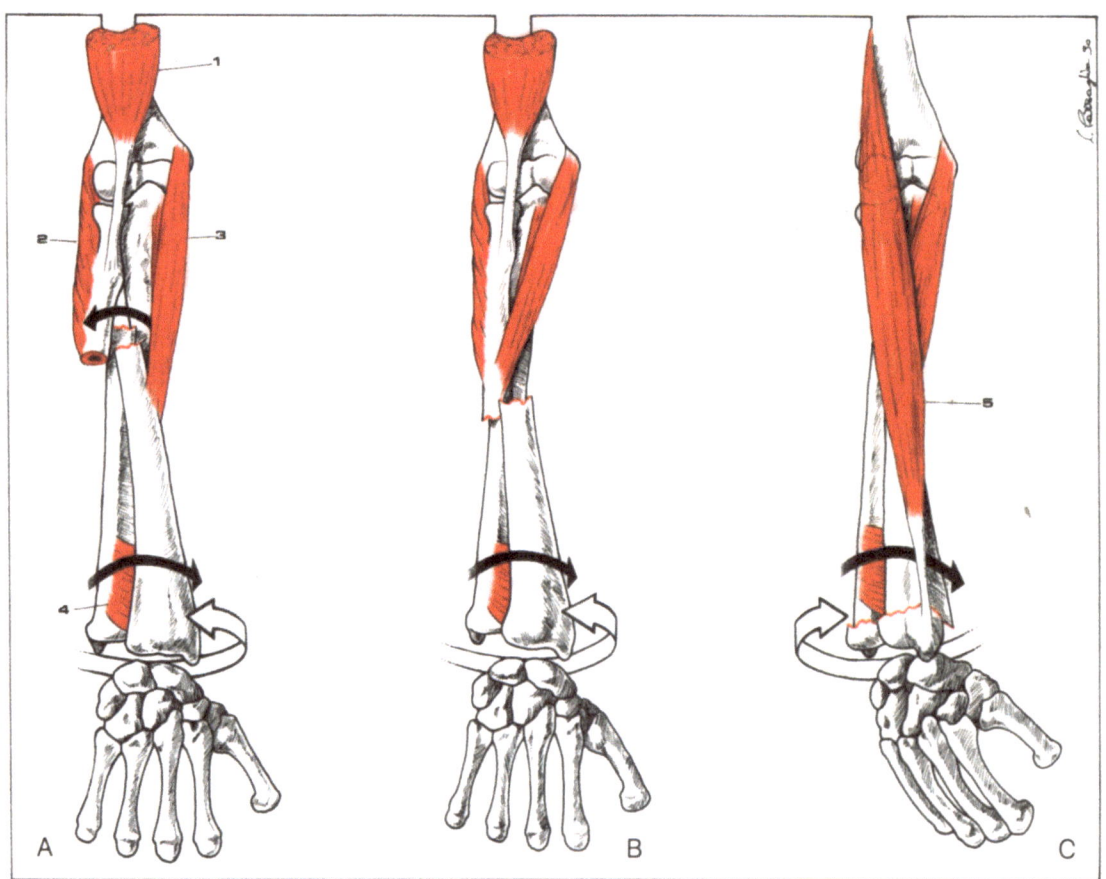

Fig. 12. - Modalities of displacement of forearm fractures at various levels: A) at the proximal insertion of the pronator teres, B) at the distal insertion of the pronator teres, C) at an extreme distal level (from Lanz - Wachsmuth: *Anatomia Pratica* [9]). Legend: 1. biceps, 2. supinator, 3. pronator teres, 4. pronator quadratus, 5. brachioradialis.

In fractures of the distal third, the proximal fragment is pronated while the distal fragment is pulled in a dorso-radial direction and slightly supinated by the brachioradialis (Fig. 12C).

Reduction and cast immobilization of these fractures must be performed with the limb in pronation.

CONCLUSIONS

The elbow is an anatomically and functionally complex joint, a condition that is fully justified by its important responsibility: the spatial orientation of the hand. This complexity explains both the repercussions of traumatic lesions on movement and the sometimes difficult physiopathologic interpretation.

The fundamental anatomical aspect seems to be the orientation of the distal head with respect to the proximal epiphysis of the bone, a result of the torsion involved in the evolution from a stooped quadriped to an upright biped.

An example of unsuccessful torsion of the humerus is the pronated position of obstetrical lesions of the upper limb, in which supination is possible only with surgical intervention such as capsulotomy or syndesmotomy in slight lesions and derotation osteotomy in more severe lesions.

The elbow's ability to flex and extend depends not only on the integrity of the osteoarticular and musculoligamentous structures, but also on the orientation of the distal humeral head with respect to the shaft on the frontal plane, which allows perfect alignment of both olecranon and coronoid with their respective humeral fossae.

The integrity of the two bones of the forearm and their respective proximal and distal joints is indispensible to the rotational movements of the elbow.

A fracture of the radial head can provoke elbow stiffness; this can be counteracted with resection, but such treatment is rarely without complications.

A corollary that is essential for joint function is the stability supplied by the integrity of the ligaments, in particular the collateral ones, as well as the relative coordination of the muscle levers.

Finally, the evaluation of muscular traction is very important in the treatment of two-bone fractures of the forearm: depending on the location of the fracture in relation to the insertions of the muscles, reduction must be performed with the bones in different degrees of rotation. Otherwise, the direction of the muscular forces prevents accurate reduction and restoration of the normal relationship between the two bones, which is indispensible to the movements of pronation and supination.

REFERENCES

1) BASMAJIAN J.V., LATIF A.: Integrated action and functions of the chief flexors of the elbow. *J. Bone Jt Surg.* 1957; **39A**, 1106.

2) BASMAJIAN J.V.: Spurt and shunt muscles: an electromyographic confirmation, *J. Anat.* 1959; **93**, 551.

3) BERNHANG A.M., DEHNER W., FOGARTY C.: Tennis elbow: a biomechanical approach. *J. Sports Med.* 1974; **2**, 235.

4) BUNNEL S.: Retoring flexion to paralytic elbows. *J. Bone Jt Surg.* 1951; **3-A**, 556.

5) CASTAING J., DELPLACE J.: Bilans articulaires. *Encycl. Med. Chir.*, Paris, (Kinesiterapie), 26008, A-10, 4.1.10.

6) CASTAING J.: *La pronosupination*. Edition VIGOT.

7) CELLI L., BALLI A., DE LUISE G., D'ARIENZO M., PAVOLINI B.: Fisiopatologia ed evoluzione naturale delle paralisi ostetriche. *Riv. Chir. Mano* 1985; **22**: 1-13.

8) CHIARUGI G.: *Istituzioni di anatomia dell'uomo*. Società Editrice Libraria, Milano.

9) LANZ T., WACHSMUTH: *Anatomia pratica*. Piccin Editore, Padova.

10) KAPANDJI I.A.: *Fisiologia articolare*. Edizioni DEMI, Roma, 1974, vol. 1.

11) KENDALL O.H., KENDALL F.P., WADSWORTH G.E.: *Muscles. Testing and function*. William and Wilkins Company, 1971.

12) RAY R.D., JOHNSON R.J., JAMESON R.M.: Rotation of the forearm: an experimental study of pronation and supination. *J. Bone Jt Surg.* 1951; **33**, 993.

13) STEINDLER A.: Tendon transplantation in upper extremity. *Am. J. Surg.* 1939; **44**, 260.

14) STEINDLER A.: *Kinesiology of the human body under normal and pathological conditions*. Charles C. Thomas., Springfield 1955.

15) TESTUT L., LATARJET A.: *Trattato di anatomia umana*. Edizioni UTET, 1967.

16) WADSWORTH THOMAS G.: *The elbow*. Churchill Livingstone, Edinburgh, 1982.

17) WALLER T.J.: *The mechanism of elbow flexion*. In: *Resident Papers*. Downey, California: University of Southern California, Department of Orthopaedic Surgery, L.A.C.-U.S.C. Medical Centre, Rancho Los Amigos Hospital, vol. 3, pp. 287-294.

Overload syndromes of the elbow

F. Postacchini - G. Cinotti - E. Adriani - M. Rosa

Overload syndromes of the elbow are characterized by a series of conditions whose pathogenesis is directly or indirectly related to either excessive functional strain or repeated microtrauma. Some of these conditions affect periarticular musculotendinous structures such as the aponeuroses at the insertion points of the epicondylar and epitrochlearis muscles, the distal biceps brachii tendon, and the triceps tendon. Diseases affecting the osteoarticular structures of the elbow feature purely articular clinical manifestations.

medical history, can result in local microcirculatory system damage or avascular necrosis. Repeated microtrauma can be caused by endogenous factors or exogenous factors, as in the case of the tennis player whose racquet strings are too tight. The former can be sectoral or heterogenous muscle strains due to incorrect movement. Even functional overloading, which occurs in athletes or manual laborers who repeatedly carry out the same movement, can be considered endogenous factors. The importance of occasional functional overloading is shown by the high

LATERAL AND MEDIAL EPICONDYLITIS

Anatomy: the distal humerus widens proximally at the elbow to form the lateral and medial epicondyles. The "extensor-supinator" and "flexor-pronator" muscle groups, repectively, originate from these structures. Laterally these muscles are closely attached to each other, connected to the epicondyle by a common tendinous lamina, the antebrachial fascia, and the intermuscular septa. This connection is less evident on the medial side, as the epitrochlearis muscles originate from a wider bone surface (Fig. 1). This anatomical situation and the fact that most hand functions are executed in slight extension explain the high incidence of epicondylar muscle pathology.

Etiology and pathogenesis: although these are controversial, the mechanical and diathetic components are probably the determining factors.

The mechanical component can be direct trauma, repeated microtrauma, or excessive functional strain. Direct trauma, often the only possible cause found in the patient's

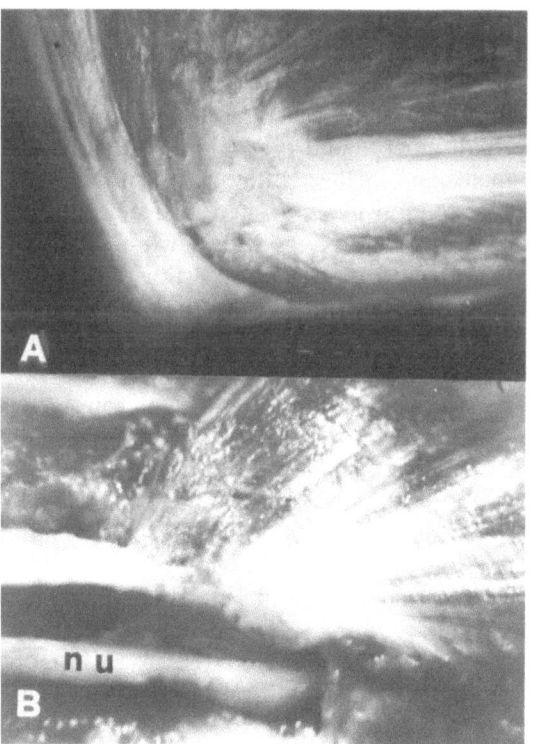

Fig. 1. - A) The insertion of the epicondylar muscles. B) The insertion of the epitrochlearis muscles; the epitrochlear and olecranal insertions of the flexor carpi ulnaris are evident — between them runs the ulnar nerve.

incidence of these tendonopathies, as well as others of mechanical origin, among beginners at a particular athletic or occupational activity and people who resume activity after a relatively long absence.

The constitutional idiopathic element is especially important in patients who have never engaged in sports or manual labor. Some patients exhibited distinct reactivity of the mesenchymal tissues as well as degenerative changes in both the bone-tendon junctions and the joint cartilage (14). These changes are sometimes so closely related that they may have a common etiology, consisting of a degenerative tendency of the cartilaginous tissue involving the hyaline cartilage in arthritis and the fibrocartilage in insertional pathology.

These etiologic and pathogenetic interpretations are supported by the periodic operative discovery of partial tears in the tendinous lamina of the insertion (10) and by the histopathologic investigations that, in the cases of epicondylitis we studied, revealed degenerative changes in both the tendinous tissue and the bone-tendon junction. The changes in the tendinous tissue consisted primarily of hyaline degeneration and occasionally of mucoid and fibrinoid phenomena and small tears in the tendinous tissue. Near the bone-tendon junction there were often areas of granulation tissues with newly-formed capillaries and perivascular histiocytic infiltrations, fragmentation of the "blue line", and a microcystic cavity filled with necrotic material (11).

Clinical picture: the chief symptom is epicondylar pain, which usually arises gradually and returns and intensifies according to the functional involvement. The pain can be exacerbated by tensing up the bone-tendon junction through flexion or extension of the wrist against resistance. This movement evokes pain on the affected side of the elbow. In lateral epicondylitis, wrist extension opposed by the middle finger often evokes acute pain in the epicondyle (Fig. 2). Also in lateral epicondylitis, intensification of the symptoms is typically brought on by prehension movements, such as those required for lifting or carrying a heavy object. Palpation of the affected epicondyle reawakens pain.

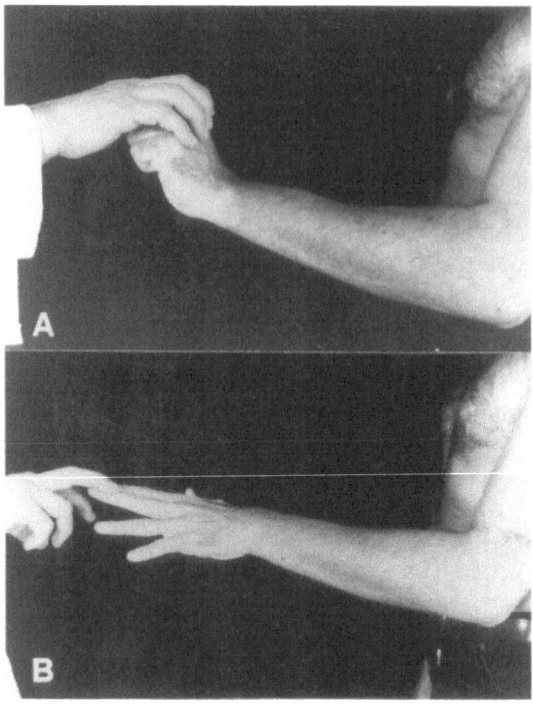

Fig. 2. - Extension of the wrist (A) and the middle finger (B) carried out against resistance evoke pain in the epicondyle.

The differential diagnosis for lateral epicondylitis should be made with arthritis, synovitis, radial neuropathy, and other diseases of the humeroradial joint. In humeroradial joint diseases, pain is localized in the joint space and can be exacerbated by flexion, extension, pronation, or supination. Radial nerve disease can be caused by arthritis of the cervical spine or compression of the superficial, sensory branch of the nerve in the proximal forearm, where it passes between the supinator and the extensor carpi radialis brevis muscles. This syndrome is most commonly caused by accretions between the humeroradial joint capsule and the nerve or hypertrophy of the aponeurosis of the muscles touching the nerve branch (13).

In medial epicondylitis, which is rarer, the differential diagnosis is made with ulnar nerve pathology, which is attributable to cervical spine arthritis or peripheral involvement of the nerve.

The natural course of the disease is generally benign; if left untreated, it often goes into remission after a couple of months.

Preventive measures have been studied

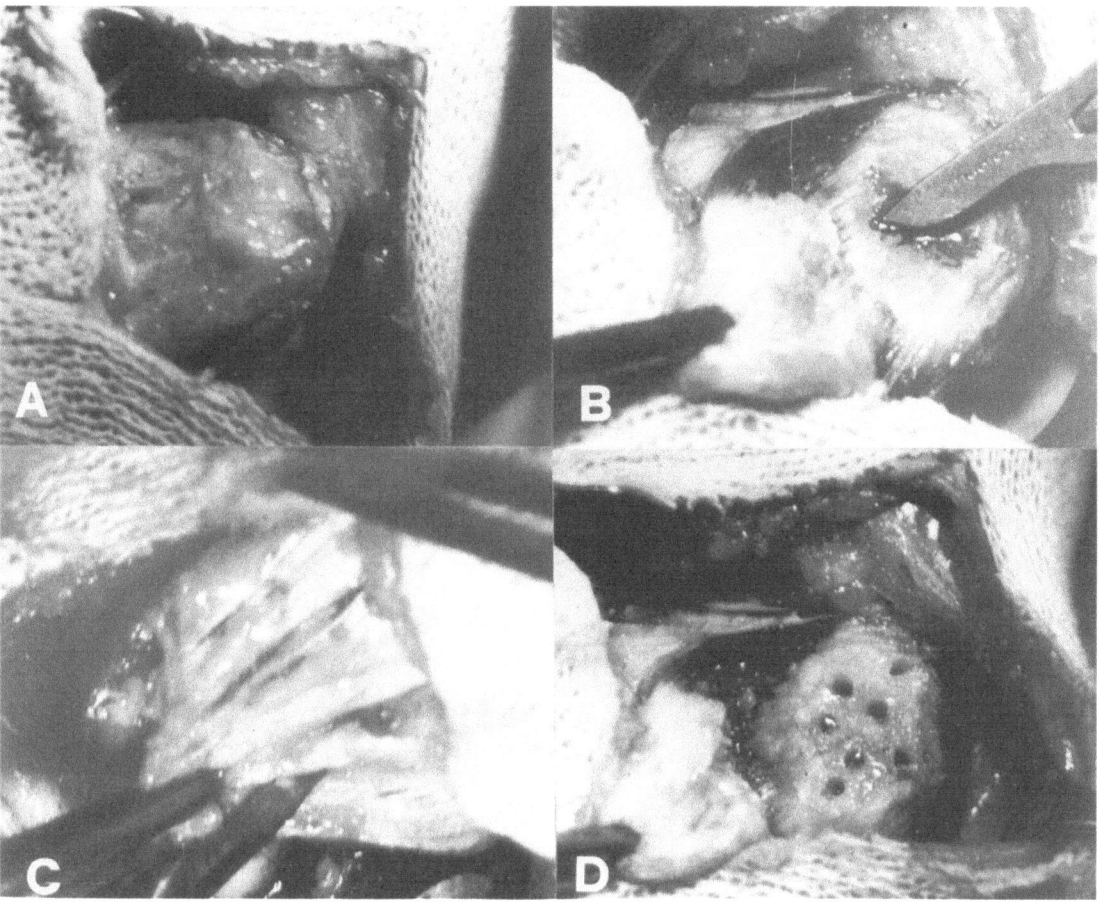

Fig. 3. - Surgical treatment of epitrochleitis. The exposed tendinous lamina (A) is detatched from the epitrochlea (B). Longitudinal scarifications are then made in the tendinous lamina (C) and perforations in the epitrochlea (D).

in tennis players with lateral epicondylitis. Electromyographic and biomechanical studies show the stretching of the extensor muscles at the moment that the racquet hits the ball (4). Incorrect movements as well as defects in the racquet such as excessive weight, high string tension, or undersized grip should be avoided.

Treatment: treatment consists of medical, orthopedic, surgical, and physical therapy. The first is based on general and/or local administration of antiphlogistic drugs. Local infiltration of slow-absorbing cortisone is by far the most effective medical therapy. From one to three infiltrations should be done between the tendinous insertion and the subcutaneous tissue, taking care not to infiltrate the medication into the tendon itself, which might cause necrosis and/or degenerative changes.

Physical therapy makes use of laser, diathermy, and ultrasound. Orthopedic treatment is supposed to reduce the functional strain on the forearm musculature with casts or orthoses that immobilize the elbow at 90 degrees and the wrist in neutral position. In acute cases immobilization may last for 2-4 weeks.

In surgical treatment various techniques are adopted, testifying to the incomplete knowledge we possess of the pathogenesis of these diseases. The chief objective of our surgical intervention is to reduce the tension on the bone-tendon junction. This is achieved by sectioning the aponeurotic lamina of the insertion just under its origin. The degenerated tissue is then excised and multiple perforations are made in the epicondyle at the bone-tendon junction to promote vascularization and regeneration of the fibrocartilaginous junction. The affected tendons are then scarified to aid tissue regeneration (Fig. 3).

The outcome of surgical treatment is usually satisfactory, even though many weeks often pass before relief of pain and recovery of force of the epitrochlearis and epicondylar muscles are complete.

RUPTURE OF THE DISTAL BICEPS BRACHII TENDON

Anatomy: the distal biceps brachii tendon originates just above the bend of the elbow and is slightly flattened in an anteroposterior direction. It heads distally and, rotating on its axis, takes a sagittal course. Having reached the anterior side of the radial biceps tuberosity, it circles around to the back and inserts on the posterior side of the tuberosity by means of a serous bursa (Fig. 4).

Etiology and pathogenesis: lesions of this tendon represent 3% of biceps tendon ruptures (5). The typical patient is a manual laborer in his 40's or a younger person who engages in a sport such as gymnastics or body-building.

In most of these patients a histologic exam reveals degenerative changes in the tendinous tissue, which reduce the tendon's resistance to functional strain and make it vulnerable to rupture. Nevertheless, some studies have shown that even a healthy tendon can rupture when sudden stretching of the muscle-tendon unit is accompanied by a violent muscular contraction (1). This can happen as a result of an uncoordinated movement in which the tendon is pulled away from its anatomical axis. Therefore, although most lesions occur in the presence of tendinous changes, some ruptures or bone-tendon detachments can occur in structurally healthy tendons.

In most cases the lesion consists of detachment of the tendon from the biceps tuberosity of the radius. Rupture of the tendon belly as well as tenomuscular disjunction are rare, yet associated rupture of the lacertus fibrosus is common.

Clinical picture: sudden pain in the bend of the elbow with a sensation of muscle strain and functional limitation. Swelling is commonly observed in the proximal half of the arm, due to the rising up of the muscular belly, as well as a depression just below this.

Both are exacerbated by active elbow flexion. Diagnosis is usually easy, except in rare cases of partial tendinous lesion or when the lacertus fibrosus is not ruptured.

Treatment: unlike cases of lesion of the long head of the biceps, in this instance surgical treatment is the only feasible option. The goal of surgery is to either suture the ruptured tendon to the anterior brachialis tendon or reinsert it onto the biceps tuberosity of the radius. The latter offers few functional advantages compared to the former and can injure the deep branch of the radial nerve (8). The reinsertion of the loose end onto the anterior brachialis does not restore the supination capacity of the biceps, yet compensa-

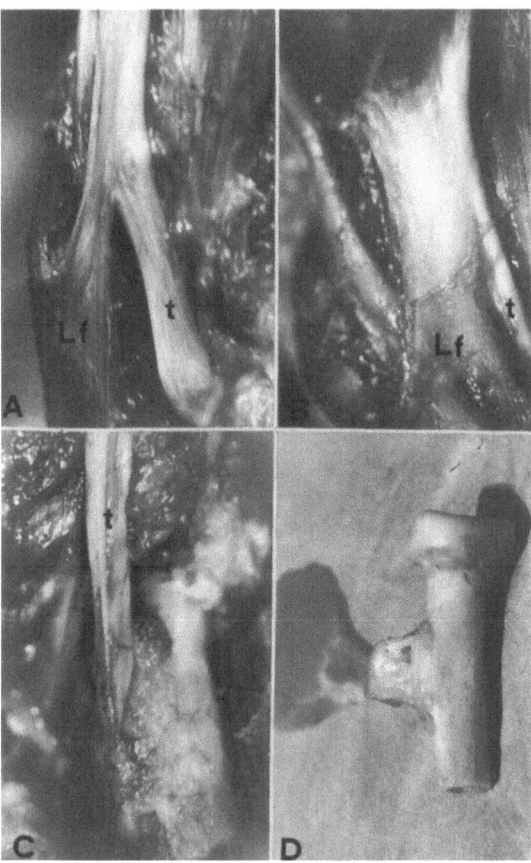

Fig. 4. - Anatomy of the distal biceps brachii tendon. The tendon is flattened in an anteroposterior direction near the bend of the elbow (A), where it gives origin to the lacertus fibrosus (B). Proceeding distally it takes a sagittal course (C) and circles around the radial tuberosity to its insertion (D). Lf = lacertus fibrosus; t = biceps tendon.

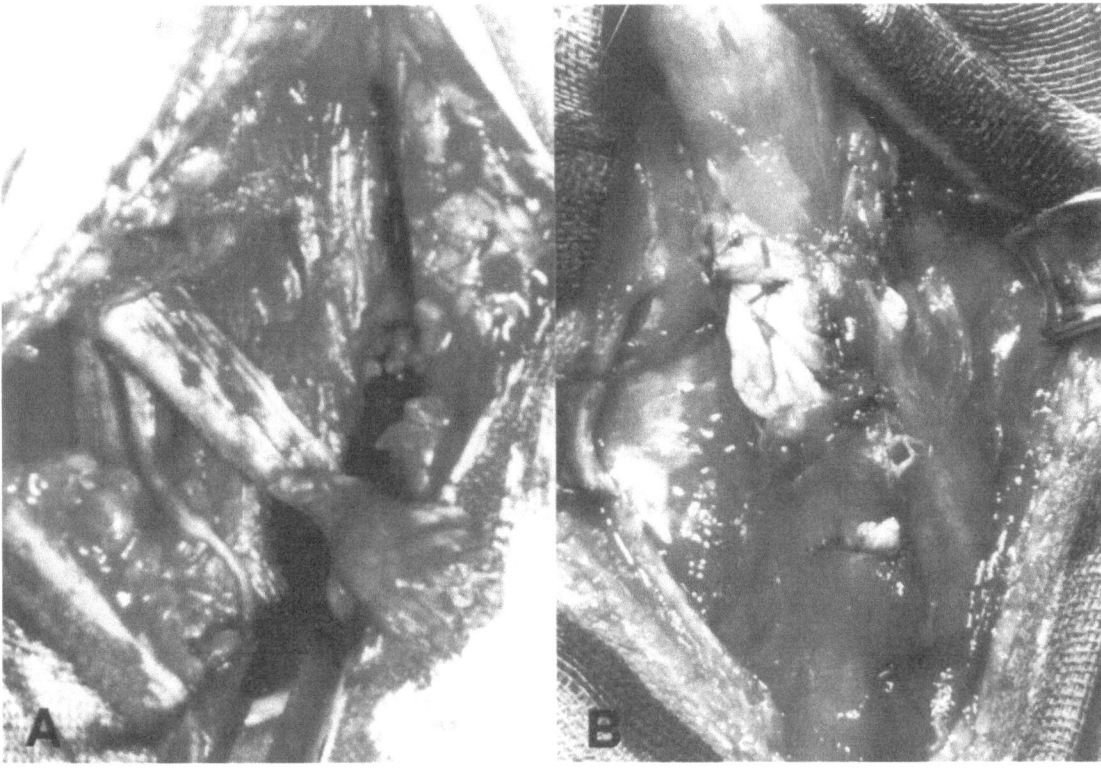

Fig. 5. - Detachment of the distal biceps brachii tendon. The end of the tendon resembles a club (A). The biceps tendon has been sutured to the anterior brachialis tendon (B).

tion is provided by the hypertrophy of the other supinator muscles of the forearm.

The evaluation of the muscular tension of the biceps during suturing is very important in this type of operation and is done by flexing the elbow to 30 degrees and pulling the loose end of the tendon until the lower end of the muscle belly is within two fingers' width of the bend of the elbow (Fig. 5).

LESIONS OF THE DISTAL TRICEPS BRACHII TENDON

Anatomy: the tendon originates where the three heads of the triceps converge, and its insertion is on the superior and posterior surfaces and the edges of the olecranon. At its insertion the tendon is protected by two bursae mucosae, subtendinea and subcutanea, of the olecranon.

Insertional pathology: this is an uncommon syndrome that occurs primarily in patients who subject the triceps tendon to excessive functional strain. It usually strikes ma-

nual laborers or athletes (especially gymnasts).

Besides the usual degenerative changes, an olecranal spur with calcifications or ossifications can also be found in the affected tendon. The spur comes up proximally through the tendon on the upper corner of the olecranon. It is either whole or split and narrower at the top than at the bottom (Fig. 6).

The *clinical picture* features pain in the olecranon that can spread proximally along the muscular belly of the triceps.

Treatment is generally conservative. In re-

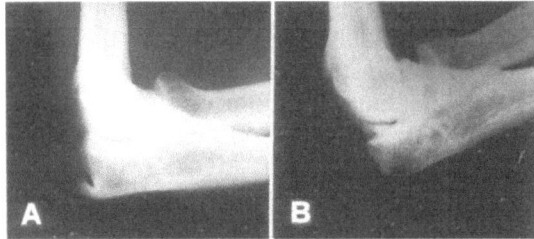

Fig. 6. - A) Insertional pathology of the triceps brachii featuring a large olecranal spur. B) The same case after surgical removal of the spur.

sistant forms, either removal of the degenerated tissue or excision of the olecranic spur is indicated.

Subcutaneous rupture. This lesion is rare and almost never solely tendinous. As a matter of fact, due to the sturdiness of the triceps tendon, most cases of subcutaneous rupture are accompanied by fracture-separation of a bone chip from the olecranon.

This lesion is generally provoked by direct trauma to the olecranon region when the elbow is partially flexed.

The clinical manifestion of the rupture is ecchymotic swelling on the extensor surface of the elbow, which tends to extend along the dorsal surface of the forearm. There is also a palpable transverse depression along the tendon. Acute pain and limited active range of motion are always present.

The *radiographic examination* is instrumental in differentiating fracture-separation from pure separation. In the former, the detached bone fragment seems to have shifted proximally due to tendon retraction.

The *treatment* is surgical. In cases of pure separation or rupture of the tendon belly, the operative technique consists of either an end to end suture or a bone-tendon synthesis using transosseous sutures. In cases of fracture-separation, the removal of small bone fragments is followed by bone-tendon synthesis, while larger fragments are treated with internal fixation.

OSTEOCHONDROSIS DISSECANS

This is a rare pathological condition that involves the joint cartilage of the subchondral bone and can produce intraarticular loose bodies.

The knee is by far the most commonly affected joint, followed by the elbow, the ankle, and the hip. More than one joint can be affected simultaneously. It occurs in people between the ages of 10 and 50, with a peak at 15. Although there is some evidence for heredity, a genetic etiology for osteochondrosis dissecans has not yet been proven (12).

Etiology and pathogenesis: a direct or indirect, slight or moderate trauma is often present in the medical history of the patient. In cases of repeated trauma, it has been hypothesized that the first episode provokes retardation of bone growth or avascular necrosis, while the subsequent episodes cause detachment of the affected osteocartilaginous region (6).

Other studies have demonstrated the importance of a change in the epiphyseal ossification process even without trauma (2). If this situation persists during growth, it can provoke osteochondrosis dissecans.

A third mechanism, ischemia, has also been proposed. It could act alone or in conjunction with previous occurrences through changes in the microcirculatory system due to systemic and/or local factors. Some authors (7) have discovered the presence of a poor anastomotic network in the subchondral bone that would explain the high incidence of avascular necrosis following vessel occlusion. Subsequent trauma would cause the fracture and then the detachment of the overlying cartilage which, nourished by the synovial liquid, remains viable in the joint, unlike the bone tissue.

Clinical picture: most patients have a limited range of motion and pain after intense activity (Fig. 7). In other cases the onset is more insidious, with years passing before diagnosis. In the presence of loose bodies, joint block is common.

The humeral condyle and the radial head are the most commonly affected areas (Fig. 8). In the early stages a standard AP x-ray can be negative, while the lateral view reveals a flattened area of the humeral profile. This can be better documented by a tomographic exam, revealing a characteristic crateriform formation with a sclerotic border which may contain the loose fragment. Besides, the only radiographically shown pathologic element is very often one or two intraarticular loose bodies (Fig. 9). Widening of the radial head and premature closure of the joint cartilage can sometimes be seen in growing patients (15).

A differential diagnosis should be made with other diseases, such as arthritis and osteochondromatosis, capable of causing the formation of intraarticular loose bodies. The physician should keep in mind that arthritis is by far the most common cause of intraarticu-

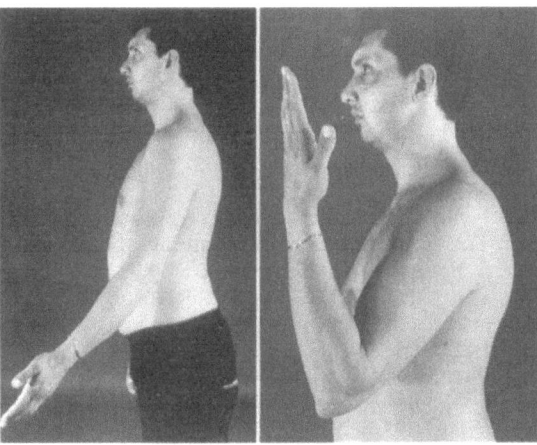

Fig. 7. - Patient with intraarticular loose bodies. Range of flexion and especially extension is reduced.

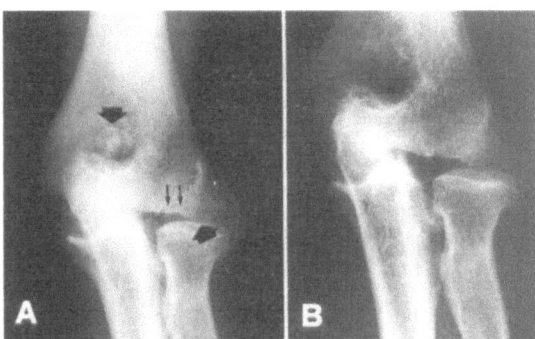

Fig. 8. - A) Osteochondrosis dissecans of the capitulum humeri. Numerous loose bodies are present in the olecranon fossa and proximal to the radial head (large arrow). The capitulum appears flattened and hollow near the affected area (small arrows). B) X-ray after removal of the loose bodies.

lar loose bodies in the elbow (9,3). The differential diagnosis should also be made with osteochondrosis of the capitulum humeri, or Panner's disease, which affects children between the ages of 5 and 10 and is characterized radiographically by fragmentation and the deformity of the epiphyseal plate of the capitulum humeri. In this case, conservative treatment guarantees adequate reconstruction of the growth plate (15).

Treatment: the treatment is conservative except in cases of symptomatic intraarticular

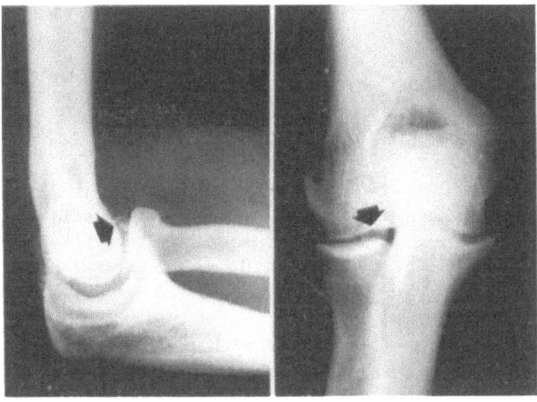

Fig. 9. - Isolated loose body (arrow) in the joint without evident areas of osteochondrosis.

loose bodies. When the patient has joint block or limited elbow mobility, removal of the loose bodies, by arthroscopy if possible, is recommended.

ARTHRITIS

The elbow is rarely the site of marked arthritic changes, except those caused by joint fracture. Primary arthritis can be observed in manual laborers and, less frequently, in middle-aged or elderly people who are long-time participants in sports that place a particular strain on the elbow. Besides, in these cases functional overload is almost never the only *etiologic and pathogenetic factor,* but is usually accompanied by a constitutional predisposition to degenerative joint changes, which explains the high incidence of arthritis in other joints as well. Secondary arthritic changes are common, however, in patients with osteochondrosis dissecans or intraarticular loose bodies.

The *clinical picture* features pain and limitation of flexion-extension and pronation-supination. *Treatment* is generally conservative. Considering that the results achieved with prosthetic replacement of the elbow are often only partially satisfactory, this is indicated only in instances of very severe arthritic changes.

REFERENCES

1) BARFEDT: Experimental rupture of the Achilles tendon. Comparison of various types of experimental rupture in rats. *Acta Orthop. Scand.* 1971; **42**: 528.

2) BARRIE H.J., Osteocondritis dissecans 1887-1987. A centennial look at Konig's memorial phrase. *J. Bone Jt Surg.* 1987; **69-B**: 693.

3) BELL M.S.: Loose body in the elbow. *Br. J. Surg.* 1975; **62**: 921-24.

4) BERNHANG A.M., DEHNER W., FOGARTY C.: Tennis elbow: a biomechanical approach. *J. Sports Med.* 1974; **2**: 235.

5) BIANCHIERI T.M.: Sulla rottura sottocutanea del bicipite brachiale. *Chir. Org. Mov.* 1925; **9**: 580.

6) CODMAN E.A.: The formation of loose cartilages in the knee joint. *Boston Med. Surg. J.* 1903; **149**: 427.

7) ENNEKING W.F.: *Clinical Musculoskeletal Pathology.* Gainesville, Sorter Printing Co., 1977, p. 141.

8) FRIEDMAN E.: Rupture of the distal biceps brachii tendon. *J. Am. Med. Ass.* 1963; **184**: 60.

9) MILGRAM J.A.: The classification of loose body in human joints. *Clin. Orthop. Rel. Res.* 1975; **110**: 35.

10) NIRSCHL R.P., PETTRONE F.A.: Tennis elbow. The surgical treatment of lateral epicondylitis. *J. Bone Jt Surg.* 1979; **61-A**: 833.

11) PERUGIA L., POSTACCHINI F., IPPOLITO E.: *I tendini: biologia, patologia, clinica.* Masson Ed., 1981.

12) PETRIE P.W.R.: Aetiology of osteochondritis dissecans. *J. Bone Jt Surg.* 1977; **59-B**: 366.

13) ROLES N.C., MANDSLEY R.H.: Radial tunnel syndrome. Resistant tennis elbow as a nerve entrapment. *J. Bone Jt Surg.* 1972; **54-B**: 499.

14) SCHNEIDER H.: *Die Abnutzungserkrankungen der Sehnen und ihre Therapie.* Thieme, Stuttgart, 1959.

15) WOODWARD A.H., BINACO A.J.: Osteochondritis dissecans of the elbow. *Clin. Orthop. Rel. Res.* 1975; **110**: 35.

Nerve tunnel syndromes in the elbow

L. Celli - G. de Luise - C. Rovesta - M. Marinelli

PREMISE

Repetitive and physically demanding athletic or occupational activity, depending on the modalities of execution, can cause overwork syndromes of the articular and periarticular musculotendinous structures. The terms lateral and medial epicondylalgia define the painful syndromes of the elbow located medially (internal compartment) or laterally (external compartment) and caused by microtraumatic stress.

In these pathologies, the etiology and pathogenesis of the pain and functional limitation generally refer to three possible causes that can act either alone or together:

1) phlogistic-degenerative-type musculotendinous pathology in the muscles that insert on the epicondyles;

2) osteoarticular pathology with lateral (radial dome and capitulum) or medial (trochlea and olecranon) articular chondromalacia;

3) nerve tunnel pathologies affecting the radial nerve on the lateral side of the elbow and the ulnar nerve on the medial side.

During clinical observation of a painful elbow, precise location of the damage is often difficult; in these cases conservative and surgical treatment are ineffective and both pain and functional limitation resist therapy (resistant tennis elbow).

It is therefore necessary to use a clinical approach that takes not only the joint and musculotendinous disease into consideration, but also the neurologic pathology.

Use of specific tests and preoperative examinations should lead to the identification of the three local syndromes, either alone or combined, and their differentiation from the proximal pathologies such as vertebrocervical syndrome and neurovascular disease at the cervico-axillary passage.

THE COMPARTMENT CONCEPT

In order to distinguish nerve tunnel pathology from osteoarticular and musculotendinous syndromes in cases of epicondylalgia, it may be useful to introduce the compartment concept in diagnosis of the painful elbow.

By compartment we mean that external or internal, anterior or posterior anatomical sector where the osteoarticular, capsuloligamentous, musculotendinous, and neurologic structures can be simultaneously affected by microtraumatic overwork pathologies (Fig. 1).

We consider this concept to be important not only for the classification of microtraumatic pathology in one sector, but also because the structures in that compartment are often contemporaneously involved in the physiopathological mechanism, the clinical pictures, and the therapeutic choices.

As a matter of fact, nerve tunnel syndromes almost always occur as a result of nearby osteoarticular or musculotendinous changes. In these cases the clinical manifestations appear all together, and only with a careful semeiologic exam can the physician evaluate the pathological role of all the anatomical components of that compartment. The treatment must therefore take into account not only the neurologic damage, but also the pathology of the surrounding structures responsible for the compression.

Here is a breakdown of the structures contained in the elbow:

A) *in the external compartment*

— the humeroradial joint;

— the joint capsule, the radial collateral and orbicular ligaments;

— the lateral epicondylar muscles (extensor carpi radialis longus and brevis, supinator, and extensor digitorum communis);

— the radial nerve and its two terminal

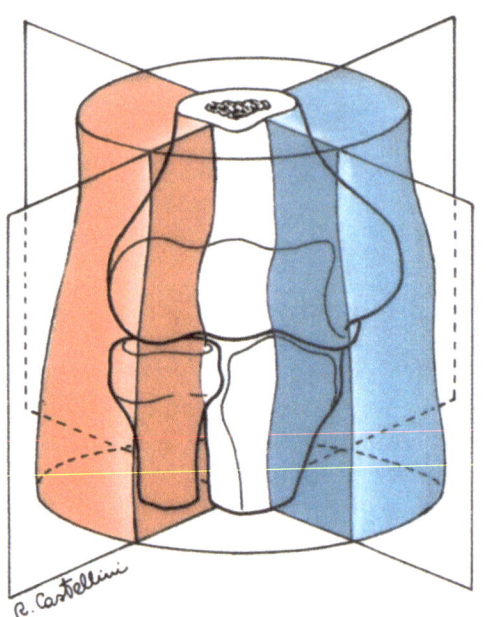

Fig. 1. - Schematic representation of the elbow compartments.

branches (motor and sensory) (Fig. 2).

B) *In the internal compartment*
— the humerocubital joint;
— the joint capsule and ulnar collateral ligament;
— the epitrochlear muscles (flexor carpi radialis and ulnaris, pronator teres, and flexor digitorum superficialis);
— the ulnar nerve (Fig 3).

C) *In the anterior compartment*
— the anterior humerocubital joint;
— the pronator teres, flexor digitorum superficialis, and flexor carpi radialis muscles;
— the median nerve.

D) *In the posterior compartment*
— the posterior humerocubital joint;
— the triceps muscle.

Among the functional activities of the upper limb are some common movements that overload the structures contained in the compartments.

The external compartment is used more heavily in activities involving shoulder external rotation, elbow extension, forearm supination, or wrist extension.

Overloading of the internal compartment occurs, however, in activities involving shoulder internal rotation, elbow flexion, forearm pronation, or wrist flexion.

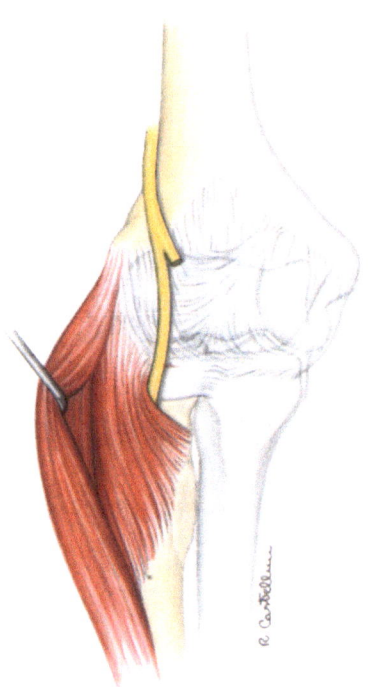

Fig. 2. - The main structures of the external compartment.

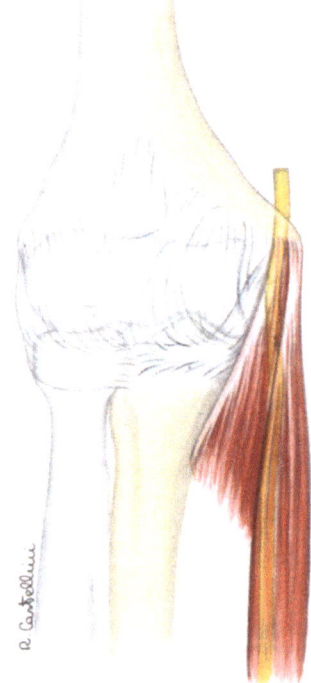

Fig. 3. - The main structures of the internal compartment.

Strain on the anterior compartment occurs in activities requiring repeated shoulder intrarotation, elbow flexion, forearm pronation, wrist extension, and finger flexion.

The posterior compartment is overworked in functional activities requiring repeated elbow extension with the shoulder internally rotated and the forearm supinated.

Functional overloading in one compartment often affects other nearby compartments whose structures are functionally associated to those initially damaged.

It is therefore easy to clinically observe how phlogistic-degenerative pathologies often occur in two compartments at once, with a combination of either the external and posterior or the internal and anterior compartments.

The purpose of this study is therefore to isolate and describe the diagnostic value of the clinical features and imaging study findings that can indicate nerve tunnel syndrome in the painful elbow. Specifically, compression syndromes of the radial nerve in the external compartment and the ulnar nerve in the internal compartment will be examined.

EXTERNAL COMPARTMENT PATHOLOGY: RADIAL TUNNEL SYNDROME

This syndrome, known to physicians for over a century (40,13) and described by numerous Italian (3, 10, 18, 20, 23) and foreign (4, 17, 19, 27, 33, 39) authors, is considered uncommon (5-8% of cases of lateral epicondylalgia) (42). Nevertheless, in our experience the damage to the posterior interosseous nerve (PIN) in cases of chronic lateral epicondylalgia, which is resistant to the usual medical treatment and physical therapy, is surely more frequent than the above percentage, even though it is difficult to quantify.

In prescribing surgery for this pathology, the possible neurologic damage as well as nearby chronic osteotendinous or joint disease must be taken into consideration.

Different combinations of the following three lesions can constitute chronic lateral epicondylalgia:

1) insertional pathology of the lateral epicondylar muscles,

2) humeroradial joint disease,

3) compression pathology of the radial nerve in the radial tunnel.

The radial tunnel

The "radial tunnel" (33) in the elbow is a possible site for nerve tunnel compression syndromes. The radial tunnel is considered to be the space that begins proximally near the external bicipital groove and ends distally at the emergence of the motor branch of the radial nerve from the supinator muscle. The radial tunnel can be divided into three levels: upper, middle, and lower.

In the upper portion (tunnel entrance) the nerve is located medially at the brachialis muscle and occupies the bottom of the lateral bicipital groove. After the nerve splits into its sensory and motor branches, the latter, which takes the name of posterior interosseous nerve, heads posteriorly towards the capitulum and the joint capsule. In this area the nerve runs in a wide space and is insheathed by loose connective tissue which binds it to nearby muscles, the joint capsule, and the radial collateral ligament (anterior bundle).

If microtrauma occurs, this loose connective tissue can be transformed into adherent and relatively inelastic fibrous tissue. The nerve then sticks to the joint capsule and may be compressed by the adherent bridles during elbow movement (5, 6, 8, 10, 30, 33, 36).

In the middle portion, the posterior interosseous nerve is engaged below the extensor carpi brevis, whose arched free edge, which spans from the lateral epicondyle to the deep antibrachialis bundle and the aponeurosis of the flexor digitorum muscles, can be inspissated and fibrotic (Fig. 4).

Many variations in form and thickness of this fibrous septum which passes over the motor branch of the radial nerve have been described. Forearm pronation tightens the aponeurosis as does the opposing wrist extension. Under such conditions, if this fibrous arcade is inspissated and inelastic it can compress the nerve (5, 6, 8, 17, 19, 27, 28, 30, 33, 37, 39).

Neurolysis is mandatory in surgical treatment of lateral epicondylar pathologies with radial nerve compression. In chronic lateral epicondylalgia, the success of surgical treatment consisting solely of the detachment of the extensor carpi radialis brevis from the lateral epicondyle depends not only on the treatment of the insertional pathology, but also on the release of the fibrous insertional arcade of this muscle, which in itself reduces the compression of the posterior interosseous nerve.

In the lower portion, the motor branch overtakes the arcade of the extensor carpi radialis brevis and then penetrates between the bundles of the superficial and deep heads of the supinator brevis muscle (8, 17, 19, 25, 33, 37). The upper edge of the superficial head of the muscle is fibrous in about 30% of adults, yet in the newborn this arcade is always muscular (37). The fibrous arcade of the supinator brevis muscle is called the arcade of Frohse (11) after the anatomist who de-

scribed it in 1908 (Fig. 5).

In the adult this arcade can be extensively fibrotic or not, often depending upon whether the patient repeatedly pronated and supinated the forearm resulting in supinator brevis muscle overload. Pronation tightens the arcade and produces nerve compression while supination releases it (30).

The superficial head of the supinator, and in particular its often fibrotic proximal bundles, insert on the anterior surface of the lateral epicondyle, under the tendon of the extensor carpi radialis brevis and the radial collateral ligament (anterior bundle), and on the lateral surface of the orbicular ligament. Considering this anatomical arrangement, it is easy to understand the role of the supinator brevis muscle, and especially its superficial head, in the pathogenesis of lateral epicondylalgia. In fact, an insertional pathology in that area can

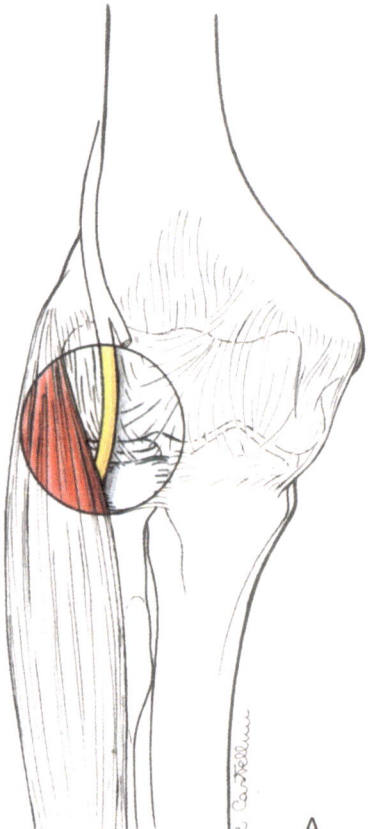

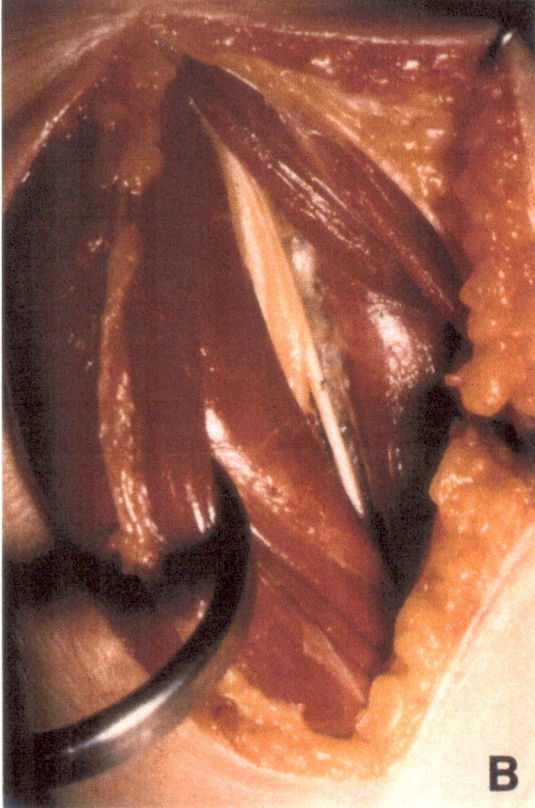

Fig. 4. - A) The schematic drawing shows the upper (joint capsule) and middle (arcade of the extensor carpi radialis brevis) sites where PIN compression is possible; B) operative photograph showing the middle compression site.

affect the entire external compartment of the elbow, with clinical manifestations attributable to syndromes of the lateral epicondyle, the motor branch of the radial nerve, and the capsuloligamentous structures of the humeroradial joint.

The final possible point of compression of the motor branch of the radial nerve is in its passage between the bellies of the superficial and deep heads of the supinator brevis muscle (5, 6, 8, 37, 39). Such an instance is rare, and may happen when the deep head is congenitally underdeveloped ("exposed" area of the radial neck in 25% of cases according to Spinner) (38) or, as in one of our cases, completely absent.

In conclusion, it should be emphasized that nerve damage in the radial tunnel can occur in several places, but predominantly happens:

a) in the fibrous arcade of the extensor carpi brevis;

b) in the fibrous arcade of the supinator brevis muscle.

Clinical diagnosis

The clinical diagnosis of posterior interosseous nerve compression in the radial tunnel is based on the presence of motor deficit in the dependent muscles, featuring radiated pain from the elbow to the forearm and the hand without objectively evident sensory loss.

Two clinical pictures are possible. The first, which is less common, features pain, in the presence of which it is often difficult to distinguish a mild motor deficit. Paresis is also difficult to observe, and the differential problems of disassociated radial nerve paresis should address possible more proximal

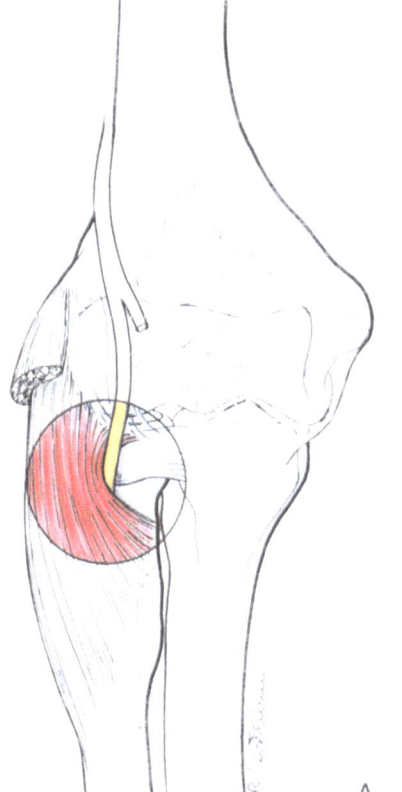
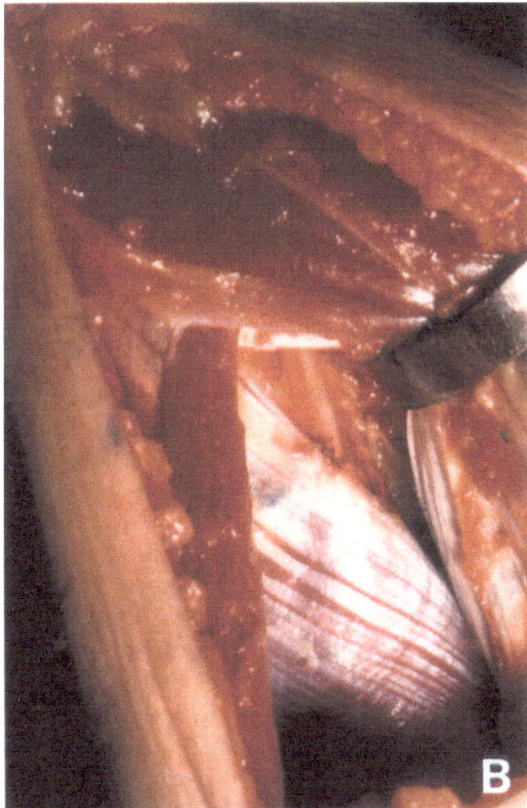

Fig. 5. - A) The schematic drawing shows the lower site (either arcade of supinator or arcade of Frohse) where PIN compression is possible; B) operative photograph of the same site.

nerve compression or neuropathies of other origin, rather than referring to lateral epicondylalgia. In instances of nerve tunnel syndromes of the posterior interosseous nerve that are primarily irritative to the elbow, the diagnosis is more difficult, since it questions the participation of nerve compression in lateral epicondylalgia and because the clinical picture is the same as in epicondylitis. In these cases the diagnosis is based on the character of the spontaneous or evoked pain, the presence of motor deficit, the limitation of active and passive elbow movement, and the preoperative examinations (x-ray, myelogram, thermography, MRI, etc.).

Pain leads the patient to consult a specialist: it is localized in the lateral epicondylar region and often radiates down the posterolateral surface of the forearm to the wrist. Many authors consider this feature important for the diagnosis of nerve compression. The pain is diurnal, but does not subside with rest and intensifies at night (1, 6, 8, 22, 33, 35, 37). We consider neither the localization, the radiation, nor the rhythm of the spontaneous pain important for the diagnosis of nerve compression, because the posterior interosseous nerve is a muscular nerve whose sensory component is proprioceptive.

Pain in such cases is dull, poorly localized, and affects the lateral epicondyle and its muscles in the distribution of the proprioceptive receptors, assuming a character similar to that of musculotendinous and osteoarticular disease.

Pain evoked by pressure on the supinator canal at the radial head is considered to be a specific sign, differentiated from lateral epicondylar pain, which is evoked by pressure on the lateral epicondyle. Likewise, the pain produced by opposing supination with elbow extension is considered specific since the nerve, tensed up by the elbow extension, is compressed by the forced contraction of the supinator muscle. The pain that is reawakened by passive pronation with the elbow extended has the same meaning. In that case the shifting of the radius together with the tension of the fully extended supinator can cause nerve compression.

These three tests that evoke lateral epicondylar pain are considered typical for nerve tunnel syndrome by many authors (6, 8, 19, 32, 35). In our experience they are reliable, but not specific signs of posterior interosseous nerve compression in patients with lateral epicondylalgia. In fact, we believe that nerve tunnel syndrome is often associated with pathology of the musculotendinous structures of the external compartment, and therefore all tests that engage this compartment evoke pain, as they always affect the nearby muscular and osteoarticular structures as well as the nerve.

Roles' sign is considered specific for nerve tunnel syndrome by many authors (8, 19, 24, 33). As to this test, which is based on the pain evoked by opposed extension of the third finger, we are in agreement with Allieu (1), Comtet (6), Howard (14), and others that it is aspecific, given its presence in many routine lateral epicondylar syndromes. It does not, in fact, as Roles thought, indicate motor branch compression below the extensor carpi radialis brevis arcade, but simply insertional pathology of this muscle and the extensor digitorum communis. The involvement of the extensor digitorum muscle in the lateral epicondylar insertion is proven by the pain evoked in this structure during the opposed extension of the third and fourth fingers when no pain is induced by the extension of the second and fifth fingers, which have a separate extensor. The character of the spontaneous and evoked pain in itself is not enough for a diagnosis of nerve tunnel syndrome of the PIN. The clinical manifestations become typical of this pathology when pain is accompanied by functional limitation and paresis of the muscles innervated below the point of compression (individual or common extensors, thumb extensors, etc.). This paralysis is progressive and does not feature a sensory deficit in the radial nerve dermatome.

The patient complains of weakening of metacarpo-phalangeal extension as well as thumb extension and abduction.

Wrist extension is preserved in order to protect the integrity of the nerve branches directed to the extensor muscles of the radius, but it is achieved with radial deviation due to extensor carpi ulnaris insufficiency (40).

The EMG confirms the presence and site of neuromuscolar damage, and is therefore important for the differential diagnosis. Nevertheless, in instances of spontaneous paralysis of the PIN and serious paretic damage, it is always advisable to consider other causes of neurologic lesions, caused by multiple neuropathies of metabolic, toxic, or infective origin. In their primary phases these forms may affect only a single nerve and localize themselves where microtraumatic damage can be done (nerve tunnel syndromes), but the neurologic damage will subsequently manifest itself in various and often symmetrical sites.

The favorable local anatomical conditions should also be considered: a tendinofibrous arcade of Frohse, an "exposed" area of the radial neck (25% of the cases according to Spinner), local neoformations such as lipomas (21, 24) or ganglia (9).

Discussion

At the Clinica Ortopedica dell'Università di Modena the clinical and therapeutic interest in nerve tunnel syndromes of the PIN goes back more than 20 years (3, 20).

From our experience with lateral epicondylar pathology, we find it useful to analyze the current pathogenetic and therapeutic problems in diagnosis of nerve tunnel syndromes of the PIN.

Lateral epicondylalgia must be considered a syndrome without a definite cause and whose pathogenesis remains obscure (28).

It can follow an isolated trauma or repeated microtrauma inflicted during athletic or occupational activity. Functional overloading causes pathological changes in all structures that make up the external compartment. Three types of lesions, either alone or combined, can cause lateral epicondylalgia:
  1) insertional pathology,
  2) humeroradial joint disease,
  3) compression syndromes of the PIN.

Insertional pathology is the most frequent cause of lateral epicondylalgia. The involvement of the anatomical structures surrounding the diseased osteotendinous junction is very important. These can in turn be affected, giving the primary pathology peculiar clinical and pathological aspects (31).

These facts help us understand the pathogenesis of lateral epicondylalgia. If the initial pathology affects the osteotendinous structures, it may subsequently involve both the humeroradial joint and the PIN.

The clinical picture then becomes confused, and a superficial clinical evaluation is unlikely to reveal all the various pathological aspects. This is often the case in lateral epicondylalgia, in which the insertional pathology can be the necessary condition for the development of nerve tunnel syndromes (Table 1). This is true because of the relationship between the tendinous arcade that forms the proximal insertion of the extensor carpi radialis brevis and the PIN, and also because of the role of the supinator brevis muscle in the external compartment.

The extensor carpi radialis brevis muscle inserts on the lateral epicondyle and has a thick fibrous lamina that inserts on the joint capsule and the orbicular ligament. The PIN is connected to this insertional arcade. Our observations of both living patients and cadavers show how this thick fibrous lamina tenses up in full forearm supination, and then relaxes in pronation. The nerve is compressed in supination, and the resulting damage may be aggravated by the presence of fibrotic changes causing hardening and retraction of the tendonous lamina. It is necessary to consider how the extensor carpi radialis brevis carries out its action unaided by the extensor carpi radialis longus in manual labor done with elbow flexed, forearm supinated, and wrist extended. The supinator brevis muscle bears the entire responsibility of forearm supination, and is thus overworked in manual labor requiring repeated forearm supination against resistance. The nearby muscles do not participate in supination when the elbow is extended, yet when it is flexed, supination is aided by the contraction of the biceps and the supinator muscles. Pronation, however, is carried out by the pronator teres with the help of the wrist flexors, and in particular the flexor carpi ulnaris muscle, through the entire range of elbow flexion and extension. The supinator brevis muscle is therefore overworked in the normal functional positions of the upper limb.

For this reason we believe that insertional

Table 1
COMBINED FORMS

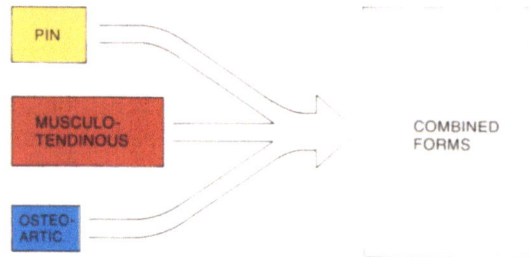

Table 2
EPICONDYLALGIA

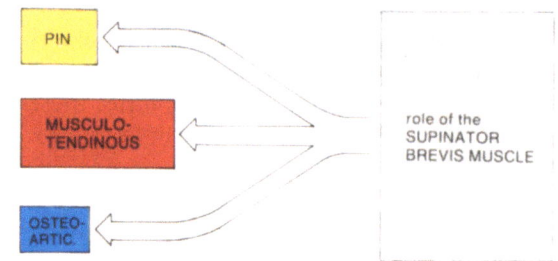

syndromes are frequent, and could be the common pathogenetic factor in all types of lateral epicondylalgia, the symptoms of which are determined by nerve tunnel syndromes caused by musculotendinous and osteoarticular syndromes (Table 2). The superficial head of the supinator brevis muscle inserts on the lateral epicondyle, the capsule, and the radial collateral ligament, and has a direct relationship with the PIN (Fig. 6). Therefore, a osteotendinous pathology of the supinator brevis can eventually provoke neurologic, musculotendinous, and joint disease. In these cases, lateral epicondylalgia is often resistant to the usual medical and physical therapy and must therefore be subjected to surgery, which should aim to treat the osteotendinous, osteoarticular, and neurologic pathologies all at once.

Surgical intervention consists of isolating and freeing the portion of the radial nerve inside the radial tunnel. Exploration can be done through either a parallel or a zig-zag incision (8). Either a posterior or an anterolateral approach can be used to expose the radial nerve and the arcade of Frohse (30). Using a posterior approach, the nerve is reached by passing through the extensor carpi radialis brevis anteriorly and the extensor digitorum communis posteriorly (8). In instances of possible compression near the extensor brevis, the nerve can also be reached by passing through the extensor carpi radialis longus and brevis. Such an incision can be lengthened proximally in case of possible lateral epicondylar muscle detachment (11, 27, 30, 33). The anterolateral approach requires a rectilinear, zig-zag, or S-shaped incision dis-

tally at the bend of the elbow and medially at the brachioradialis. The advantage of this approach is that it isolates the nerve proximally, facilitating mobilization. The approach does, however, require the isolation of numerous intramuscular neurovascular bundles along the course of the nerve and leaves a prominent scar. The incision in the arcade of the extensor radialis brevis muscle is transverse, while the section of the arcade of Frohse is longitudinal and parallel to the nerve.

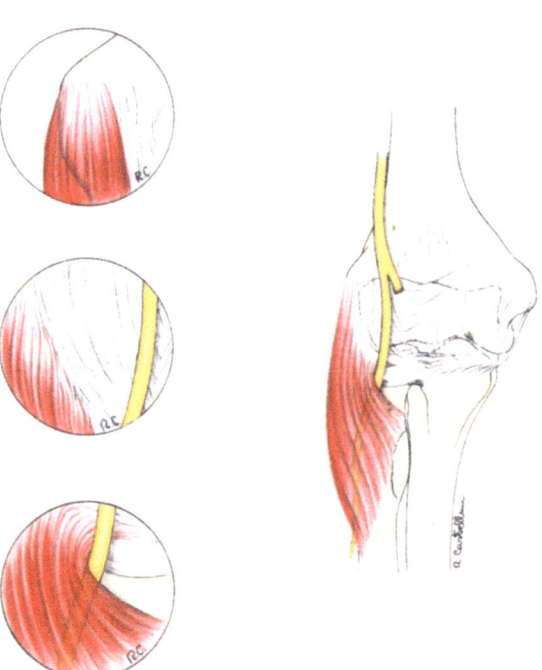

Fig. 6. - The superficial head of the supinator muscle inserts on the lateral epicondyle, the capsule, and the radial collateral ligament, then comes into direct contact with the PIN. It may therefore be the common element in neurologic, musculotendinous, and joint pathology.

In this operation we have used the following procedure for over five years:

1) anesthesia (local or general) without curarization,

2) limb ischemia with a tourniquet,

3) 5 cm lateral incision starting at the lateral epicondyle and heading distally toward the radial styloid process (Fig. 7),

4) isolation of the lateral cutaneous nerve of the forearm in the subcutaneous tissue above the antebrachial fascia (Fig. 8),

5) recognition of the passage between the extensor carpi radialis longus and brevis muscles (Fig. 9),

6) singling out of the two terminal branches, sensory and motor, of the radial nerve and isolation of the nervous branch that innervates the extensor carpi radialis brevis,

7) recognition of the fibrous tendinous arcade of the extensor carpi radialis brevis and its section or detachment from the lateral epicondyle (Fig. 10),

8) singling out of the arcade of Frohse, the PIN, and the anterior recurrent vein and artery of the elbow (Fig. 11),

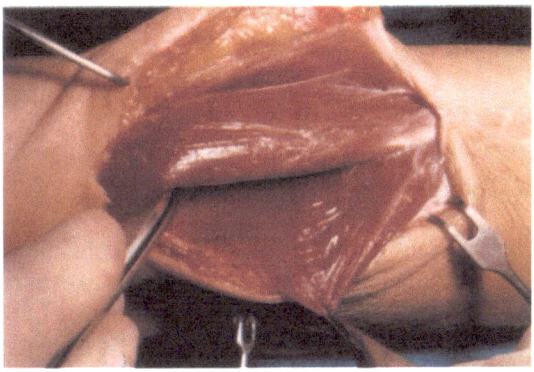

Fig. 9. - View of the passage between the extensor carpi longus and brevis.

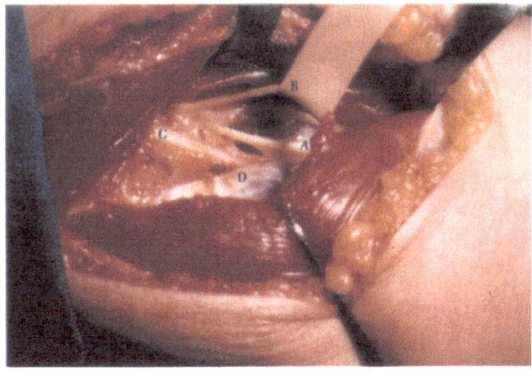

Fig. 10. - View of the branches of the radial nerve: A) sensory; B) headed for the extensor carpi radialis brevis; C) motor; and D) headed for the arcade of the supinator muscle, or arcade of Frohse.

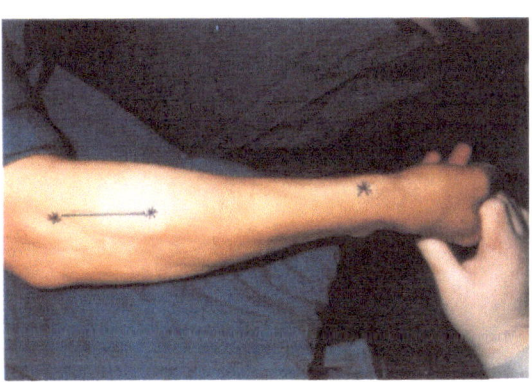

Fig. 7. - Lateral incision.

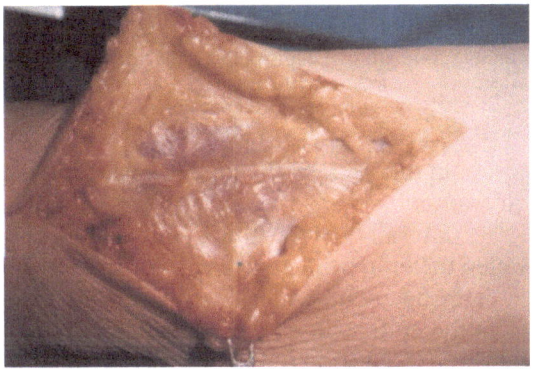

Fig. 8. - Isolation of the lateral cutaneous nerve of the forearm in the subcutaneous tissue.

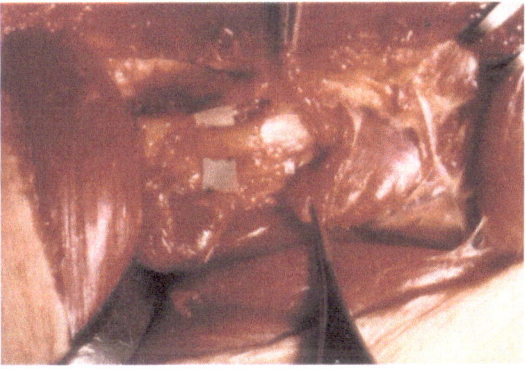

Fig. 11. - Isolation of the PIN and section of the arcade.

9) section of the fibrous arcade of the supinator brevis and possible detachment of the supinator from the lateral epicondyle. This allows the exploration of the humero-radial joint (Fig. 12),

10) neurolysis of the PIN with the aid of optics.

PATHOLOGY OF THE INTERNAL COMPARTMENT: ULNAR NERVE TUNNEL SYNDROME

The numerous studies dedicated to ulnar nerve tunnel syndrome over the last 50 years have given us a thorough knowledge of its physiopathogenetic and clinical aspects. Starting from the first observations of Panas (1878) and Andrae (1889), both foreign (51, 52, 64, 67, 68, 70, 71, 40, 73, 74) and Italian (44, 46, 47, 62) physicians have described the different pathological and clinical aspects as well as those of surgical treatment (43, 45, 48, 49, 50, 53; 55, 56, 57, 59, 60, 51, 65, 63; 66, 67, 68, 69). Nevertheless, there are still some unresolved clinical and surgical problems. The differential diagnosis with C8-T1 spinal compression and compression of the primary lower trunk and the secondary medial trunk at the interscalenic and costo-clavicular passage is difficult in some cases.

Surgical neurolysis is unanimously considered the most suitable treatment, yet the choice of method is still controversial.

The cubital tunnel

The ulnar nerve passes from the posterior portion of the arm to the medial portion of the forearm inside the cubital tunnel, an osteo-fibrous canal where true kinetic anatomy is achieved (64), allowing the nerve to change its position according to the different movements of the elbow.

The osteofibrous tunnel that carries the ulnar nerve is split into two anatomical parts with different functional characteristics (Fig. 13).

The proximal portion is a true triangular osteofibrous canal bordered:

— in the front by the posterior surface of the epitrochlea;

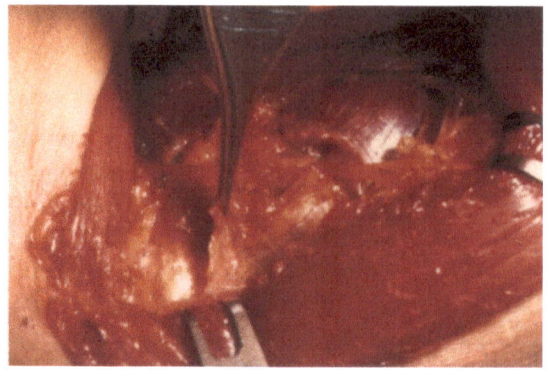

Fig. 12. - Detachment of the supinator and possibly the extensor carpi radialis brevis from the lateral epicondyle.

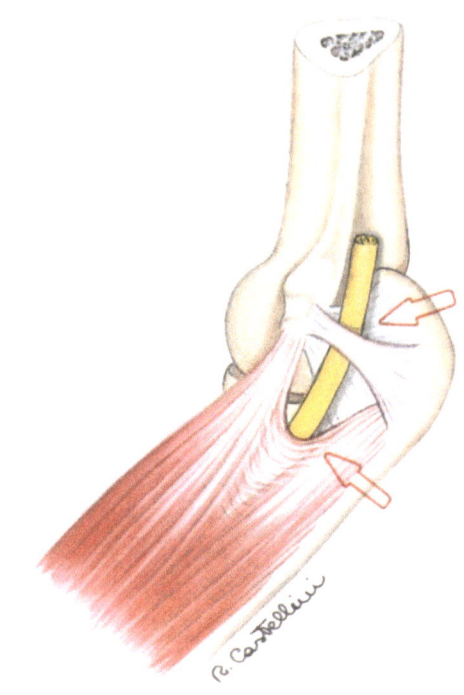

Fig. 13. - Schematic drawing showing the two segments of the cubital tunnel (epitrochlear-olecranal ligament, arcade of the flexor carpi ulnaris) where ulnar nerve compression is possible.

— in the back by the medial surface of the olecranon;

— laterally by a thick fibrous bundle called the epitrochlear-olecranal ligament.

This ligament, which is transversely tense from the epitrochlea to the olecranon, is a rudimentary epitrochleoulnar muscle that is present in many mammals and even sometimes in humans, where it is categorized as a regressive anomaly (Gruber's muscle). In the proximal tract of the cubital tunnel, the nerve is surrounded by loose cellular tissue and accompanied by the posterior recurrent ulnar artery. A small serous bursa allows the nerve to slide over the posterior surface of the epitrochlea and thus avoid traction or compression during elbow movement.

In the distal portion of the tunnel the nerve exits from the elbow region and continues down the forearm. This portion of the tunnel is an osteofibrous opening with a floor formed by the olecranon and the ulnar collateral ligament and a roof formed by the fibrous arcade that joins the two heads of the flexor carpi ulnaris that insert on the epitrochlea and olecranon (Fig. 14). Anglo-Saxon physicians call this fibrous arcade, that becomes the epitrochlear-olecranal ligament, Osborne's arcade, after the author who discovered its pathogenicity and coined the term "cubital tunnel syndrome". Osborne (67, 68) describes the structure of this fibrous membrane, pointing out the potential harmfulness of the transversal fibers that close the opening of the canal, since the position of the ulnar nerve varies during elbow flexion and extension. Mansat (64) describes the dynamic anatomy of the ulnar nerve in elbow flexion (Fig. 15). During these movements the nerve tightens and lengthens about 5 mm for every 45 degrees of flexion; it also shifts toward the anteromedial portion of the groove and tends to dislocate anteriorly (Fig. 16). This shift is

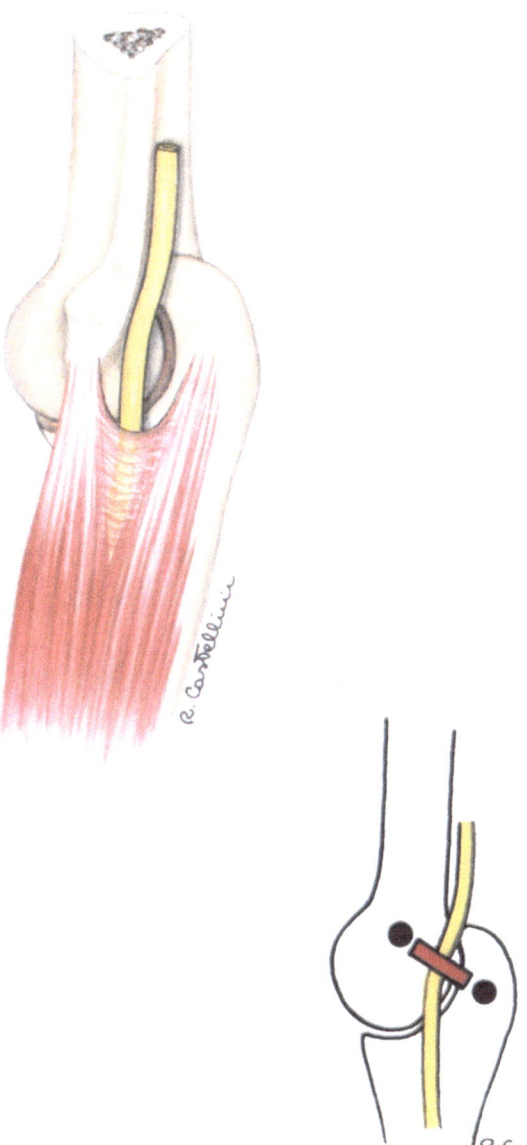

Fig. 15. - In elbow extension the ulnar nerve is located centrally in the groove and under the loose arcade of Osborne.

possible in the proximal part near the epitrochlear-olecranal groove, but becomes critical in the distal part near the cubital tunnel. In fact, the two heads of the flexor carpi ulnaris that insert on the epitrochlea and the olecranon move apart, putting stress on the fibrous arcade that joins them (67, 68, 74, 64). The epitrochlear head then compresses and hooks the ulnar nerve. This harmful mechanism is aided by the decrease in height (about 2.5 mm) and volume of the cubital tunnel and the three to sixfold increase in intraneural

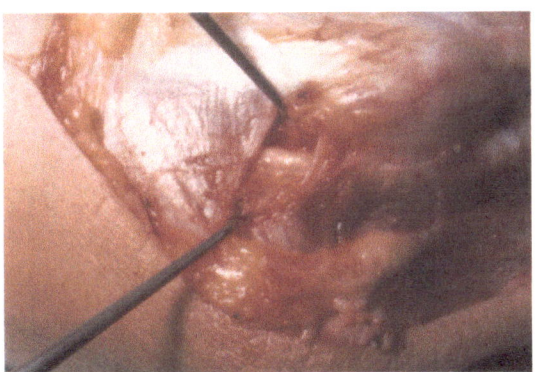

Fig. 14. - Operative photograph showing the fibrous arcade (held taut by the hooks) that joins the two heads of the flexor carpi ulnaris that insert on the epitrochlea and olecranon.

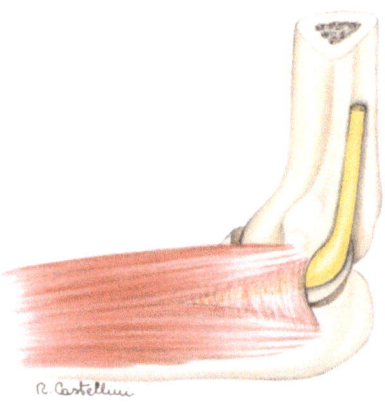

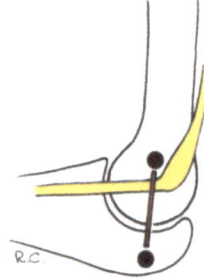

Fig. 16. - During elbow flexion the nerve tends to dislocate anteriorly, coming into contact with the epitrochlear head of the flexor carpi ulnaris.

pressure. These observations indicate that true primary ulnar nerve tunnel syndrome occurs near the arcade of the flexor carpi ulnaris. In fact, even under normal conditions this area subjects the nerve to compression, strain, and intraneural hemodynamic changes during elbow flexion that can lead to neuropathy with peri- and intraneural fibrosis. Elbow flexion can also be used as a clinical test (cubital maneuver). In nerve compression pathologies occurring in the arcade of the flexor carpi ulnaris, simply flexing the elbow is enough to bring on paresis in the parts of the hand near the ulnar nerve. This maneuver can be facilitated by completely abducting the shoulder and hyperextending the wrist to pull the nerve taut. Compression pathology of the ulnar nerve in the internal compartment of the elbow can therefore occur in two locations:

A) the epitrochlear-olecranal groove,

B) the fibrous arcade of the flexor carpi ulnaris.

The epitrochlear-olecranal groove is predisposed to this pathology because of congenital and/or acquired factors. In this area the nerve is free and insheathed by loose, well-vascularized cellular tissue (72). In many cases the looseness of the epitrochlear-olecranal bundle allows the nerve to dislocate in front of the epitrochlea (70). The most common congenital factors capable of changing this space are constitutional cubital valgus deformity, epitrochlear-olecranal ligament hypertrophy, epitrochlear and anconeus muscle persistence, and congenital overlooseness of the ligament.

The most common acquired factors that can encourage the onset of ulnar neuropathy are traumatic (Fig. 17) and degenerative lesions that cause valgus deformity in the elbow as well as the formation of bone spurs in the groove. Both articular synovial diseases, especially in rheumatoid arthritis, and local disease with reactive bursitis can occupy the epitrochlear-olecranal space and cause nerve compression. Yet currently the structure most likely to cause compression of the ulnar nerve in overwork syndromes of the internal compartment is considered to be (1, 67, 68) the arcade of the flexor carpi ulnaris. The specific etiology is caused by repeated occupational or athletic movements that produce hypertrophy of the flexor carpi ulnaris and thickening of the proximal insertional arcade, resulting in chronic compression of the ulnar nerve. Even though the arthritic changes in the humerocubital joint do not cause compression in the groove, they may encourage primary

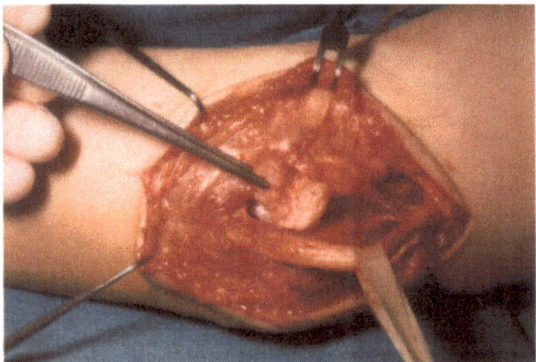

Fig. 17. - Operative photograph of a bone fragment inside the groove as a result of a fracture.

neuropathy in the flexor carpi ulnaris since they limit the movement of the nerve during elbow flexion and extension. This leads Allieu (1) to declare that the elderly patient's hand made thin by interosseous muscle hypotrophy is partially a result of compression pathology of the ulnar nerve, which over time is exacerbated by arthritis and repeated microtrauma.

Clinical diagnosis

The clinical picture features sensory and motor deficit of the ulnar nerve. McGowan (65) distinguishes three successive phases. The first is characterized by subjective sensory deficit with episodic paresis most often in the little finger. Slight hypesthesia may be present. In the second phase the paresis becomes painful, the hypesthesia is more severe, and an initial muscular deficit appears with mild hypotrophy of the hypothenar and interosseous muscles.

Amyotrophy of the first interosseous space is often the first sign (1) (Fig. 18). The patient exhibits a weakened grip, especially between the thumb and forefinger (first-degree Froment sign). In the third phase the sensory and motor deficits are more significant. The clinical picture becomes typical and features all signs of ulnar nerve paresis in the hand. The marked hyposthenia is accompanied by muscular deficits and either hypotrophy or atrophy. Nevertheless, the "ulnar hand" is inconstant and often mild compared to what is caused by traumatic nervous lesions. Local signs may be revealed, such as the search for the ulnar pain focal point through palpation or percussion at the cubital tunnel and the positivity of the cubital maneuver (awakening of pain during passive elbow flexion), which is similar to the Phalen test used for carpal tunnel syndrome. The complementary examinations are based above all on EMG, which shows not only the neurogenic damage to the intrinsic hand muscles dependent on the ulnar nerve (potential for denervation), but especially the decrease in conduction time, which can help localize the compression site. It should be pointed out that, in cases of primary pathology, the decrease in conduction time may become evi-

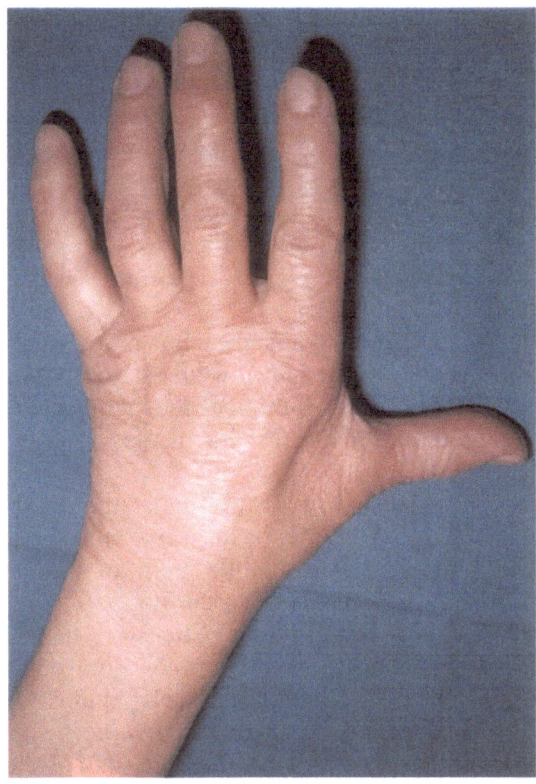

Fig. 18. - Marked amyotrophy of the 1st interspace.

dent after stress tests of the flexor carpi ulnaris (Mansat, 1981). Both routine and tangential x-rays can show possible epitrochlear-olecranal groove changes. MRI, which is used infrequently at present, may provide useful information on the movement of the nerve and its relationship with the nearby tissues in different degrees of elbow flexion.

The differential diagnosis should be made with other possible sites of nerve compression in the upper limb. The spinal character of C8-T1 compression and irritative pathologies in cervicobrachialgia as well as the typical peripheral motor character of ulnar nerve compression in Guyon's canal are elements that allow easy differentiation of these pathologies from nerve compression in the elbow. The differential diagnosis with the outlet syndrome is more difficult. The following clinical observations facilitate this diagnosis:

1) Compression syndrome of the ulnar nerve in the elbow is more common in males and in those who suffer repeated microtrauma in athletic or occupational activity. Outlet syndrome is more common in females

who exhibit hyperkyphosis during shoulder adduction. Painful subacromial pathology may also be present.

2) In ulnar nerve compression, hand paresis can be evoked by passive elbow flexion. In the outlet syndrome, however, it can be brought on by upper limb abduction and dynamic tests that modify the costo-clavicular and interscalenic spaces (Adson, Wright, etc.).

3) In elbow syndromes the paresis primarily affects the hand, while in the outlet syndrome the distribution of the medial cutaneous nerve of the forearm is also affected (Fig. 19).

4) The Tinel sign is present at the proximal insertion of the flexor carpi ulnaris in elbow syndromes and in the supra- or subclavicular region in the outlet syndrome.

5) Sensory and motor deficits are typical of the ulnar nerve in compression syndromes of the elbow. While the intrinsic hand muscles almost always experience deficits, the flexor carpi ulnaris and the flexor profundus of the little finger are rarely affected. In costo-clavicular syndromes, however, there is a sensory-motor deficit in the entire C8-T1 distribution.

6) In the diagnosis of compression neuropathy of the elbow, the EMG is the most indicative exam, while in costo-clavicular compression syndrome diagnosis the EMG result can be confirmed by hemodynamic exams (phlebogram, Doppler, arteriogram).

Treatment

The primary stages of nerve tunnel syndrome (McGowan's phase 1) can be treated conservatively. Curtailment of manual labor, use of an orthosis, and local and general medical treatment can curb the evolution of the disease. Surgical treatment is indicated in the subsequent stages, however, due to the clinical and instrumental evidence of nervous damage (phases 2 and 3).

Treatment should have two main objectives:

1) nerve decompression;

2) improvement of peri- and intraneural circulatory conditions.

Many different techniques have been proposed to achieve these aims in the 70 years since Platt (70) described the nerve anteposition technique. All authors, however, tend to emphasize the importance of the following three stages of surgery: the section of the epitrochlear-olecranal ligament, the section of the arcade of the flexor carpi ulnaris, and the lateral neurolysis with epinerviotomy. The proposed techniques can be divided into three groups:

A) those which include only the above three stages;

B) those which add anteposition of the nerve;

C) those which add medial epicondylectomy (49, 57, 59). Foster (53), Lugnegard (61), and Adelaar (43) compared the studies in which these methods were used, concluding that the results are influenced very little by the choice of technique.

In light of our experience, we do not believe that a standard surgical technique can be identified. We do not consider anteposition necessary in all cases. The essential elements

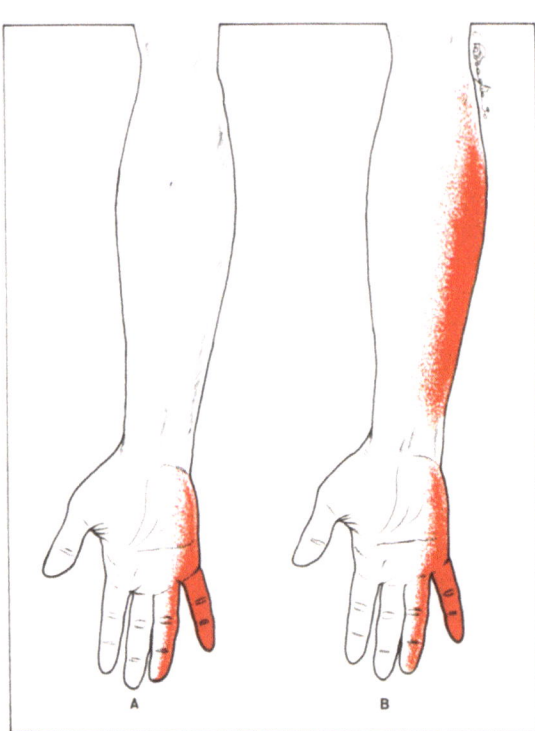

Fig. 19. - Schematic drawing showing the distribution of paresis in A) tunnel syndromes of the elbow and B) outlet syndrome.

are the section of both the arcade of the flexor carpi ulnaris and the epitrochlear-olecranal ligament in order to check the condition of both the nerve and the perinervous tissue in the space behind the epitrochlea. Therefore, if there are no congenital or acquired malformations of the epitrochlear-olecranal groove and the compression is identified at the arcade of the flexor carpi ulnaris, the following procedure should be followed:

– section of the arcade of the flexor carpi ulnaris, which should be wide and lengthened distally (Fig. 20). Care must be taken not to injure it at the collateral nervous branch, headed for the muscle, that detaches from the posterior wall of the nerve and is therefore protected by the head of the muscle that inserts on the olecranon.

– Section of the epitrochlear-olecranal ligament.

– Anterior longitudinal epinerviotomy with the aid of optic magnification, taking care not to cut off the arterial and venous perinervial circulation. It is often necessary to perform the epinerviotomy near the arcade of the flexor carpi ulnaris, where the nerve compression can be observed, rather than in the epitrochlear-olecranal groove.

Anteposition is necessary in cases of cubitus valgus, bone spurs inside the groove, inability of the groove to hold the nerve which tends to dislocate during elbow flexion, or further surgery to treat inveterate neuropathy. Anteposition must be accurately performed; the main stages are as follows:

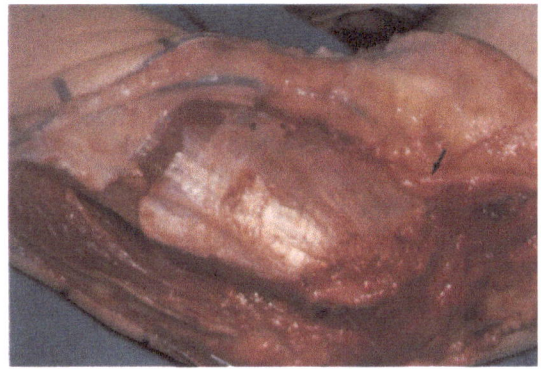

Fig. 21. - Anteposition of the ulnar nerve (arrow) into the flexor carpi ulnaris.

– isolation of the nerve by opening the groove and widely sectioning the proximal (arcade of Struthers) and distal (arcade of the FCU) fibrous structures;

– detachment of the nerve from the bottom of the groove while attempting to save the loose perinervous tissue that contains venous and arterial vessels;

– the anteposition should place the nerve in well-vascularized tissue protected by the bone surface. For this reason we prefer to perform anteposition in the flexor carpi ulnaris belly (Fig. 21) rather than the subcutaneous tissue.

The detachment of the epitrochlear head of this muscle is done at the tendinous insertion, even if some authors (49, 57, 59) prefer to chip off a piece of bone from the epitrochlea. At the end of the operation, elbow flexion and extension should cause no compression of the muscle-covered nerve.

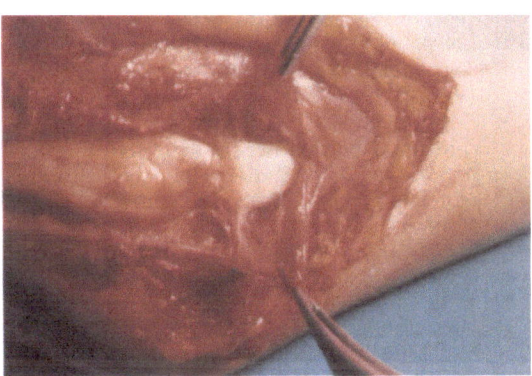

Fig. 20. - The section of the arcade of the flexor carpi ulnaris should be wide and lengthened distally.

CONCLUSIONS

Among the painful pathologies of the elbow, tunnel syndromes with nerve compression must be generally considered a product of regional musculotendinous inflammation (1).

Ulnar nerve pathology in the elbow is common, although diagnosis is often difficult. In its primary phases, the arcade of the flexor carpi ulnaris is the true site of compression. The Tinel sign in that area indicates nerve damage, and the EMG can confirm the diagnosis. The success of surgical treatment depends on both its timeliness and a correct choice of technique, which is based on the presence of congenital or acquired malformations of the epitrochlear-olecranal groove. Whatever method is chosen, it should aim to free the nerve in the osteofibrous groove of the flexor carpi ulnaris.

Isolated pathology of the motor branch of the radial nerve in the elbow is very rare. Lateral epicondylalgia may be manifested by pathologic and clinical signs of either radial tunnel syndrome of the PIN plus lateral epicondylar insertional disease, or the former plus humeroradial joint disease. Since the supinator muscle is anatomically connected to the lateral epicondylalgia (at its insertion point),

the posterior interosseous nerve (in the arcade of Frohse), and the humeroradial joint (on the radial collateral and orbicular ligaments), in case of microtraumatic phlogistic pathology it may be the pathogenetic element that explains the different tendinous, neurologic, and articular manifestations of many types of lateral epicondylalgia. Surgical treatment should be reserved for forms with clinical signs of peripheral nerve damage that are resistant to the usual therapy. A lateral approach provides an anatomical route to the supinator muscle that runs between the extensor carpi longus and brevis muscles. In this way insertional, compression, and osteoarticular syndromes can all be treated simultaneously.

REFERENCES

External compartment pathology

1) ALLIEU Y.: *Compressions nerveuses non traumatiques du membre supérieur. Cahiers d'enseignement de la SOFCOT. Conferences d'enseignement 1976 sous la direction di J. Duparc.* Expansion Scientifique Francaise Paris.

2) BAUMGARD S.H., SCHWARTZ D.R.: Percutaneous release of the epicondylar muscles for humeral epicondylitis. *Am. J. Sports Med.* 1982; **10**: 233-236.

3) BEDESCHI P., CELLI L.: Lesioni dei nervi periferici da sport. *G.I.O.T.* 1979; 5, Suppl. 323-329.

4) CAPENER N.: The vulnerability of the posterior interosseous nerve of the forearm. *J. Bone Jt Surg.* 1966; **48-B**: 770.

5) COMTET J.J., CHAMBAUD D., GENETY J.: La compression de la branche postérieur du nerf radial. *Nouv. Presse Med.* 1976; **5**: 1111-1114.

6) COMTET J.J., LALAIN, MOYEN B., GENETY J., BRUNET-GUEDJ E., LAZO-HENRIQUEZ R.: Les epicondylalgies avec compression de la branche postérieure du nerf radial. *Rev. Chir. Orthop.* 1985; Suppl. 2, **71**: 89-93.

7) DURANDEAU A., GENESTE R.: Un syndrome canalaire rare: la paralysie du nerf interosseux postérieur. A propos de 10 cas. *Rev. Chir. Orthop.* 1988; Suppl. 2, **74**: 156-157.

8) EVERSMANN W.W.: Entrapment and compression neuropathies. In: *Operative hand surgery* (Green D.P. ed.). Churchill Livingstone, 1988.

9) FERRINI L.: Paralisi dissociata parziale del nervo radiale al gomito da ganglio artrogeno. *Chir. Org. Mov.* 1974; **63**: 153-157.

10) FRIGNANI R., MARCHETTI N.: Sulla sindrome dissociata del nervo radiale nella doccia di torsione del gomito. *Riv. Chir. Mano* 1967; **6**: 38-41.

11) FROHSE F., FRANKEL M.: *Die Muskeln des menschlichen Armes.* Iena Fischer, 1908.

12) FROIMSON A.I.: Tenosynovitis and tennis elbow. In: *Operative hand surgery* (Green D.P. ed.). Churchill Livingstone, 1988.

13) HEYSE-MOORE G.H.: Resistant tennis elbow. *J. Hand Surg.* 1983; **9-B**: 64-66.

14) HOWARD F.M.: Controversies in nerve entrapment syndromes in the forearm and wrist. In: *Controversies in hand surgery.*

15) KAPLAN P.E.: Posterior interosseous neuropathies: Natural history. *Arch. Phys. Med. Rehabil.* 1984; **65**: 399-400.

16) KENESI CL., FICAT C.: Traitement chirurgical de l'epicondylalgie. *Rev. Rhum.* 1973; **40**: 347-351.

17) KOPELL H.P., THOMPSON W.A.L.: *Peripheral entrapment neuropathies.* Williams and Wilkins Company, Baltimore, 1963.

18) LAUS S., GALLI G.: Paralisi dissociate del nervo radiale da compressione nel muscolo breve supinatore. *Riv. Chir. Mano* 1976; **4**: 166-170.

19) LISTER G.D., BELSOLE R.B., KLEINERT H.E.: The radial tunnel syndrome. *J. Hand Surg.* 1979; **4**: 52-59.

20) LUPPINO T., CELLI L., VACCARI A.: Ulteriore contributo alla conoscenza delle sindromi compressive del nervo radiale alla doccia di torsione del gomito. *Boll. Soc. Med. Chir. di Modena* 1971; 71.

21) MALCAPI C., GRASSI G.: I lipomi profondi degli arti e la sindrome di compressione del nervo radiale da lipoma dell'avambraccio. *Min. Ortop.* 1975; **26**: 551-570.

22) MANSAT M.: Syndromes canalaires et des defilés. *Enc. Med. Chir.* 1986; Paris, 15005, A10, 11.

23) MARCHETTI N. ET AL.: *Sindromi nervose*

canalicolari degli arti ad eziologia non traumatica. Liviana Ed., Padova, 1978.

24) MOSS S.H., SWITZER H.E.: Radial tunnel syndrome: a spectrum of clinical presentations. *J. Hand Surg.* 1983; **8**: 414-420.

25) MOSSER J.J., DEFLASSIEUX M., AUPECLE P., PIGANIOL G.: Compression de la branche postérieure du nerf radial par un tumeur benigne de la region du coude. *J. Chir.* 1978; **115**: 515-522.

26) MULHOLLAND R.C.: Non traumatic progressive paralysis of the posterior interosseous nerve. *J. Bone Jt Surg.* 1966; **48-B**: 781-785.

27) NARAKAS A.: Epicondylite et nerf radial. *Med. Hyg.* 1974; **22**: 2067.

28) NARAKAS A.: Le traitment chirurgical de l'epicondylalgie. In: *Coude et médecine de rééducation.* Masson, 1979, 129-139.

29) NIRSCHL R.P., PETTRONE F.A.: Tennis elbow. The surgical treatment of lateral epicondylitis. *J. Bone Jt Surg.* 1979; **61-A**: 832-839.

30) PALAZZI S., PALAZZI C., RAIMONDI P., ARAMBURO F.: Syndromes compressifs du nerf radial. In: *Syndrome canalaire du membre supérieur.* Monographie du G.E.M. Expansion Scientifique Francaise, Paris, 1983, pp. 41-54.

31) PERUGIA L., POSTACCHINI F., IPPOLITO E.: Tendinopatia inserzionale degli estensori della mano (epicondilite-«tennis elbow»); Tendinopatia inserzionale dei flessori della mano e pronatori dell'avambraccio (epitrocleite-epicondilite mediale). In: *I tendini. biologia/patologia/clinica.* Masson Italia Ed., Milano, 1981.

32) RITTS G.D., WOOD M.B., LINSCHEID R.L.: Radial tunnel syndrome. A ten-year surgical experience. *Clin. Orthop. Rel. Res.* 1987; **219**: 201-205.

33) ROLES N.C., MAUDSLEY R.H.: Radial tunnel syndrome. Resistant tennis elbow as a nerve entrapment. *J. Bone Jt Surg.* 1972; **54-B**: 499-508.

34) SCARAGLIO C., PISU G., BIGNOTTI B.: La sindrome da compressione del nervo radiale all'arcata di Frohse. *Min. Ortop. Traum.* 1988; **39**: 55-58.

35) SERRE H., SIMON L., CLAUSTRE J.: L'origine canaliculaire de certains syndromes du membre supérieur. *Rev. Rhum.* 1966; **33**: 231-246.

36) SHARRAD W.J.W.: Posterior interosseous neuritis. *J. Bone Jt Surg.* 1966; **48-B**: 777-780.

37) SPINNER M.: The arcade of Frohse and its relationship to posterior interosseous nerve paralysis. *J. Bone Jt Surg.* 1968; **50-B**: 809-812.

38) SPINNER M.: The radial nerve. In: *Injuries to the major branches of peripheral nerves of forearm.* Philadelphia, W.B. Saunders, 1972.

39) SPONSELLER P.D., ENGBER W.D.: Double-entrapment radial tunnel syndrome. *J. Hand Surg.* 1983; **8**: 420-423.

40) SUNDERLAND S.: *Nerves and nerve injuries.* Livingstone, London, 1968.

41) VAN ROSSUM J., BURUMA O.J.S., KAMPHUISEN, ONVLEE G.J.: Tennis elbow- A radial tunnel syndrome? *J. Bone Jt Surg.* 1978; **60-B**: 197-198.

42) WERNER C.O.: Lateral elbow pain and posterior interosseous nerve entrapment. *Acta Orthop. Scand.* 1979; Suppl., **174**: 1.

Internal compartment pathology

43) ADELAAR R.S., FOSTER W.C., MC DOWEL C.: The treatment of the cubital tunnel syndrome. *J. Hand Surg.* 1984; **9-A**: 90-95.

44) ALTISSIMI M., PECORELLI F., PIMPINELLI G.: La compressione del nervo ulnare al gomito. *G.I.O.T.* 1986; **12**: 413-418.

45) BENOIT B.G., PRESTON D.N., ATACK D.M., DA SILVA M.D.: Neurolysis combined with the application of a silastic envelope for ulnar nerve entrapment at the elbow. *Neurosurg.* 1987; **20**: 594-598.

46) CALANDRIELLO B., COLÌ G., PEDEMONTE P.: *Patologia del nervo ulnare alla doccia epitrocleare.*

47) CATALANO F., DI LAZZARO A., DE SANTIS E.: La neuropatia del nervo ulnare alla doccia epitrocleare. *Arch. Putti* 1980; **30**: 143-153.

48) CHAISE F., BOUCHET T., SEDEL L., WITVOET J.: Résultats de la liberation chirurgicale du nerf cubitale dans les syndromes du défilé retro-epitrochléen. *J. Chir.* 1983; **120**: 251-255.

49) CRAVEN P.R., GREEN D.P.: Cubital tunnel syndrome. Treatment by medial epicondylectomy. *J. Bone Jt Surg.* 1980; **62-A**: 986-989.

50) DIMOND M.L., LISTER G.D.: Cubital tunnel syndrome treated by long-arm splintage. *J. Hand Surg.* 1985; **A-10**: 430.

51) DURANDEAU A., CHAVOIX J.B., GENESTE R.: A propos de 91 compressions du nerf cubital au niveau du coude. *Rev. Chir. Orthop.* 1986; Suppl., **2**: 240-242.

52) FEINDEL, STRATFORD: Cubital tunnel compression in tardy ulnar palsy. *Can. Med. Ass. J.* 1958; **78**: 351.

53) FOSTER R.J., EDSHAGE M.D.: Factors related to the outcome of surgically managed compressive ulnar neuropathy at the elbow level. *J. Hand Surg.* 1981; **6**: 181-192.

54) FRAGIADAKIS E.G., LAMB D.W.: An unusual cause of ulnar nerve compression. *The hand* 1970; **2**: 14-15.

55) FROIMSON A.I., ZAHRAWI M.D.: Treatment of compression neuropathy of the ulnar nerve at the elbow by epicondylectomy and neurolysis. *J. Hand Surg.* 1980; **5**: 391-395.

56) KAMHIN M., GANEL A., ROSENBERG B., ENGEL J.: Anterior transposition of the ulnar nerve. *Acta Orthop. Scand.* 1980; **51**: 475-478.

57) KING T., MORGAN F.P.: Late results of removing the medial humeral epicondyle for traumatic ulnar neuritis. *J. Bone Jt Surg.* 1959; **41-B**: 51-55.

58) HARRELSON: Hypertrophy of the FUC as a cause of ulnar nerve compression in the distal part of the forearm. *J. Bone Jt Surg.* 1975.

59) JONES R.E., GAUNTT C.: Medial epicondylectomy for ulnar nerve compression syndrome at the elbow. *Clin. Orthop.* 1979; **139**: 174-178.

60) LEARMONTH J.K.: A technique for trasplanting the ulnar nerve. *Surg. Gynec. Obstet* 1942; **75**: 792-793.

61) LUGNEGARD H., JUHLIN L., NILSSON B.J.: Ulnar neuropathy at the elbow treated with decompression. *Scand. J. Plast. Reconstr. Surg.* 1982; **16**: 195-200.

62) LUPPINO T., CELLI L., VACCARI A.: Considerazioni anatomo-cliniche sulle sindromi compressive canalicolari del nervo ulnare al gomito e al polso. *Boll. Soc. Med. Chir. di Modena* 1971; **71**: 1-11.

63) MACNICOL M.F.: The results of operation for ulnar neuritis. *J. Bone Jt Surg.* 1979; **61-B**: 159-164.

64) MANSAT M., GUIRAUD B., CIANET M., TESTUT M.F.: *Le tunnel cubital et les paralysies cubitales idiopathiques au niveau du coude. Pathologie des nerfs périphériques.* P. Fabre, 1978.

65) MC GOWAN A.J.: The results of transposition of the ulnar nerve for traumatic neuritis. *J. Bone Jt Surg.* 1950; **32-B** 293-301.

66) OGATA K., MANSKE P.R., LESKER P.A.: The effects of surgical dissection on regional blood flow to the ulnar nerve in the cubital tunnel. *Clin. Orthop.* 1985; **193**: 195-198.

67) OSBORNE G.: The surgical treatment of tardy ulnar neuritis. *J. Bone Jt Surg.* 1957; **39-B**: 1-82.

68) OSBORNE G.: Compression neuritis of the ulnar nerve at the elbow. *The hand* 1970; **2**: 10-13.

69) PAYAN J.: Anterior transposition of the ulnar nerve: an electrophysiological study. *J. Neurol. Neurosurg.* 1970; **33**: 157-165.

70) PLATT H.: The pathogenesis and treatment of traumatic neuritis of the ulnar nerve in post condylar groove. *Br. J. Surg.* 1926; **13**: 409-413.

71) ROULLET J.: *Syndrome compressif du nerf cubital au coude.* Monografia GEM, 1983, pp. 74-95.

72) TESTUT L.: *Anatomia umana.* Utet, 1923.

73) VANDERPOOL D.W., CHALMERS J., LAMB D.W., WHISTON T.B.: Peripheral compression lesions of the ulnar nerve. *J. Bone Jt Surg.* 1968: **50-B**: 792-803.

74) WADSWORTH T.G.: The external compression syndrome of the ulnar nerve at the cubital tunnel. *Clin. Orthop.* 1977; **124**, 189-204.

Fractures and joint injuries in children

G.E. Jacchia - M. D'Arienzo - M. Innocenti - L. Ciampalini

Elbow fractures and joint injuries in children are reported in order of frequency (Table 1) according to the Gui classification.

Table 1

1) Supracondylar fracture
2) Lateral condylar fracture
3) Medial epicondylar fracture
4) Trochlear fracture
5) Lateral epicondylar fracture
6) Complete epiphyseal fracture

FRACTURES

Fractures not involving the epiphyseal growth plates can be supracondylar, radial neck, or olecranon fractures, the first being by far the most common.

Supracondylar fractures

These constitute about 75% of all traumatic elbow lesions in growing patients.

The mechanism of injury is usually a fall on the outstretched, hyperextended hand; in this case the proximal fragment is displaced anteriorly away from the distal fragment, thus forming a posteriorly facing angle.

Only rarely is this fracture caused by direct trauma to the posterior side of the elbow, and in such a case displacement occurs in the opposite direction.

Vascular and/or neurologic lesions may result from the anterior dislocation of the proximal fragment, which occurs quite frequently.

Vascular lesions involve the brachial artery and usually take the form of a contusion with resulting spasm or thrombosis. Laceration occurs very rarely thanks to the protection of the anterior brachialis muscle.

Neurologic lesions usually involve the radial and median nerves, and less often the ulnar nerve; these lesions, however, occur very seldom.

Clinical observations include pain, swelling, and functional limitation in proportion to both the displacement of the fragments and, after several hours, the edema in the hand and fingers, the tension of which makes movement difficult.

In radiographic examination, the normal conformation of a child's elbow must be kept in mind. This may be done by measuring Baumann and Sandegard's "alpha" and "beta" angles (Fig. 1).

The alpha angle is formed by the line a, perpendicular to the humeral shaft, and the line b, which passes through the growth cartilage of the capitulum humeri. This angle, which normally measures 20 degrees, defines the radiographic valgus deformity of the elbow. Even though this value does not correspond to the absolute clinical valgus, it can be considered a reliable index of the clinical variations.

The beta angle, which is measured by a lateral x-ray, is formed by the humeral shaft and the line passing through the growth cartilage of the capitulum humeri. It normally measures 40 degrees and is an index of the alignment of both the capitulum and the epiphysis in the sagittal plane.

Rotatory deviation may be difficult to ascertain with an AP x-ray since our technique requires immobilization of the elbow at 90 degrees, so we suggest evaluation using a lateral x-ray, examining the radiotransparent space that is normally seen between the capitulum and the olecranon in children.

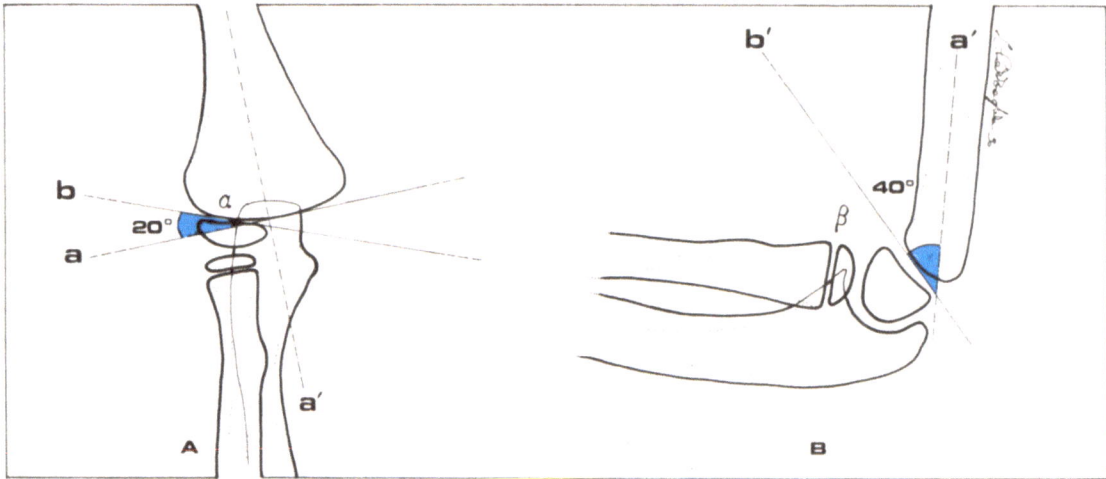

Fig. 1. - A) Baumann and Sandegard's α angle: formed by line *a*, which is perpendicular to the humeral shaft, and line *b*, which passes through the growth plate of the capitulum humeri. Its normal value is 20 degrees. B) Flexion β angle: formed by *a'*, the humeral shaft, and *b'*, a line that passes through the growth plate of the capitulum. Its normal value is 40 degrees.

The disappearance of this space, defined as a sign of "eclipse" (Fig. 2), indicates rotatory deviation of the distal fragment.

In the treatment of these fractures, both the possibility of these immediate complications and the possible long-term outcome must be considered.

At our institution, treatment with normal skeletal traction followed by closed reduction and cast immobilization has proved capable of satisfying both of these requirements.

While traction protects the fractured limb from immediate complications, reduction must restore the normal angular alignment of the elbow of the growing patient.

Materials and methods

Four hundred and forty-two patients who were treated at the Istituto di Clinica Ortopedica C.T.O. of Florence from 1963 to 1985 were reviewed.

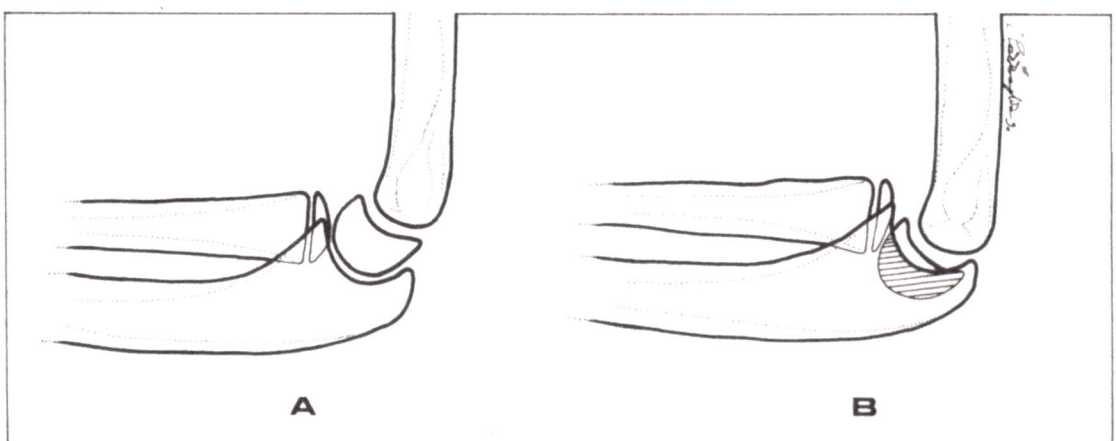

Fig. 2. - A) Lateral x-ray of a normal child's elbow shows a radiotransparent space between the capitulum and the olecranon. B) The image of the capitulum overlaps that of the olecranon, which is a sign of "eclipse" and indicates internal rotation of the distal fragment.

The patients were between 1 and 5 years old, 68% male and 32% female; 64% had fractures in the right elbow and 36% in the left.

Three hundred and sixty-four of these were treated with traction for an average of 5 days, followed by reduction under general anesthesia and immobilization in a shoulder spica for an average of 5 weeks (range 4-7 weeks) (Fig. 3).

Forty-three patients with only slight displacement were immediately immobilized in a long-arm cast for 4 weeks.

In 35 cases the fracture required open reduction and internal fixation with Kirschner wires or other fixation devices. Nineteen of these fractures were severely displaced and therefore could not be reduced by the usual method; the other 16 had neurovascular complications.

The choice of treatment was not based on the extent of the original displacement, since closed reduction and cast immobilization were attempted, if possible, even in severely displaced fractures. Instead, this choice depended upon the tendency of the individual orthopedic surgeon; some colleagues with whom we compared research tended toward open reduction and minimal fixation in both severely and mildly displaced fractures.

As mentioned above, we used open reduction in cases of neurovascular complications when alignment was not achieved within the first few hours of skeletal traction, as well as in irreducible fractures or relatively rare dia-supracondylar fractures.

Temporary circulation problems were the only frequent vascular complications, yet there were two cases of Volkmann's syndrome. Both patients had sustained serious

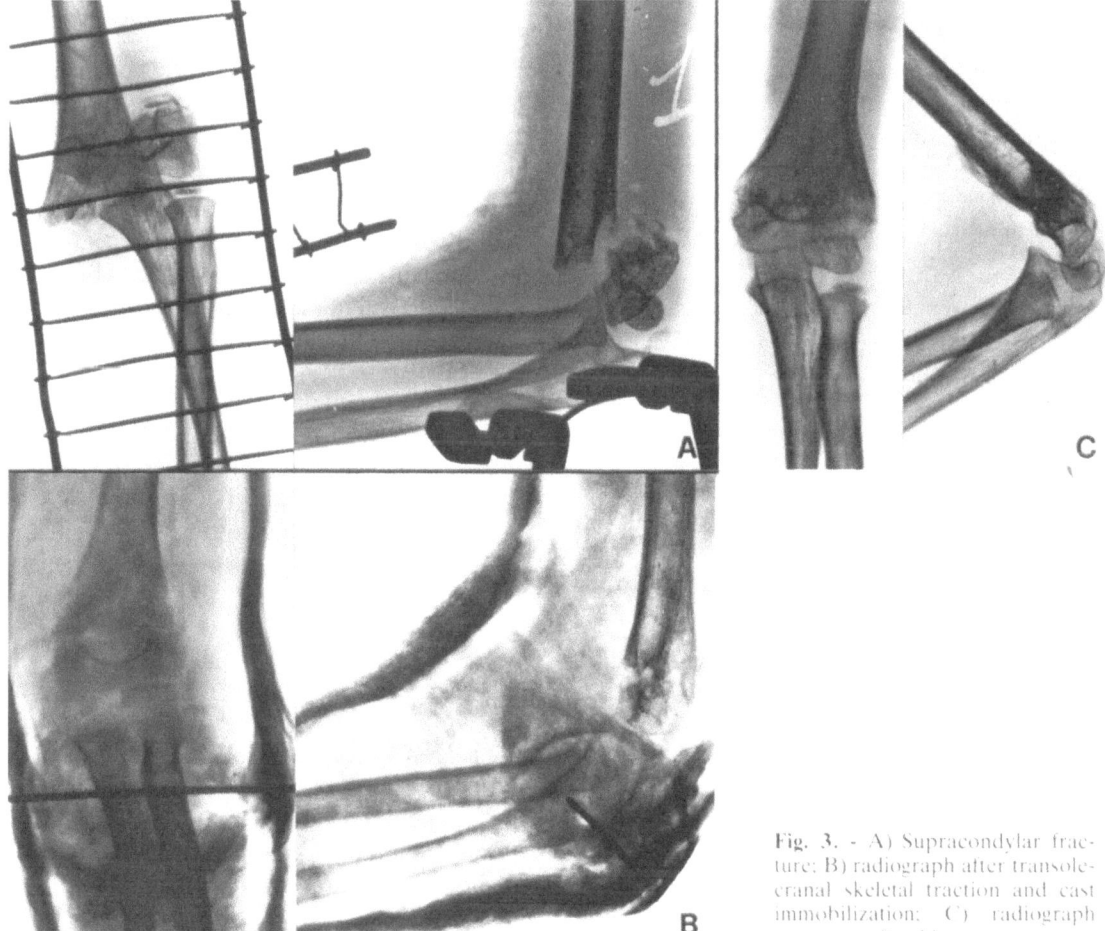

Fig. 3. - A) Supracondylar fracture; B) radiograph after transolecranal skeletal traction and cast immobilization; C) radiograph after 1 years.

injury to the brachial artery, causing ischemia in spite of revision and fasciotomy.

Thirty-six patients suffered neurologic lesions: the radial nerve was involved in 15 cases, the ulnar nerve in 7, and the median nerve in 6; in the other 8 cases various combinations of the nerves of the upper limb were involved.

Full recovery was achieved in 28 of these cases, after simple skeletal traction in 20 patients and revision in 8. Despite surgical revision, the remaining 8 cases suffered permanent neurologic damage: to the median nerve in 3 cases, the ulnar nerve in 2 cases, the radial nerve in 1 case, and more than one nerve in 2 cases.

Two hundred and thirty-six patients were reviewed after an average of 8 years, and the results were rated excellent, good, fair, or poor on the basis of the criteria shown in Table 2.

Table 2

EXCELLENT: full joint mobility, alignment the same as contralateral elbow, no pain or neurovascular complications.
GOOD: overall joint mobility loss ≤ 20°, slight elbow varus or valgus, no pain or neurovascular complications.
FAIR: overall joint mobility loss of 20°-50°, 10°-20° angular deviation (consisting usually of varus deformation), no neurovascular lesions, possible pain after exertion.
POOR: overall joint mobility loss > 50°, angular deviation > 20°, possible pain and neurovascular lesions.

The outcome was excellent in 189 cases, good in 28, fair in 13, and poor in 6 (Table 3).

The poor results were all due to either vascular or neurologic complications.

Table 3

EXCELLENT	189 (80.2%)
GOOD	28 (11.8%)
FAIR	13 (5.5%)
POOR	6 (2.5%)

TRAUMATIC LESIONS OF THE EPIPHYSEAL PLATE

Traumatic lesions of the epiphyseal plate may consist of fracture, separation, or a combination of both. We integrated our classification system of epiphyseal plate fractures, presented at the 1987 SIOT convention in Rome, with Salter's in order to obtain a more comprehensive view of these lesions (Fig. 4).

Type 0 Fractures

Type 0 lesions consist of pure epiphyseal separation, the most common of which in the elbow involves the epitrochlea. Epitrochlear separation is caused by the sudden tightening of both the ulnar collateral ligament and the epitrochlear muscles when the elbow is forced into valgus angulation. Watson-Jones described 4 anatomical types of this lesion as shown in Fig. 5.

The clinical manifestations are pain, swelling, and ecchymosis on the medial side of the elbow. Palpation and strain on the valgus elbow intensify the pain. Ulnar nerve lesions ranging from simple pulls to actual tearing of the fibers are possible in the third and especially the fourth group of the Watson-Jones classification.

Undisplaced fractures should be treated conservatively (30 days in a long-arm cast with elbow and wrist flexed), while the other cases, and all those with ulnar nerve lesion, require surgical treatment. Possible fixation devices include Kirschner wires and screws.

We prefer to use screws in patients over 10 years of age and when the fragment is relatively large. Percentage-wise, we have achieved better results with this method, since

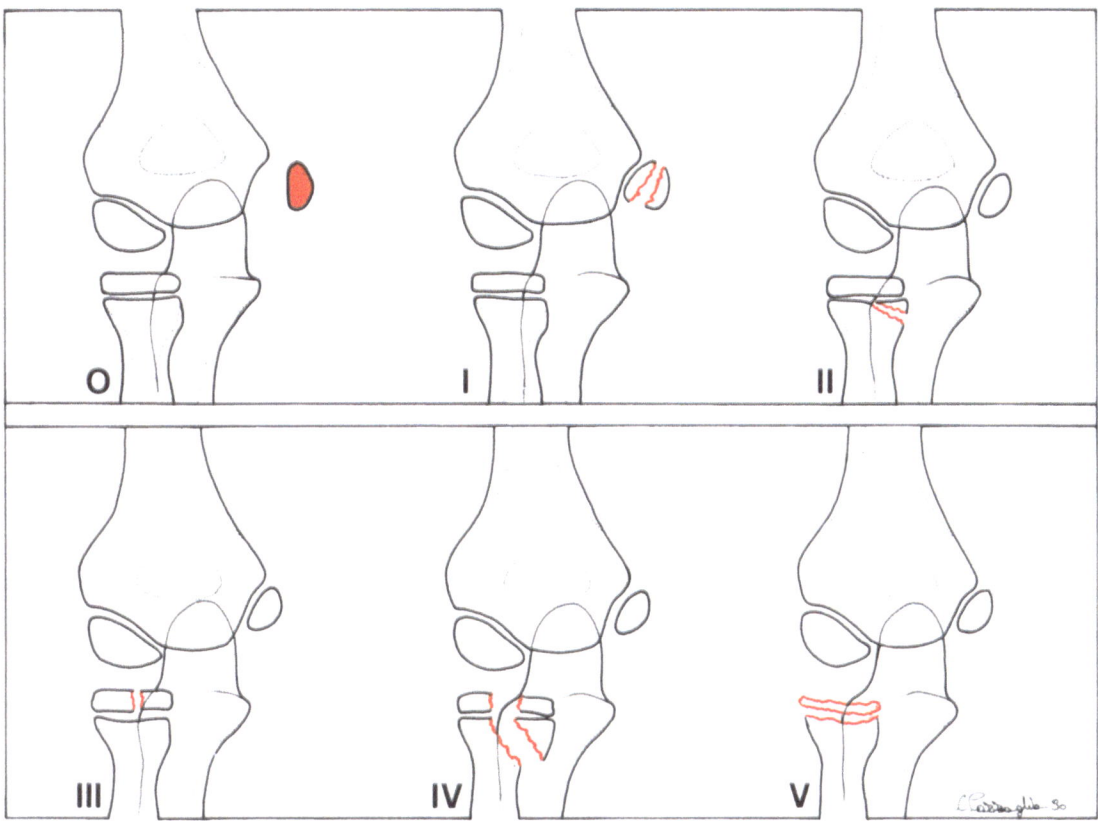

Fig. 4. - Classification of the traumatic lesions of the epiphyseal plate.

it limits immobilization to only 12-15 days.

Separation of the radial head, the lateral epicondyle, or the capitulum is very rare. Moreover, separation of the capitulum can only happen before 3 years of age, which is when the shaft inserts its triangular extension into the epiphyseal cartilage, as shown by Farabeuf.

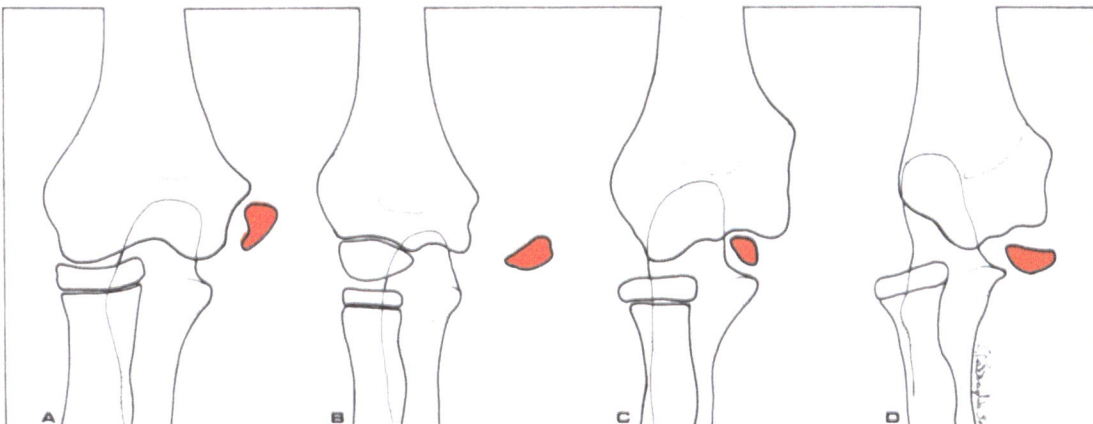

Fig. 5. - Watson-Jones classification of epitrochlear fractures: A) with simple lateral displacement; B) with displacement and rotation of the fragment; C) with entrance of the fragment into the joint space; D) with elbow dislocation.

Type I Fractures

These are pure epiphyseal fractures that do not involve the growth plate; they occur very rarely and are caused by direct trauma.

The prognosis is good.

Type II Fractures

These are lesions involving the epiphyseal plate and a metaphyseal fragment. They are rarer than type 0 lesions, and their most common site in the elbow is the radial head. The mechanism of injury is a fall on the outstretched hand.

Its clinical feature is pain that is intensified by palpation, pronation, and supination.

The treatment, as always in pure or mixed epiphyseal fractures, can be open or closed and should aim for anatomical reduction (Figs. 6-7).

Type III Fractures

In these the fracture line completely splits the epiphysis and reaches the growth plate. They are very rare in the elbow, occurring more frequently in the knee and the distal tibia.

Type IV Fractures

These fractures involve not only the epiphysis but also the metaphysis. The lateral capitulum is affected three times as often as the trochlea. They are caused by a violent collision with the radial head combined with the pulling action of both the extensor muscles and the radial collateral ligament, which occurs as a result of sudden forearm adduction with elbow extended. Two types are possible depending upon the degree of displacement of the condyle (Fig. 8).

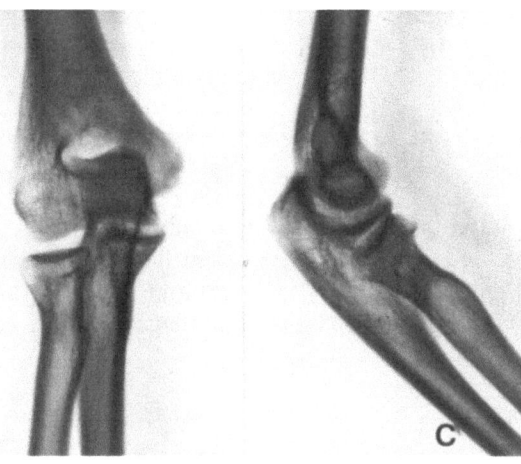

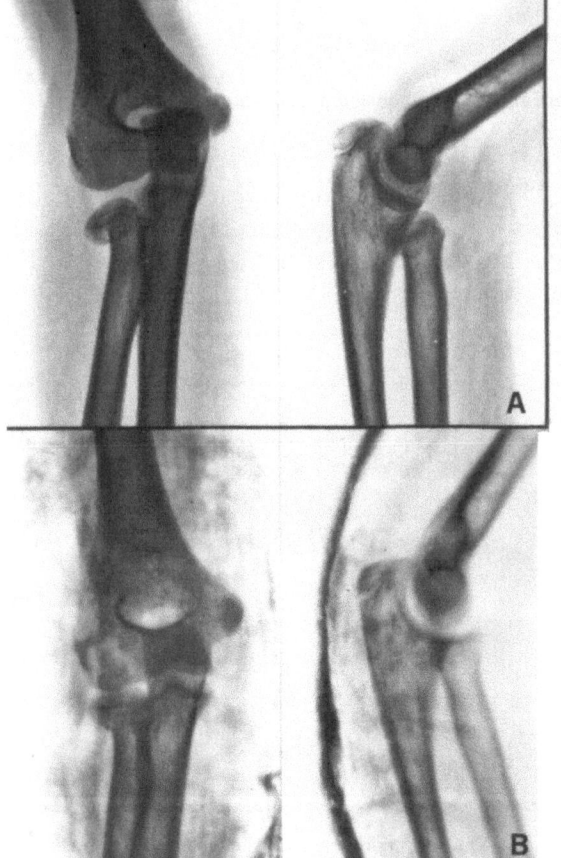

Fig. 6. - A) Type II detachment of the radial head from the epiphysis; B) x-ray through cast after closed reduction; C) follow-up x-ray after 5 years.

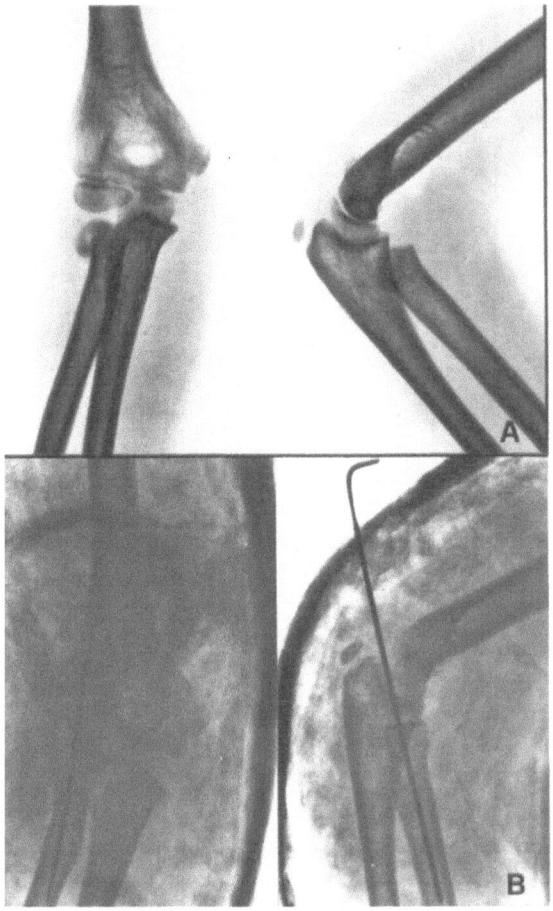
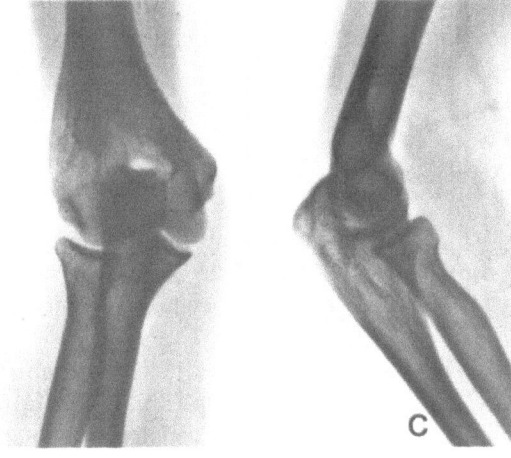

Fig. 7. - Type II separation of the radial head from the epiphysis; B) x-ray after open reduction and internal fixation with Kirschner wires; C) x-ray after 8 years.

The clinical manifestations are pain, swelling, and ecchymosis, which occurs later.

In both undisplaced fractures (Fig. 9) and displaced fractures without rotation of the capitellar fragment, conservative treatment should be attempted (long-arm cast with the elbow at 90 degrees and the forearm in zero position, for 20-25 days in patients under 8 years of age and 30-40 days in older children).

Fractures with rotation of the capitellar fragment generally require open reduction; in order to avoid further displacement, Dexon transosseous sutures, or preferably a Kirschner wire, should be used for fixation.

Type V Fractures

These involve the crushing of the epiphyseal plate. Immediate diagnosis of this le-sion is difficult, as it often manifests itself over time in the form of growth arrest or angular deviation. The prognosis is therefore poor.

Complications

The most common complications of epiphyseal fractures are avascular necrosis, nonunion, and growth arrest.

Avascular necrosis

Avascular necrosis is caused by occlusion of the blood vessels and can be very serious, as it affects growing areas. Since the unaffected areas continue to grow at a normal rate, varus or valgus deviation of the elbow can develop over time.

Avascular necrosis most often occurs in the lateral capitulum, especially in cases requiring open reduction.

Nonunion

This complication may result from either conservative or surgical treatment or failure to immobilize the limb because of incorrect diagnosis.

The most commonly affected structures are the epitrochlea and the capitulum. In the first case nonunion is not usually a problem, since the elbow retains more or less full mobility and muscle power; yet in the second case the lesion is much more serious, and can potentially cause growth arrest and angular deviation.

Growth arrest

Growth arrest in the epiphysis is usually a result of either circulatory system changes or a halt in the production of cartilage. The end result is either varus or valgus elbow depending upon which growth plate is affected, that of the trochlea or that of the humeral condyle.

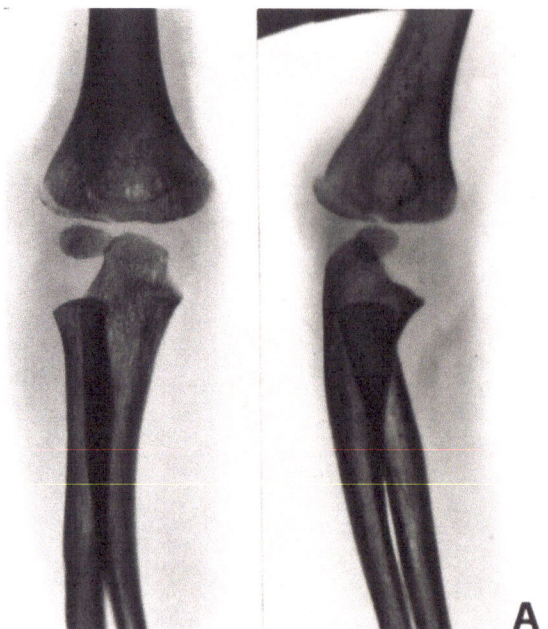

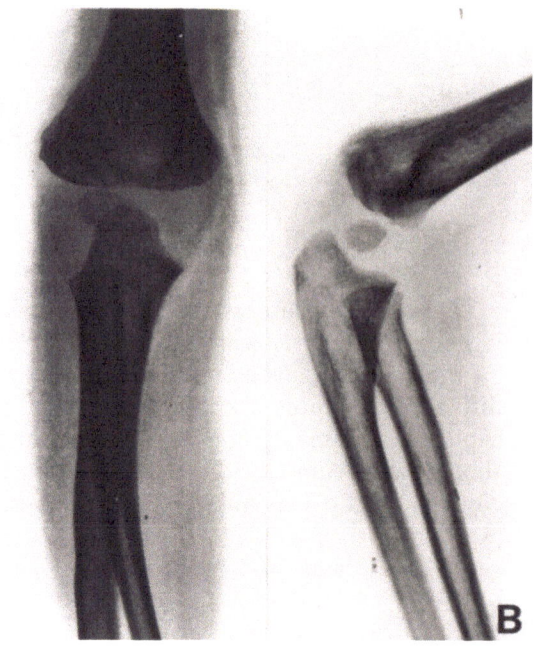

Fig. 9. - A) Undisplaced separation of the capitulum from the epiphysis; B) x-ray after 6 months.

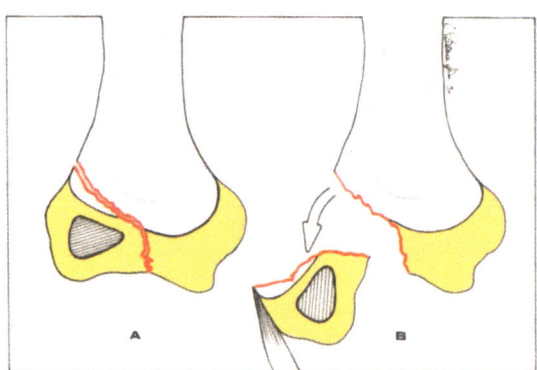

Fig. 8. - Type IV separation of the capitulum from the epiphysis: A) undisplaced; B) with displacement and rotation of fragment.

Valgus elbow

The term valgus elbow means that the angle formed by the shafts of the arm and forearm exceeds the normal range of 5-15 degrees.

It is generally caused by capitellar fracture, but can also be a result of supracondylar fracture or lesion of the lateral portion of the growth plate.

This aesthetic deformity if often compatible with normal joint function, yet at times it can be complicated by functional problems of the ulnar nerve, abnormally stretched in the epitrochlear-olecranal groove. Such cases require anteposition of the nerve or even, depending on the degree of the valgus angulation, osteotomy to correct the deformity.

Varus elbow

Varus elbow is less common than valgus elbow and is only rarely accompanied by functional limitation. It is usually caused by supracondylar fracture, other times by separation of the trochlea. Corrective osteotomy is done purely for aesthetic purposes.

REFERENCES

1) ARINO V.L., LLUCH E.E., RAMIREZ A.M., FERRER J., RODRIGUEZ L., BAIXAULI F.: Percutaneous fixation of supracondylar fractures of the humerus in children. *J. Bone Jt Surg.* 1977; **59-A** (7): 914-916.

2) ARNOLD J.A., NASCA R.J., NELSON C.L.: Supracondylar fractures of the humerus. The role of dynamic factors in prevention of deformity. *J. Bone Jt Surg.* 1977; **59-A**: 589-595.

3) CECILIANI L., CASTELLI C., BENAZZO F.: Le fratture dei nuclei epifisari: diagnosi e trattamento. *Aggiornamento del Medico* 1984; **6**: 323-329.

4) DALE G.G., HARRIS W.R.: Prognosis of epiphyseal separation. (An experimental study). *J. Bone Jt Surg.* 1958; **40-B**: 116-122.

5) D'AMBROSIA R.D.: Supracondylar fractures of humerus. Prevention of cubitus varus. *J. Bone Jt Surg.* 1972; **54-A**: 60-66.

6) DINI P., CORRADINI C.: Il gomito varo posttraumatico. *Arch. Putti* 1971; **24**: 334-343.

7) FLYNN J.C., MATTEWS J.G., BENOIT R.L.: Blind pinning of displaced supracondylar fractures of the humerus in children. *J. Bone Jt Surg.* 1974; **56-A**: 263-272.

8) KENNETH J.G.: Percutaneous pin fixation of the lower end of the humerus. *Clin. Orthop.* 1967; **50**: 53.

9) MALLET J., REY G.C., SENLJ G.: Les traumatismes du cartilage de conjugaison: le traitement des lesions anciennes. *Rev. Chir. Orthop.* 1979; **65**: 278-286.

10) OZONOFF M.B.: *Injury to the growth plate and epiphysis in children. Early recognition and late complications.* Medcon, New York, 1974.

11) RAMPOLDI A., BONI M.: *I distacchi epifisari traumatici.* Relazione XLII Congresso S.I. O.T. 1957, pp. 1-420.

12) RAMPOLDI A., BONI M., CARRERI G.: Sulle fratture dei nuclei epifisari. Loro esiti e prognosi. *Ortop. Traumatol.* 1960; **28** (4): 523-566.

13) ROCKWOOD C.A., WILKINS K.E., KING R.W.: *Fractures in children.* Lippincott Co., Philadelphia, 1985.

14) ROGERS L.F.: The radiography of epiphyseal injuries. *Radiology* 1970; **96**; 289-299.

15) SALTER R.B., HARRIS W.R.: Injuries involving the epiphyseal plate. *J. Bone Jt Surg.* 1963; **45-A**: 587-622.

16) SANDEGARD E.: Fracture of the lower end of the humerus in children. Treatment and end results. *Acta Chir. Scand.* 1943; **89**: 1-16.

17) WATSON JONES R.: *Fractures and joint injuries.* William and Wilkins, Baltimore, 1976, vol. 2, pp. 1048-1050.

18) WEBER D.G.: *Epiphyseal injuries: internal fixation of fractures of Aitken type 2 and 3.* Proceedings of the 12th Congress. Tel-Aviv S.I.C.O.T., 9-12 oct. 1972.

Classification of fractures and dislocations in the adult elbow

M. Randelli - F. Odella - P.L. Gambrioli

INTRODUCTION

The aim of traumatological classification is to adopt criteria that are anatomopathologic, prognostic, and at the same time strategic for the choice of treatment.

In cases of fracture and fracture-dislocation of the elbow, this goal is quite hard to achieve.

The elbow is composed of three bone segments, each of which can be affected by traumatic disease either alone or together with the other segments, thus creating an array of possible combinations that often elude even the most sophisticated attempts at classification.

Moreover, the difficulty of prognostic classification lies in defining, at the moment of trauma, the periarticular (capsuloligamentous and muscular) damage, which is often primarily responsible for unsuccessful treatment.

Despite these difficulties, over time orthopedists have been able to divide the lesions into typical forms for which there are sufficiently precise indications for treatment and prognoses for recovery.

To facilitate explanation we will discuss fractures, fracture-dislocations, and pure dislocations separately.

ELBOW FRACTURES

Elbow fractures can be divided into the following categories: fracture of the distal humerus, fracture of either the proximal radius or ulna, and fracture of both the proximal radius and ulna.

Fractures of the distal humerus

Since the first classifications of these fractures, such as Boehler's (2), they have been divided into articular and periarticular types, with the capsular insertion as the anatomical boundary.

The articular portion of the humeral epiphysis consists of the capitulum humeri, the trochlea, and the coronoid and olecranon fossae. The periarticular portion comprises the lateral and medial epicondyles. The upper boundary of the articular portion of the humerus is generally considered to be the insertion of the anterior brachialis muscle, which is just above the coronoid fossa.

The periarticular fractures are not difficult to classify. The epitrochlea is the most frequently affected structure. Avulsion fractures caused by the ulnar collateral ligament during forced valgus angulation of the elbow are sometimes accompanied by elbow dislocation.

Periarticular fractures are commonly divided into 4 types (12).

The difference between types 1 and 2 is the diastasis of the fragment caused by the traction of the ulnar collateral ligament

In types 3 and 4 the epitrochlear fragment enters the joint as a result of lateral or posterolateral elbow dislocation. Reduction of the dislocation after the original trauma can trap the epitrochlear fragment inside the joint space (Fig. 1).

Lateral epicondylar fractures are rarer than epitrochlear fractures. Since the lateral epicondyle is adjacent to the capitulum, fractures of the former are often accompanied by marginal fractures of the latter, which almost places them in the category of articular fractures.

In addition to fractures of the lateral and medial epicondyles, fractures of the supracondylar segment with one or more fragments are often classified as periarticular (6, 12).

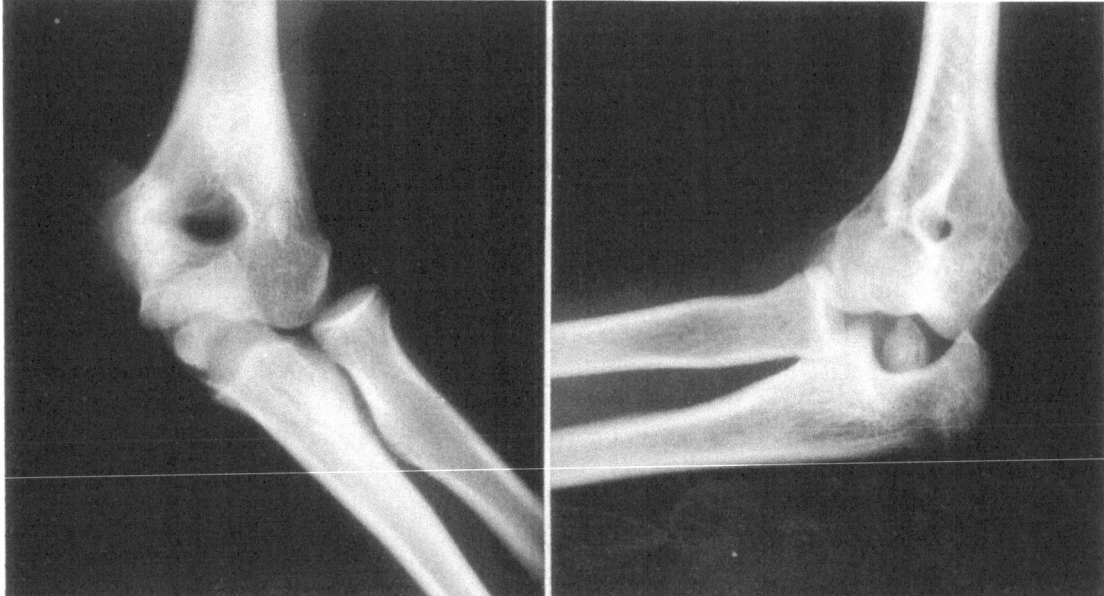

Fig. 1. - Epitrochlear fracture with lateral elbow dislocation and entrapment of the epitrochlear fragment in the joint space.

The most important element in these cases is the involvement of the coronoid and olecranon fossae.

Even marginal involvement of the olecranon fossa can limit the range of motion of the joint because either scar tissue, bone calluses, or structural changes are produced that rob both the olecranon and coronoid of the space needed for elbow flexion and extension.

Such fractures should be considered articular.

Many classifications are possible for articular fractures of the distal humerus.

In their comparison of the results of various closed management techniques, Riseborough and Radin (14) used a classification based primarily on the displacement and rotation of the fragments of classic T, Y, and V-shaped intercondylar fractures.

According to the cited authors, the displacement or rotation of the fragments was the main obstacle to closed reduction and therefore the most important criterion for classification.

When a surgical approach was preferred, however, this distinction was abandoned and the lesions were classified according to criteria that allowed the evaluation of techniques

and results of open reduction.

Of the numerous proposals (3, 4, 5, 10), only the most recent one put forth by the Associazione Osteosintesi (A.O.) in 1979 will be described in this chapter, as we find that it satisfies most of the practical requirements of documentation and planning of treatment.

The A.O. classification (Fig. 2) includes both articular fractures and periarticular fractures (epitrochlear avulsion fractures, simple and comminuted supracondylar fractures), which we have already discussed.

Articular fractures are divided into two categories: monocondylar (fracture of trochlea or capitulum, or transverse fracture of both these structures) and bicondylar (Y fracture, comminuted supracondylar Y fracture, comminuted metaphyseal fracture).

Fractures listed in the other classifications can be considered special cases of those cited in the A.O. classification.

Examples could be the Kocher fracture, in which the whole articular portion (trochlea and capitulum) is separated, and the Hahn-Steinthal fracture (Fig. 3), which involves the capitulum and the portion of the trochlea attached to it. Both of these, from a surgical and pathologic standpoint, can be considered spe-

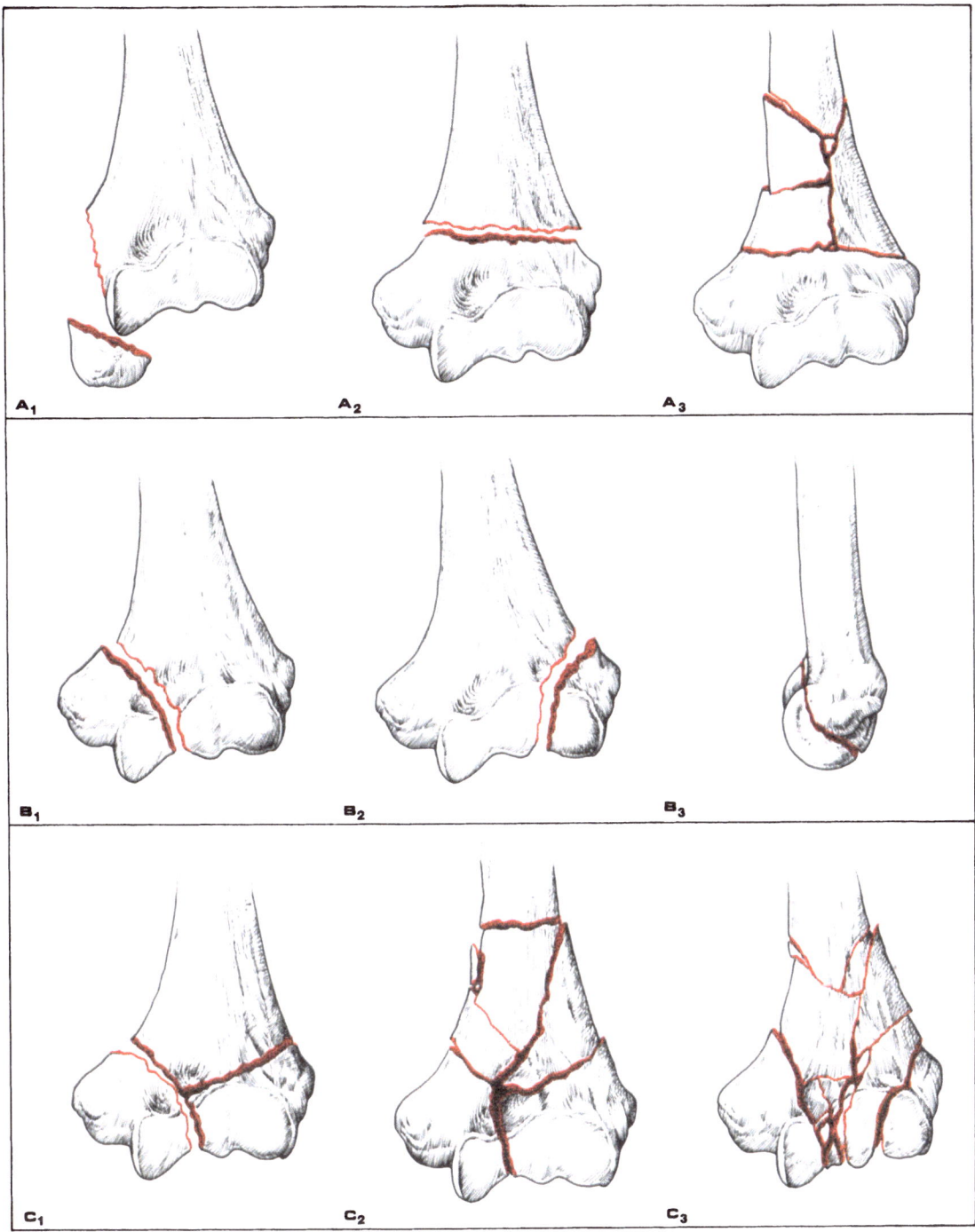

Fig. 2. - A.O. (Associazione Osteosintesi) classification of fractures of the distal humerus. *Periarticular fractures:* (A1) avulsion fracture of the epitrochlea, (A2) single transmetaphyseal fracture, (A3) comminuted transmetaphyseal fracture. *Condylar articular fractures:* (B1) transtrochlear fracture, (B2) capitellar fracture, (B3) transverse trochlear fracture. *Intercondylar fractures:* (C1) Y-shaped fracture, (C2) Y-shaped fracture with multiple supracondylar fragments, (C3) complex comminuted fracture (from: Müller M.E., Allgower M., Willeneger H., 1979).

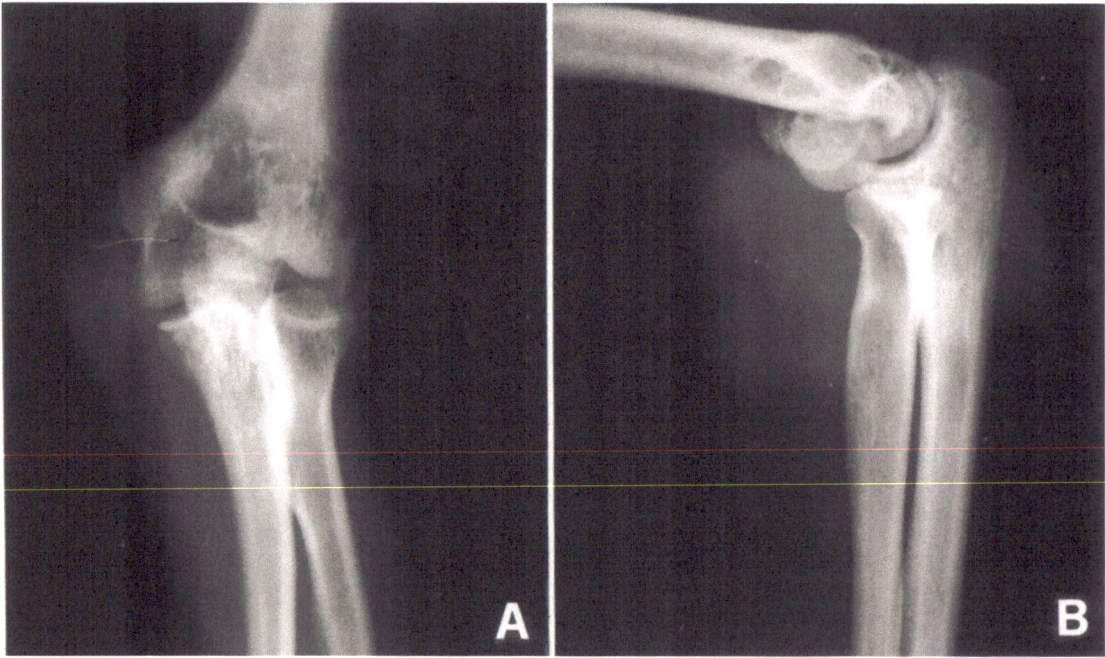

Fig. 3. - Transverse fracture of the capitulum and the trochlea, known as the Hahn-Steinthal fracture.

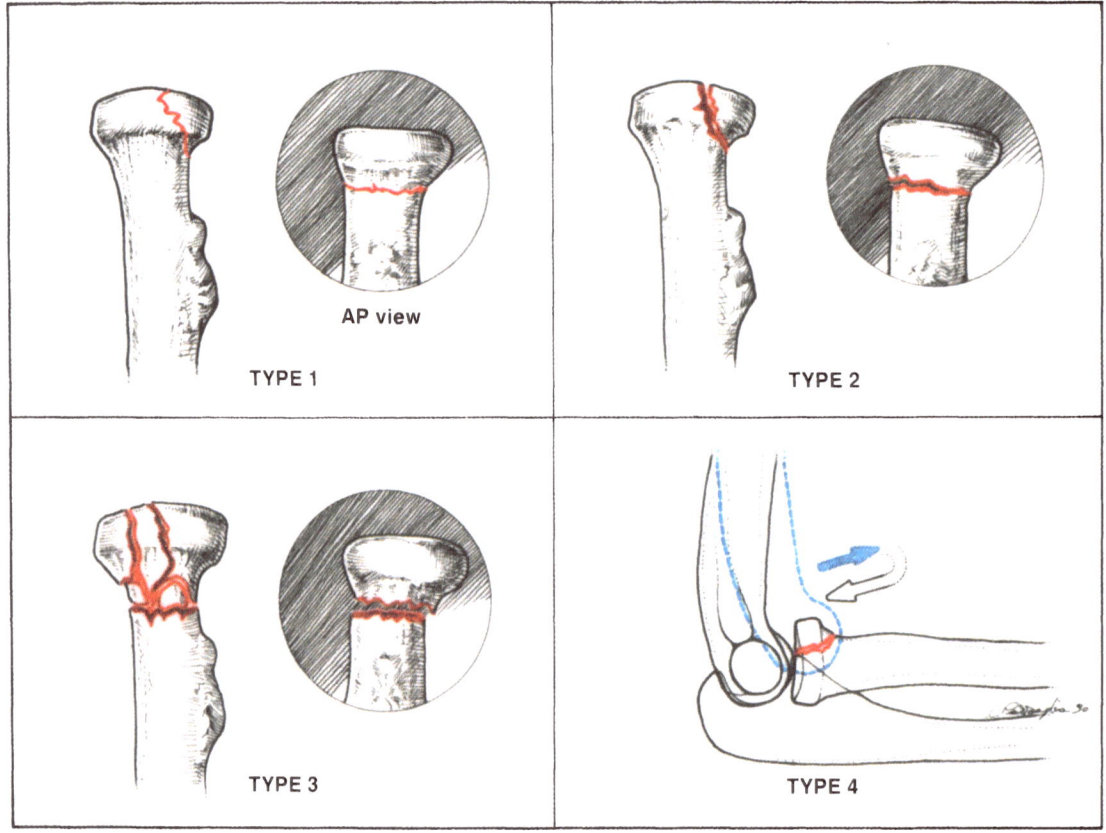

Fig. 4. - Mason classification of radial head fractures.

cial cases of the transverse fracture of trochlea and capitulum included in the A.O. classification.

The A.O. classification, therefore, may be considered comprehensive enough for current use.

Fractures of the radial head

The most well-known classification of articular fractures of the radial head was conceived by Mason (8), who divides these fractures into four categories (Fig. 4).

Both type 1 and type 2 fractures are segmental, but type 1 is undisplaced while type 2 is displaced.

Radin (13), in agreement with the most recent classification methods, divided type 2 into two subcategories that take into account the portion of articular surface involved in the fracture.

Type 3 is a comminuted fracture, while type 4 is a comminuted fracture-dislocation. The dislocation may not show up on x-rays taken after the trauma.

The radial head fracture is often the only apparent lesion, but a thorough investigation will in many cases reveal a type 4 lesion, that is, elbow dislocation at the moment of trauma with resulting periarticular soft tissue damage that cannot be seen radiologically.

Fractures of the proximal ulna

These fractures involve both the olecranon and coronoid processes.

Olecranon fractures can be divided into those with one fragment and those with two or more fragments.

Those with one fragment were divided by Merle d'Aubigné (10) into three categories (Fig. 5).

Type 1 is a periarticular fracture of the tip of the olecranon. Quite rare, it is an avulsion fracture caused by the action of the insertion of the triceps.

The type 2 fracture has a fragment lodged in the semilunar notch.

Type 3 is a fracture of the metaphyseal portion of the ulna that extends to the articular surface near the coronoid process.

The multiple fractures of the olecranon were also divided into three categories: double fractures, comminuted fractures, and

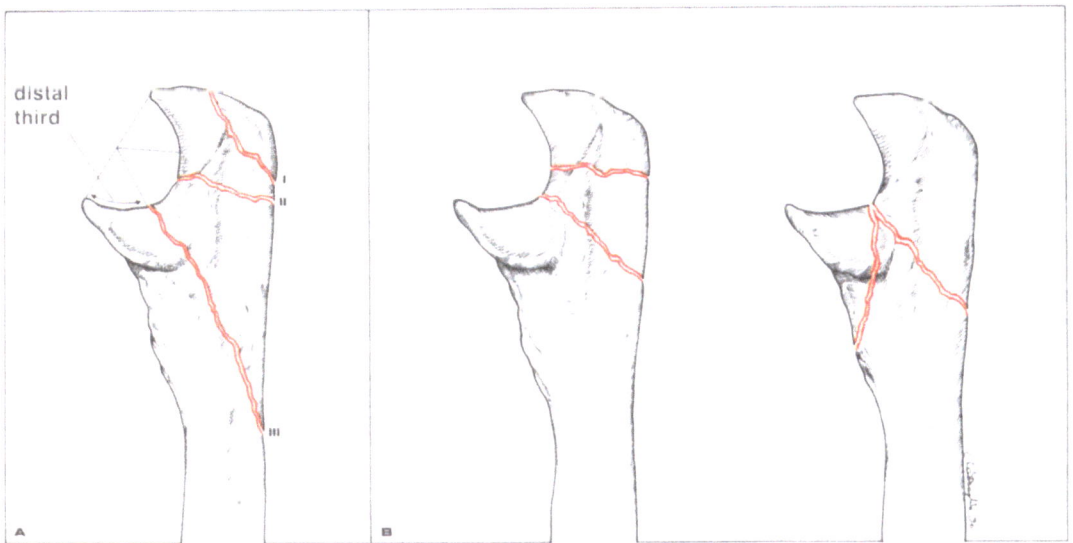

Fig. 5. - Classification of olecranon fractures. A) Fractures with only one fragment: type I, fracture of the tip of the olecranon involving no articular surface; type II, fracture involving the middle third of the articular surface; type III, metaphyseal fracture. B) Multiple fractures: double fracture and olecranon-coronoid fracture (from: R. Merle D'Aubigné, 1957).

fractures of both the olecranon and coronoid processes.

Fractures of the coronoid process alone, which are very rare except in cases of posterior dislocation of the elbow, include fractures of the tip, typical of hyperextension trauma, as well as direct fractures of the base, usually caused by a fall on the moderately flexed elbow (Fig. 6).

In coronoid fractures, the fragment is often pulled upward by the contraction of the anterior brachialis muscle.

Loss of anterior coronoid support is one of the conditions that predispose the elbow to posterior dislocation.

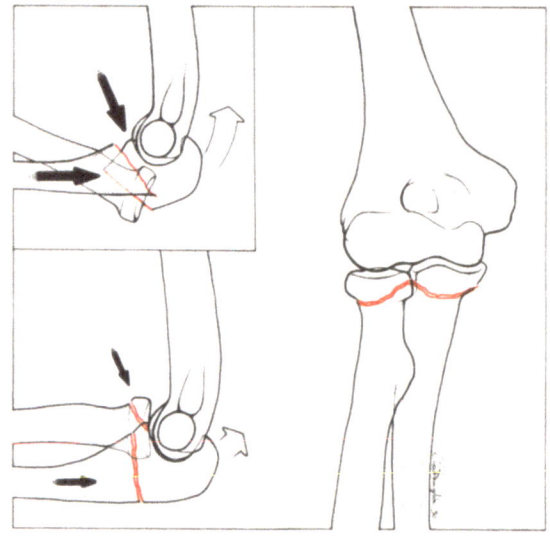

Fig. 7. - Fracture of the proximal radius and ulna with elbow "in flexion" (from J. Vidal, S. Bruel, Y. Allieu, 1970).

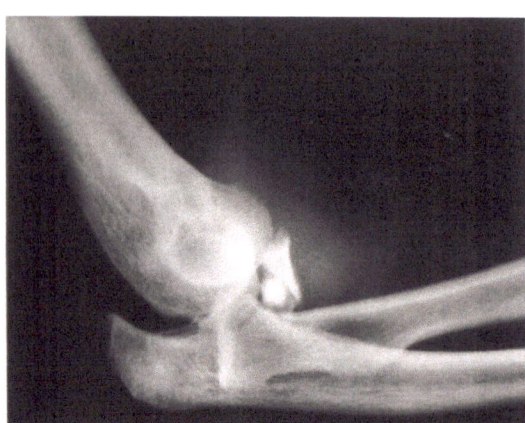

Fig. 6. - Fracture of the base of the coronoid process with posterior dislocation of the elbow.

Proximal radioulnar fractures

In addition to isolated fractures of the proximal forearm, we would like to briefly describe the situations in which the radius and ulna are fractured simultaneously (15).

These fractures seriously compromise both the function and stability of the elbow; surgical treatment is always indicated (Figs. 7-8).

Fractures can occur either in extension (olecranon-radial head or olecranon-radial neck fracture), or in flexion, in which the mechanism is similar to that of the Monteggia fracture-dislocation except that actual fracture of the radial head is involved instead of dislocation (Fig. 9).

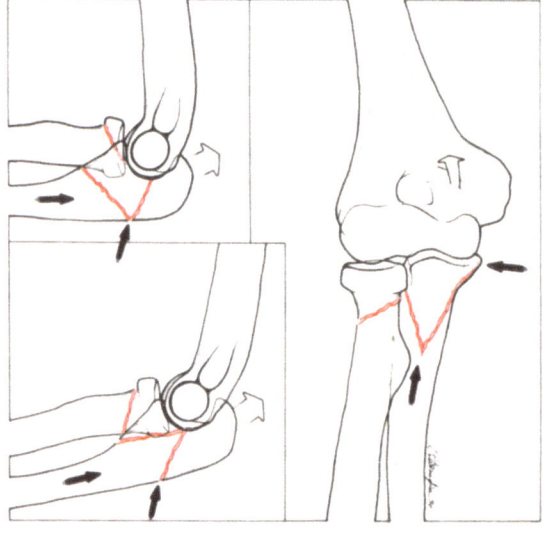

Fig. 8. - Fracture of the proximal radius and ulna with elbow "in extension" (from J. Vidal, S. Bruel, Y. Allieu, 1970).

ELBOW FRACTURE-DISLOCATION

Reference has already been made to the fact that fractures of the epitrochlea, the radial head, or the coronoid can be accompanied by elbow dislocation.

In these cases, the muscular and capsuloligamentous lesions caused by the dislocation aggravate the prognosis of the modest bone lesions.

In addition to these well-known types of elbow fracture-dislocation, two other forms of this lesion in the proximal forearm have recently been reported by several authors (1,7).

From a pathologic standpoint these lesions belong to the category of olecranon fractures, but they also involve dislocation of the two forearm bones that remain "joined" proximally by ligaments.

Several varieties have been distinguished with anterior dislocation and posterior dislocation.

Anterior fracture-dislocation of both radius and ulna, called transolecranal dislocation by Biga and Thomine (1), has been divided into two subcategories by Marotte (7): one an isolated olecranon fracture caused by an "*en cisaillement*" trauma and one a comminuted olecranon fracture caused by "*écrasement*".

The Denucé quadrate and orbicular ligaments unite the radius and ulna, allowing their anterior dislocation as if they were one structure (Fig. 10).

Different types of posterior fracture-dislocation can occur, however, depending on the level of the ulnar fracture (Fig. 11).

In case of trauma with the arm supinated and the elbow flexed, an olecranon fracture that ends at the center of the articular surface of the trochlear notch causes posterior dislocation of both radius and ulna and sometimes even fracture of the coronoid process.

If the ulnar fracture is at a more distal level near the coronoid mass, the radial head may be pushed up against the capitulum and dislocated posteriorly.

Finally, if the ulnar fracture is meta-diaphyseal or diaphyseal, besides the abovementioned two varieties of posterior fracture-dislocation of both radius and ulna we have the classic ulnar fracture with dislocation of the radial head, also known as the Monteggia fracture-dislocation.

ELBOW DISLOCATION

Dislocation represents about one-tenth of all traumatic lesions of the elbow.

This lesion has several variations, classified according to the direction of the dislocation of the two forearm bones.

Posterolateral dislocation is the most common. The degree of dislocation varies, and may result in either a total or only partial loss of contact between the articular surfaces.

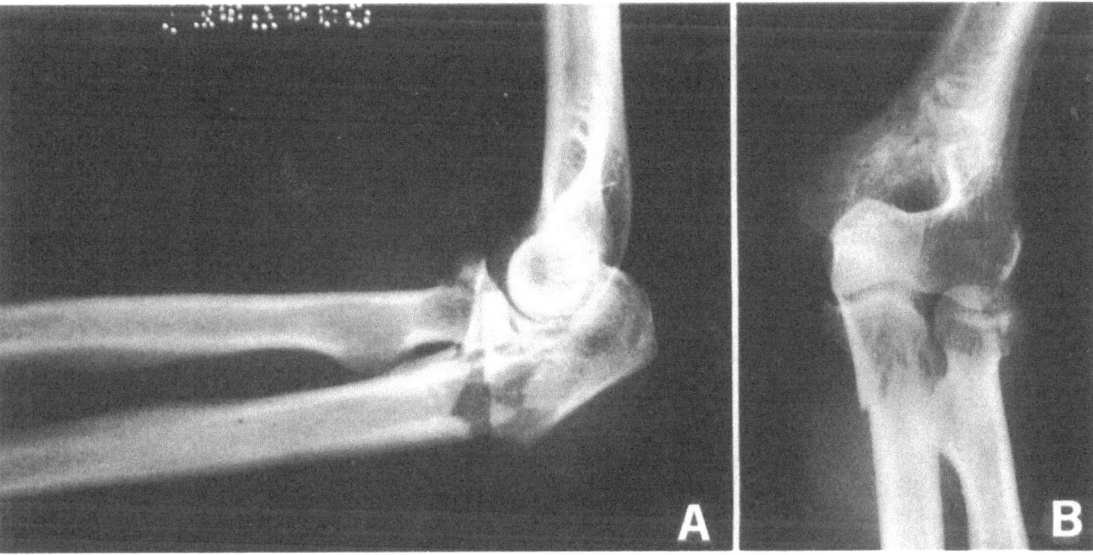

Fig. 9. - Fracture of the proximal ulna and the radial head with elbow "in flexion", according to J. Vidal.

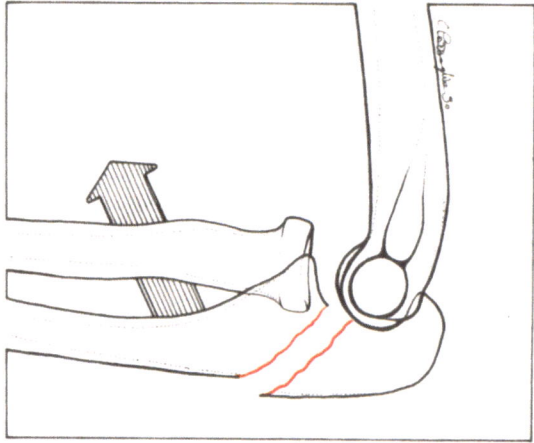

Fig. 10. - "Joined" anterior fracture-dislocation of the proximal radius and ulna (from: N. Biga and J.M. Thomine, 1974).

The severity of the capsuloligamentous lesions varies with the degree of displacement.

Lateral dislocation is rarer, and may be incomplete if the trochlear notch is in contact with the capitulum or complete if it articulates with the lateral epicondyle.

In the first case only the ulnar collateral ligament is damaged, while in the second case the radial collateral ligament is also torn.

Rarer still is anterior dislocation of both the radius and ulna, which is normally linked to either aplasia of the tip of the olecranon or joint hyperlaxity.

Divergent dislocation of the radius and ulna affects all three elbow joints. In this case the distal humeral epiphysis ruptures both the quadrate and orbicular ligaments, thus leading to the separation of radius and ulna.

Extremely rare is cruciate dislocation of the radius and ulna, often caused by reduction of a posterior dislocation with the arm pronated.

The classification of dislocation is therefore based only on its extent and direction, while a prognostic classification could be based on diagnostic methods that, at the moment of trauma, allow evaluation of the muscular and capsuloligamentous damage associated with this lesion.

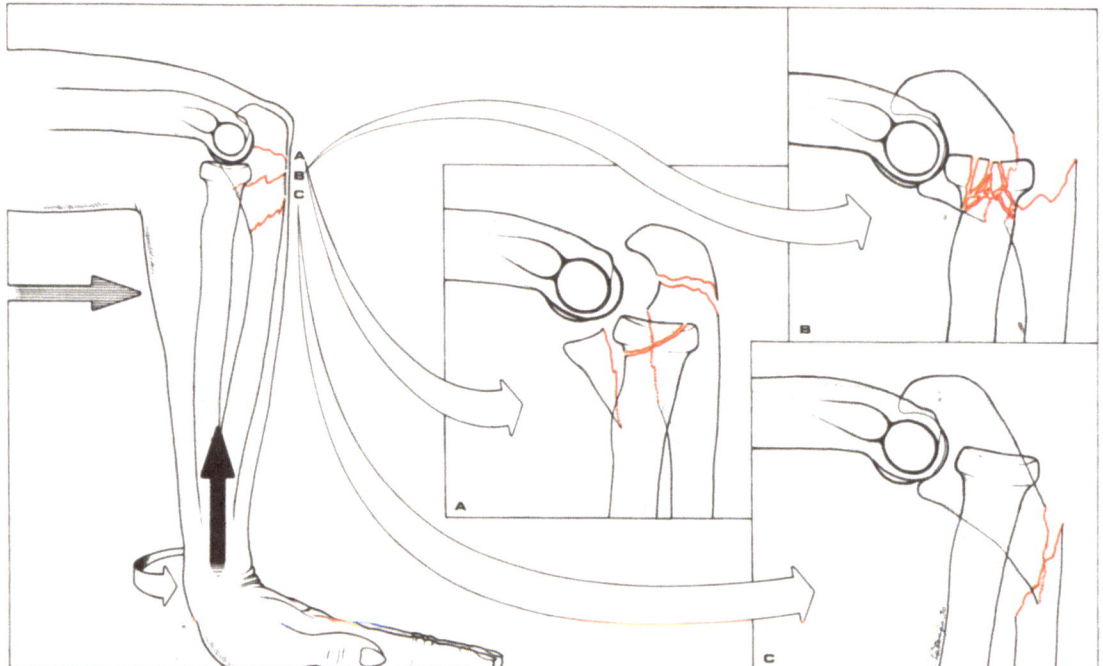

Fig. 11. - The two types of "joined" posterior fracture-dislocation of the proximal radius and ulna and the Monteggia fracture-dislocation. A) Olecranon-coronoid process fracture and posterior displacement of the radial head; B) proximal epiphyseal fracture of the ulna at the level of the coronoid mass with posterior dislocation of the radius; C) Monteggia fracture-dislocation (from: J.H. Marotte, P. Samuel, G. Lord, J.P. Blanchard, J.L. Guillamon, 1982).

CONCLUSIONS

Attempting to classify fractures and dislocations of the elbow reveals the great variety of clinical features that has forced the orthopedic surgeon to make such minute subdivisions.

Only by such an effort, however, is it possible to plan a therapeutic strategy that must be highly specific and at the same time have a precise point of reference for evaluating the results of treatment for each of the lesion combinations of this important chapter in joint traumatology.

REFERENCES

1) BIGA N., THOMINE J.M.: La luxation trans-olècrânienne du coude. *Rev. Chir. Orthop.* 1974; **60**: 557-567.

2) BOEHLER L.: *Technique du traitement des fractures*. Ed. Médicales France, Paris, 1944.

3) DECOULX P., DUCLOUX M., HESPEEL J., DECOULX J.: Les fractures de l'extrémité inférieure de l'humérus chez l'adulte. *Rev. Chir. Orthop.* 1964; **50**: 263-273.

4) GUI L.: *Fratture e lussazioni*. Aulo Gaggi Autore, Bologna, 1975.

5) JUDET R.: Le traitement des fractures de l'extrémité inférieure de l'humérus chez l'adulte. *Rev. Chir. Orthop.* 1964; **50**: 275-278.

6) LECESTRE P.: Les fractures de l'extrémité inférieure de l'humérus chez l'adulte. *Rev. Chir. Orthop.* 1980; **66** (suppl. II): 21-50.

7) MAROTTE J.H., SAMUEL P., LORD G., BLANCHARD J.P., GUILLAMON J.L.: La fracture-luxation conjointe de l'extrémité supérieure des deux os de l'avant-bras. *Rev. Chir. Orthop.* 1982; **68**: 103-114.

8) MASON M.L.: Some observations on the radial head fractures. *Br. J. Surg.* 1954; **172**: 123-132.

9) MERLE D'AUBIGNÉ R.: *Affections traumatiques*. Flammarion Ed., Paris, 1957.

10) MERLE D'AUBIGNÉ R., MEARY R., CARLIOZ J.: Fractures sus et intercondyliennes récentes de l'adulte. *Rev. Chir. Orthop.* 1964; **50**: 279-288.

11) MÜLLER M.E., ALLGOWER M., WILLENEGER H.: *Manual of internal fixations*. New York, Springer-Verlag, 1979.

12) PIDHORZ L., BEDDOUK A.: Fractures de la palette humérale de l'adulte. *Encycl. Méd. Chir.*, Paris (Appareil Locomoteur), 14041 A10, 2, 1983.

13) RADIN E.L., RISEBOROUGH E.H.: The fracture of the radial head. *J. Bone Jt Surg.* 1966; **48-A**: 1055-1064.

14) RISEBOROUGH E.H., RADIN E.L.: Intercondylar T fractures of the humerus in the adult: a comparison of operative and non-operative treatment in 29 cases. *J. Bone Jt Surg.* 1969; **51-A**: 130-141.

15) VIDAL J., BRUEL S., ALLIEU Y.: *Les fractures associées de l'extrémité supérieure des deux os de l'avant-bras*. Congrés Franco-hellénique d'orthopédie, Athénes, May 1970.

Fractures of the distal humerus in the adult

F. Catalano - F. Fanfani - G. Taccardo - A. Pagliei

INTRODUCTION

Fractures of the distal humerus are usually defined as involving the portion of the humerus distal to the origin of the anterior brachialis muscle. The mechanism of injury is either direct with the elbow flexed or, more rarely, indirect with the elbow extended. The latter is more commonly responsible for elbow dislocation in the adult.

Fractures of the distal epiphysis of the humerus, except epicondylar fractures, are articular and thus have a severe *quoad functionem* prognosis due to the probable onset of both stiffness and arthritis, the latter a result of damage to the articular surfaces.

The numerous pathologic features of fractures of the distal humerus have led authors (1, 6, 9, 10, 13) to propose various classifications in an effort to bring together anatomical, prognostic, and therapeutic criteria. This study uses Gui's classification (8), which divides the fractures as follows:
— intercondylar fractures (T, Y, and V-shaped)
 — condylar fractures
 — trochlear fractures
 — epicondylar fractures
 — capitellar fractures

The purpose of this study is to contribute to the knowledge of these lesions in order to establish an appropriate therapeutic strategy.

For a long time fractures of the distal epiphysis of the humerus received only orthopedic treatment and rare attempts at osteosynthesis, whereas today they are treated almost exclusively with surgery. This switch was made with the goal of both an anatomical reduction of the fracture to restore joint symmetry, as well as a stable fixation that would allow early mobilization.

The extension of the surgical indications in the treatment of these fractures requires a thorough evaluation.

We have therefore made a distinction between *simple* and *complex* fractures. "Simple" fractures are those of the condyle, trochlea, capitulum, and epicondyle; they are defined as such because they do not present particular therapeutic problems. Either a lateral or a medial approach can be used, and fixation, after reduction of the fracture or removal of the fragment (in case of capitulum fracture), is easy and stable and the functional outcome is usually good.

"Complex" fractures, on the other hand, present two problems: joint reconstruction and stable fixation. A lateral or medial approach cannot achieve these goals, thus a posterior or, more rarely, an anterior approach is necessary.

MATERIALS AND METHODS

From 1982 to 1988, we surgically treated 33 fractures of the distal epiphysis of the humerus in adult patients; 24 of these were complex and 9 were simple (1 condylar, 2 trochlear, 2 epicondylar, and 4 capitellar).

Twenty-one fractures were in male patients who were 38 years old on average, and 12 fractures were in female patients who were 49 years old on average (Table 1). The age discrepancy can be attributed to the fact that different kinds of trauma prevail in the two sexes: the trauma suffered by male patients occurred primarily during sports, at work, or in motor vehicle accidents, while domestic accidents prevailed as the cause of trauma in female patients, vulnerable to fracture because of age-related osteoporotic processes.

The follow-up period ranged from 1 to 6 years (average 3.8). We did however observe,

Table 1
FRACTURES OF THE DISTAL HUMERUS. DISTRIBUTION ACCORDING TO AGE IN BOTH SEXES

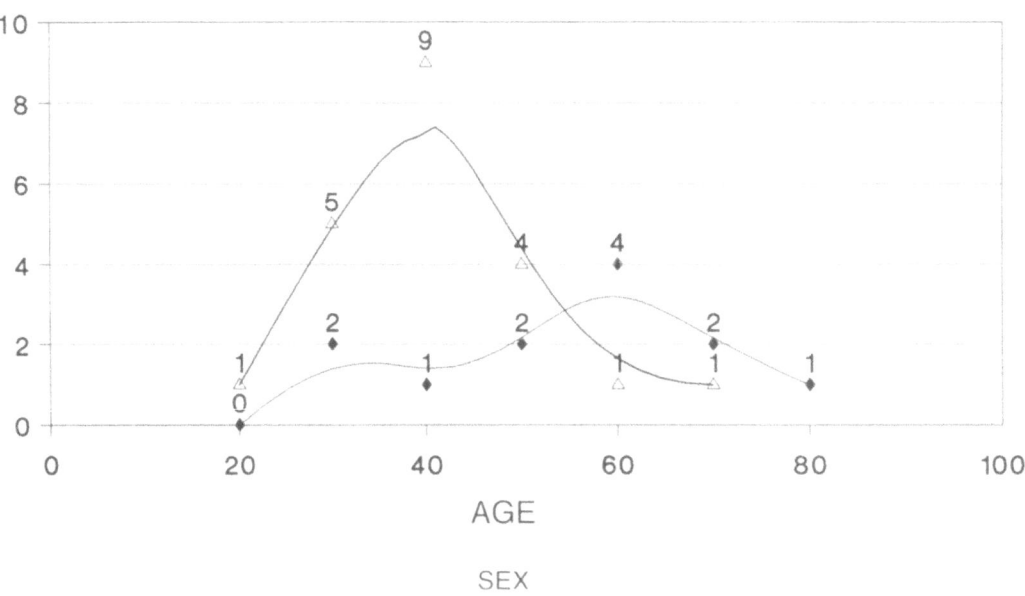

as have other authors (4), that about 6 months after surgery the result can be considered as stabilized, since it rarely deteriorates but tends rather to improve over time.

In the simple fractures (Fig. 1) a lateral or medial approach was adopted, using screw fixation or, as in the 4 cases of capitellar fracture, simply removing the osteochondral fragment.

For the complex epiphyseal fractures we used the posterior approach in most cases (22), resorting to the anterior approach in only 2 instances because of neurovascular complications which necessitated an accurate inspection of the anterior structures (Figs. 2-3).

The period of cast immobilization was minimal (average of 3 weeks) and immediately followed by physical therapy.

OPERATIVE TECHNIQUE

The posterior approach is particularly appropriate for the treatment of most of the complex fractures, since it provides the best

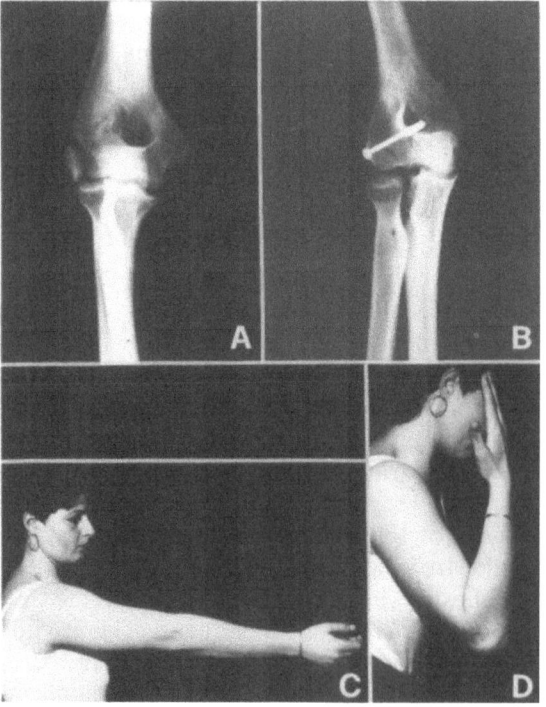

Fig. 1. - Fracture of the humeral condyle. In simple fractures, a lateral approach is adequate for reduction and fixation. A) Radiograph of the fracture. B) Radiograph after healing. C,D) Clinical outcome 4 years later.

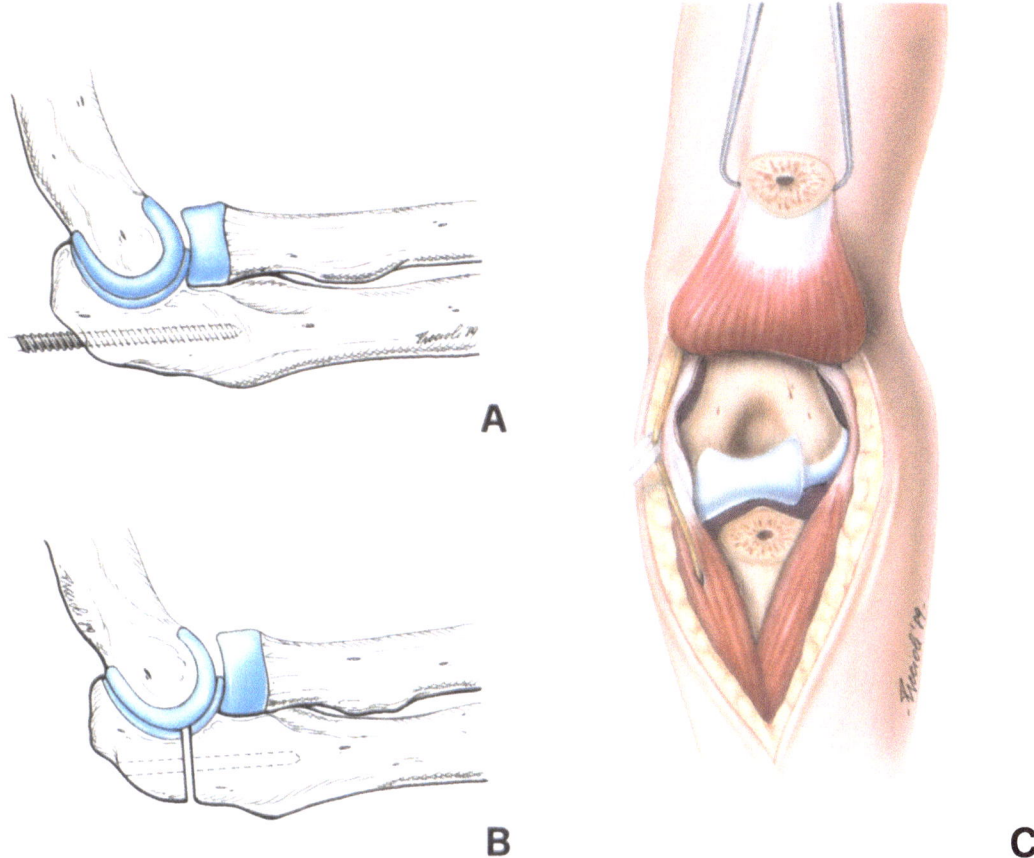

Fig. 2. - Posterior surgical approach to the elbow joint. A,B) Schematic representation of the osteotomy of the olecranon after preparation of the screw hole. C) The top of the olecranon is folded back along with the triceps tendon and belly after isolation of the ulnar nerve in the cubital groove. This allows wide exposure of the distal meta-epiphysis of the humerus, making fracture reduction possible. The final stage of the operation is fixation of the olecranon osteotomy.

exposure and facilitates reduction and fixation of the fracture (Fig. 2).

A posterior longitudinal incision exposes both the muscular surface and fascia. Before proceeding, the ulnar nerve must be isolated inside the epitrochlear-olecranon groove in order to avoid secondary damage during reduction and fixation. The next stage consists of transverse osteotomy of the olecranon. Before performing the osteotomy, however, it is a good idea to prepare the screw hole for the olecranon fixation.

Lifting back the olecranon and the attached triceps exposes the entire meta-epiphysis, making both reduction and fixation of the fracture possible. Some authors (7,11) prefer not to do the olecranon osteotomy and perform a V-shaped tenotomy of the triceps

tendon instead. We used the transtricipital approach in only a few cases (Fig. 5), and currently the transolecranon approach is preferred.

The epiphysis is usually broken into 2 or more fragments by a vertical fracture line with displacement and rotation of the fragments. After anatomical reduction, the fragments are fixed with screws: the epiphyseal fragments are fixed first with a transversally-placed lag screw, then the epiphyseal mass is reattached to the metaphysis with one or more obliquely-placed screws. After the reduction and fixation of the olecranon osteotomy, the superficial layers are reconstructed and the limb is immobilized in a plaster cast. After the removal of the cast, 2-5 weeks later depending upon the stability of the fixation,

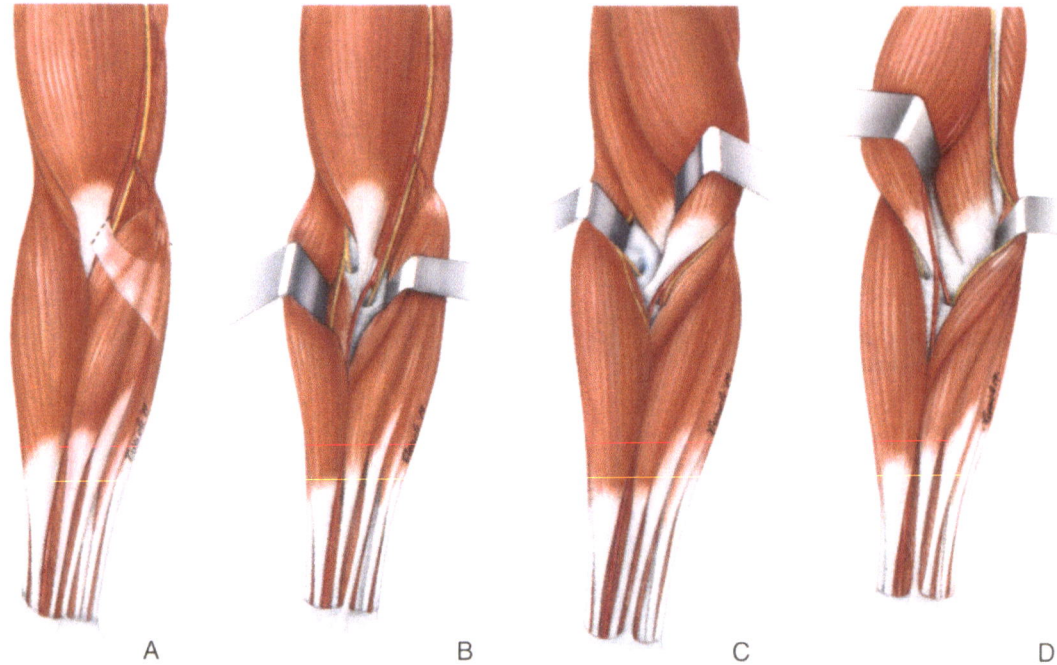

A   B   C   D

Fig. 3. - Anterior approach to the elbow joint. A) Section of the lacertus fibrosus permits isolation of the medial neurovascular bundle. B) Pulling the epitrochlear and lateral epicondylar muscles apart, the following structures are exposed: the median nerve with the brachial artery, the biceps tendon with the underlying anterior brachialis muscle, and the radial nerve with its superficial and interosseous branches. C) Pulling the biceps medially, the lateral portion of the joint capsule is exposed. D) Pulling the biceps and brachial artery laterally, the medial portion of the capsule is exposed.

the patient begins physical therapy.

The anterior approach is used very rarely, and only in cases with significant neurologic or vascular complications (Figs. 3-8).

After making a curved incision on the anterior surface of the elbow, both the fascia and the lacertus fibrosus are in turn incised. It is then possible to explore the medial neurovascular bundle (median nerve, brachial artery and veins) and the radial nerve between the anterior brachialis and brachioradialis muscles, repairing any possible damage. The capsular level is reached by way of the interstitium between the brachial artery and the median nerve. After the arthrotomy, reduction and then fixation are performed.

RESULTS

The criteria for the clinical evaluation have been recovery of joint function (range of flexion, extension, pronation, and supination), recovery of muscle strength, and presence of pain.

For the evaluation of the range of flexion and extension, we used a modified version of Merle d'Aubigné's (7) functional quotation since it was necessary to take into account the residual limitation of both flexion and extension (Fig. 4). In fact, we must remember that an overall mobility of 90 degrees, for example, does not have the same significance between 0 and 90 degrees as it does between 35 and 125 degrees. In the latter case the range, even though limited and equal to the former, allows the elbow to carry out most of the movements involved in everyday social and occupational activity.

The evaluation of pronation and supination has not yet been addressed because it did not undergo significant changes. The simple fractures (Table 2) showed full recovery of range of motion (Fig. 1), while the complex fractures had generally satisfactory results with full recovery of flexion and extension in 6 cases. In all cases the age factor together with the type of fracture obviously determined the functional result: the best results

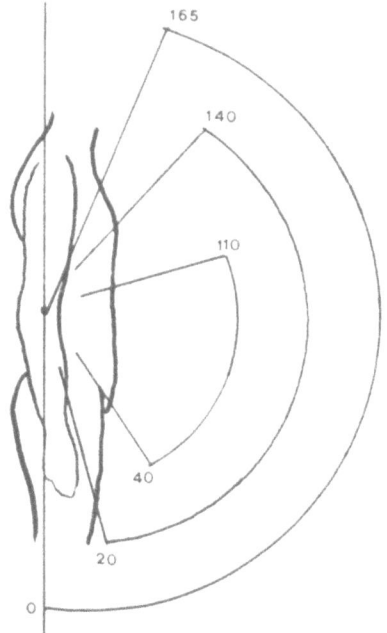

Fig. 4. - Schematic drawing of a modified version of Merle d'Aubigné's functional quotation of flexion and extension. A recovery of range of motion from 0 to 165 degrees is considered full, from 20 to 140 degrees is considered good, and from 40 to 110 degrees is considered fair.

◄

were achieved in the youngest patients, who fully cooperated in the demanding postoperative physical therapy program (Figs. 5-8).

The recovery of muscle strength was satisfactory in most cases (Table 3); only partial recovery occurred mostly with complex fractures, especially in the oldest and least motivated patients.

Pain was evaluated (Table 4) more than 1 year after the trauma. It was almost com-

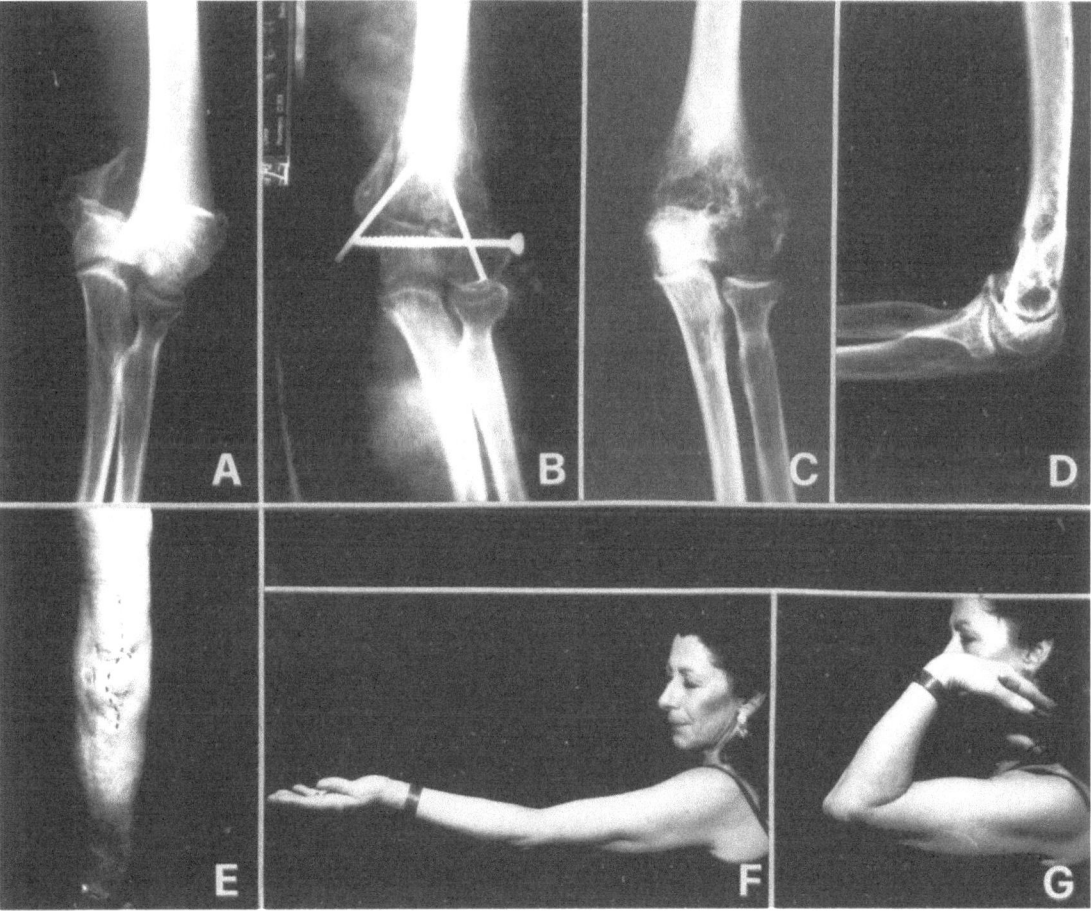

Fig. 5. - Complex comminuted epiphyseal fracture treated through a posterior transtricipital approach. A) Radiograph of the fracture. B) Radiograph after reduction and fixation. C,D) Excellent radiographic result 5 years later. E) Scar (dotted line) on the posterior side of the elbow. F,G) Good clinical outcome after 5 years.

Table 2
RECOVERY OF FLEXION AND EXTENSION

	Full	Good (20°-140°)	Fair (40°-110°)
Simple fractures	6	3	0
Complex fractures	6	15	3

Table 3
RECOVERY OF MUSCLE STRENGTH

	Partial	Full
Simple fractures	8	1
Complex fractures	18	6

pletely lacking in cases of simple fracture, and was present in only 4 cases of complex fracture, limited however to the extreme degrees of elbow movement and not severe enough to compromise normal activity or necessitate the administration of anti-inflammatory drugs.

DISCUSSION AND CONCLUSIONS

Experience in the treatment of these le-

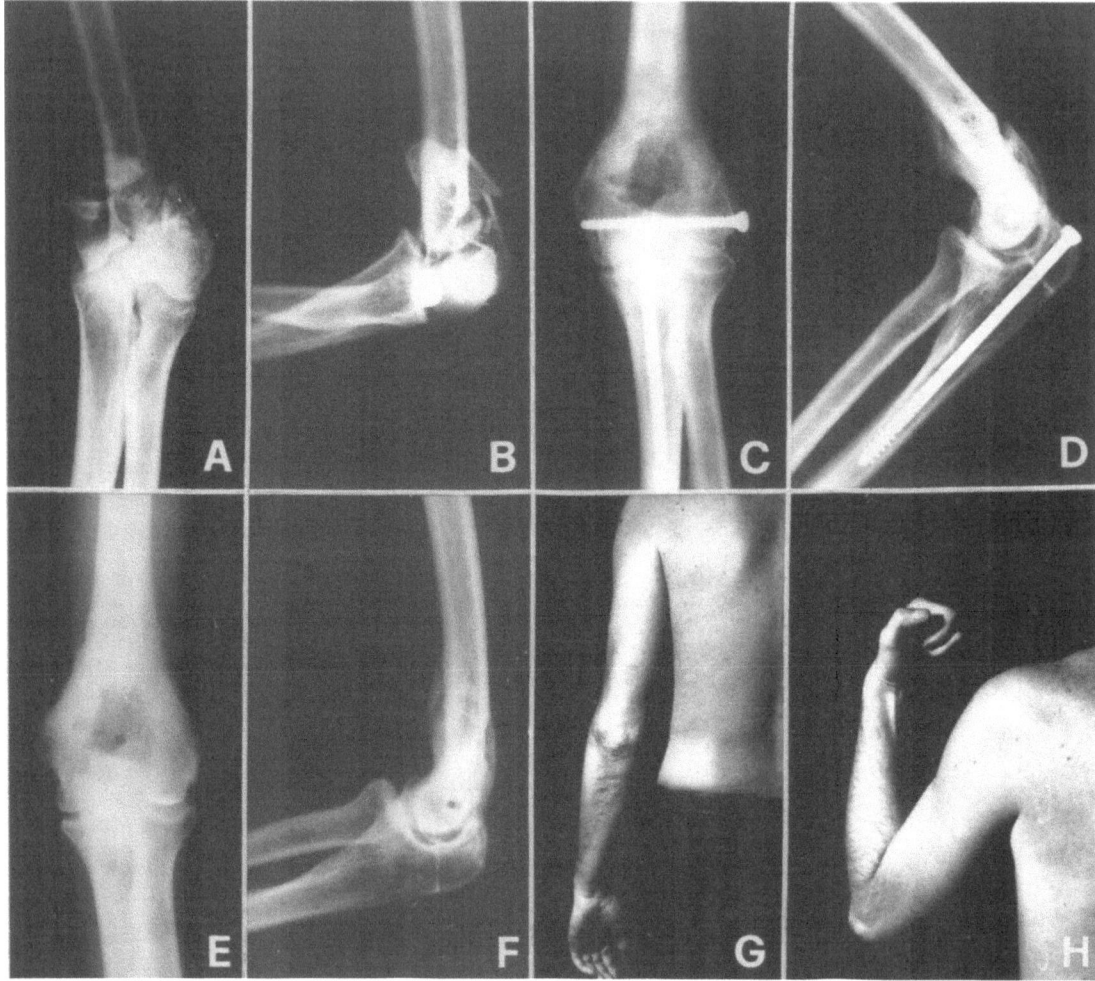

Fig. 6. - Complex epiphyseal T fracture treated with a posterior transolecranon approach. A,B) Radiograph of the fracture. C,D) Radiograph 6 months after open reduction. Note the good reconstruction of the articular surfaces as well as the union of the olecranon osteotomy. E,F) Radiograph 4 years later, all fixation devices have been removed. G,H) Good clinical outcome 4 years after surgery.

Table 4
PRESENCE OF PAIN

	Simplex fractures	Complex fractures
None	8	18
At rest	0	0
During activity	0	2
At the extreme degrees of motion	1	4

sions allows us to make some conclusions in light of the results.

From a prognostic standpoint, the fractures of the distal humerus are serious because of the possible consequences to elbow function. Rigorous treatment that takes into account the age of the patient, the type of fracture, and any possible complications is therefore needed.

Conservative orthopedic treatment cannot always solve the problems presented by these lesions, and should therefore be reserved primarily for undisplaced fractures and older patients with fewer functional needs. In displaced fractures, on the other hand, open reduction and fixation are required because of the need for good reconstruction of the articular surfaces. As a matter of fact, adequate reduction of the articular surfaces is essential for a good clinical result. Furthermore, a simultaneous stable fixation allows early mobilization with a lower risk of joint stiffness.

The lateral and medial approaches should be reserved for the simplest fractures (condy-

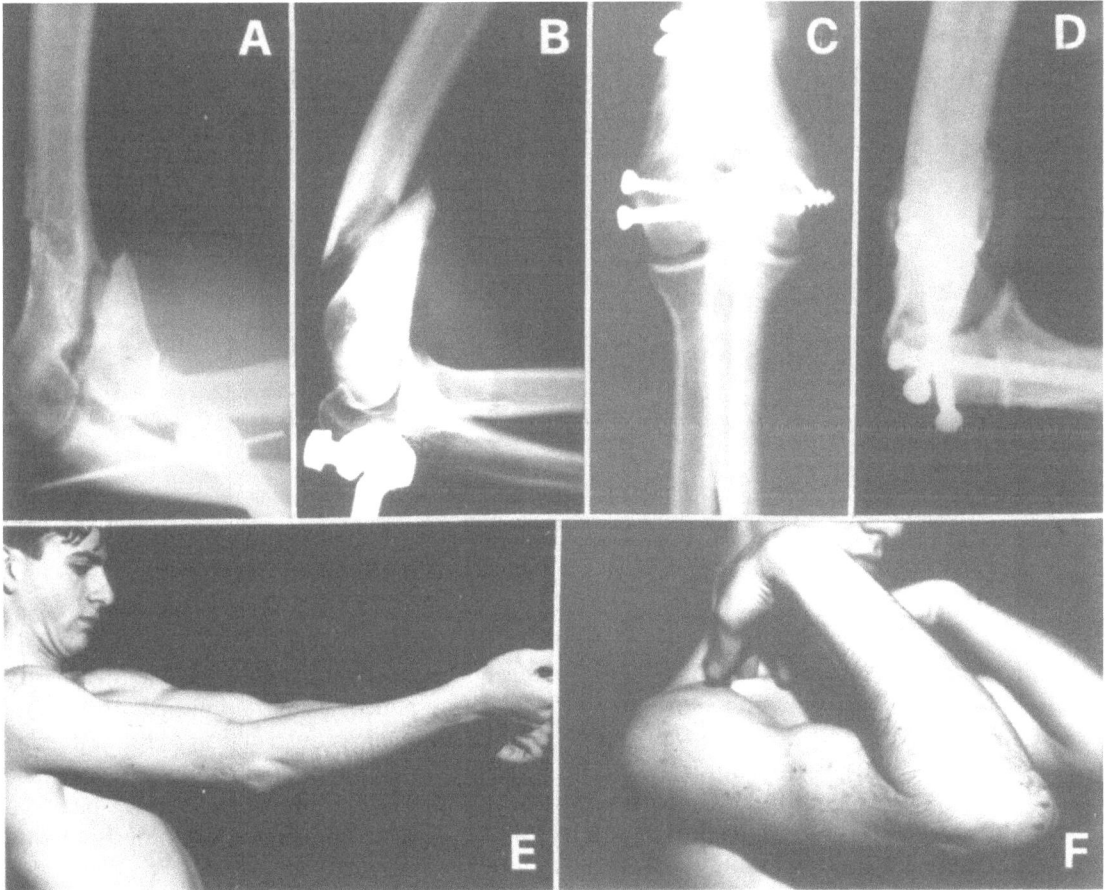

Fig. 7. - Complex epiphyseal V fracture treated through a posterior transolecranon approach. A,B) Radiograph of the fracture. C,D) Radiograph after 1 year, with excellent reconstruction of the joint rima. E,F) Good clinical outcome after 1 year.

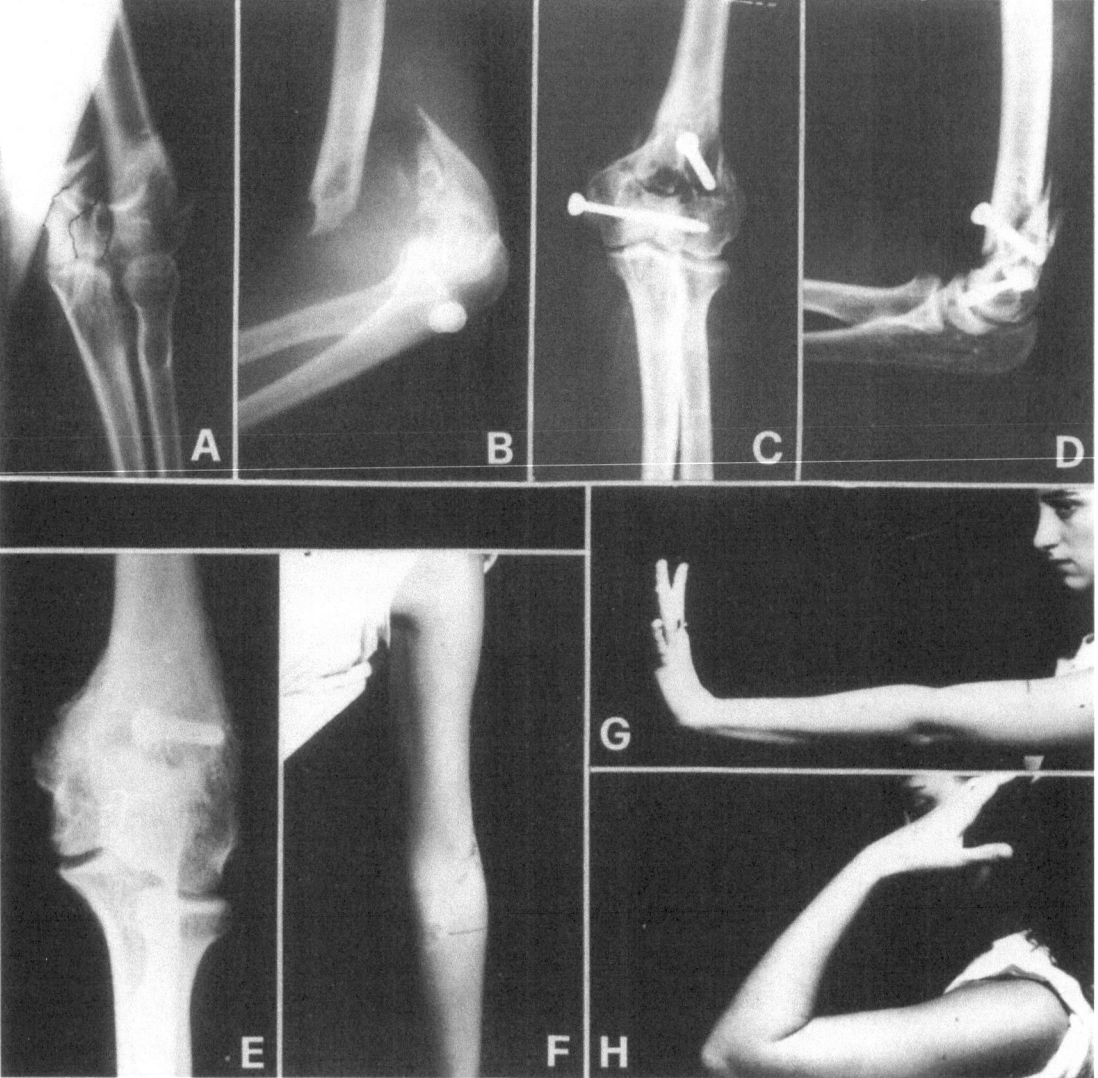

Fig. 8. - Complex multiple epiphyseal fracture with paralysis of the radial nerve treated through an anterior approach. A,B) Radiograph: note the severe displacement of the principal fracture. C,D) Radiograph after reduction and fixation. E) Radiograph after 1 year; epiphyseal screw has been removed. F) Scar on the anterior side of the elbow. G,H) Good clinical outcome after 1 year.

lar, epicondylar, trochlear, capitellar).

For the treatment of complex epiphyseal fractures, however, the posterior approach (transolecranon or transtricipital) is the most appropriate as it provides the best exposure. The only disadvantage of the transolecranon route is that it requires osteotomy of the articular portion of the olecranon. In our experience this procedure has not caused any particular problems.

The anterior approach is used more rarely, reserved in any case for fractures with significant neurovascular complications.

Anatomical reconstruction of the articular surface is a common goal in modern traumatology. This is essential for weight-bearing joints, yet also important for joints like the elbow.

The analysis of the results of surgical treatment of these fractures is especially encouraging.

Arthrolysis was necessary an average of 7

months after open reduction in the 3 cases that had a fair recovery of flexion and extension (Table 2), and in only 5 of the patients who had a good recovery, in order to address specific functional needs of these patients.

Arthrolysis resulted in significant improvement of range of motion in all cases; this result was no doubt aided by good reconstruction of the articular surfaces achieved with the initial surgery.

In fact, when arthrolysis was used for the same types of fracture in which the initial treatment had been conservative and there had not been adequate anatomical reconstruction of the joint surfaces, the results were substantially poorer.

REFERENCES

1) BOEHLER L: *Tecnica del trattamento delle fratture*. Vallardi Ed., Milano, 1955.

2) BROWN R.F., MORGAN R.G.: Intercondylar T-shaped fractures of the humerus: results in ten cases treated by early mobilisation. *J. Bone Jt Surg.* 1971; **53-B**: 425.

3) BURRI C., HENKEMEYER H., SPIER W.: Results of operative treatment of intra-articular fractures of the distal humerus. *Acta Orthop. Belg.* 1975; **41(2)**: 227.

4) CLAISSE P.: Les fractures de l'extrémité inférieure de l'humérus chez l'adulte. Casuistique. *Rev. Chir. Orthop.* 1980; Suppl. 2, **66**: 23.

5) COLLERT SVEN: Surgical management of fractures of the capitulum humeri. *Acta Orthop. Scand.* 1977; **48**: 603.

6) DECOULX P., DUCLOUX M., HESPEEL J., DECOULX J.: Les fractures de l'extrémité inférieure de l'humérus chez l'adulte. *Rev. Chir. Orthop.* 1964; **50**: 263.

7) DURIAU F.: Fractures de la palette humérale de l'adulte. Etude clinique de 60 cas. *Acta Orthop. Belg.* 1976; **42(1)**: 50.

8) GUI L.: *Fratture e lussazioni*. Aulo Gaggi Ed. Bologna, 1981.

9) JUDET R.: Le traitement des fractures de l'extrémité inférieure de l'humérus chez l'adulte. *Rev. Chir. Orthop.* 1964; **50**: 275.

10) LECESTRE P., DUPONT J.Y., LORTAT JACOB A., REMADIER J.O.: Les fractures de l'extrémité inférieure de l'humérus chez l'adulte. A propos de 66 cas dont 55 opérés. *Rev. Chir. Orthop.* 1979; **65**: 11.

11) MERLE D'AUBIGNÉ R., MEARY R., CARLIOZ J.: Fractures sus et intercondyliennes récentes de l'adulte. *Rev. Chir. Orthop.* 1964; **50**: 279.

12) MILLER W.E.: Comminuted fractures of the distal end of the humerus in the adult. *J. Bone Jt Surg.* 1964; **46-A**: 644.

13) RISEBOROUGH E.H., RADIN E.L.: Intercondylar T fractures of the humerus in the adult: a comparison of operative and non-operative treatment in twenty-nine cases. *J. Bone Jt Surg.* 1969; **51-A**: 130.

AO open reduction and internal fixation of fractures of the distal humerus in the adult

T. Luppino - A. Salsi - R. Fiocchi - T. Stefanini - A. Laganà

PREMISE

Fractures of the distal humerus require the maximum effort of the orthopedic surgeon in order to restore the original shape of the epiphysis, essential for the normal function of one of the most important anatomical sectors.

The anatomical and functional complexity of this epiphysis, the variety of possible fractures, and the difficulties involved in surgical treatment have, especially in the past, led orthopedists to prescribe conservative orthopedic treatment, the long-term results of which are almost always mediocre.

In fractures with one or more fragments that are irreducible by external means, open reduction is the only way to achieve anatomically perfect reconstruction.

We therefore agree with other authors (1, 2, 4, 7) that AO open reduction and internal fixation is the most effective surgical method, permitting anatomical reduction and early mobilization.

FRACTURES

This chapter uses the Müller classification system (6) of fractures of the distal humerus, dividing the fractures into three main categories, which are each in turn subdivided into three further categories (Fig. 1):

A - *Periarticular fractures*
A1 - epitrochlear;
A2 - transverse supracondylar;
A3 - comminuted supracondylar.
B - *Articular condylar fractures*
B1 - trochlear-epicondylar fragment;
B2 - capitellar lateral epicondylar fragment;
B3 - capitellar dome only.

C - *Articular intercondylar fractures*
C1 - Y condylar through trochlea;
C2 - Y condylar through trochlea with comminution of supracondylar area;
C3 - comminuted articular.

OPERATIVE TECHNIQUE

Approaches

We abided by the AO recommended surgical exposure time.

The patient is in a prone position with elbow flexed at 90 degrees and hanging off the bed.

Usually, the posterior transtricipital approach is used (Fig. 2). After isolating the ulnar nerve, the triceps tendon is detached with an inverted V-shaped incision, the apex of which should be about 10 cm from the olecranon.

The section is done at the musculotendinous passage, leaving a tendinous bundle attached to the muscle belly. The fold of the triceps is then folded back in order to expose the posterior aspect of the epiphysis.

Exposure can be increased by hyperflexing the elbow more than 90 degrees. Using this method we have never had to resort to preventive osteotomy of the olecranon.

We reserve the medial approach with isolation of the ulnar nerve exclusively for epitrochlear fractures.

In lateral condylar fractures, however, we prefer to use the lateral approach, with a superior incision that runs along the lateral intermuscular septum and an inferior incision between the radial extensors and the extensor communis.

This approach, which we also use for arthrolysis, gives good exposure of both the lat-

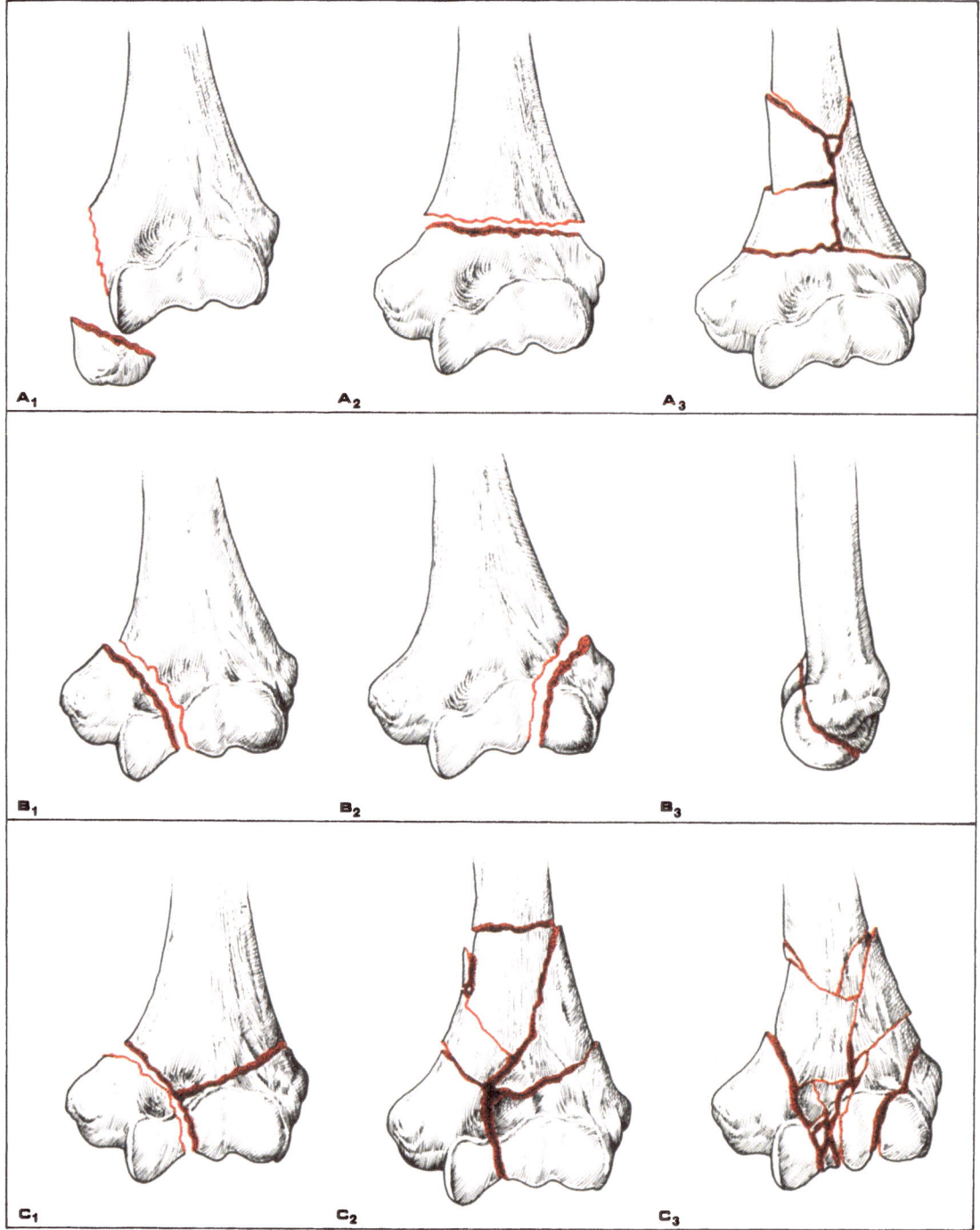

Fig. 1. - Müller classification system for distal humeral fractures: A1 – medial epicondylar fracture; A2 – transverse supracondylar fracture; A3 – comminuted supracondylar fracture; B1 trochlear-epicondylar fragment; B2 – capitellar-lateral epicondylar fragment; B3 – capitellar dome fracture; C1 – Y condylar fracture through trochlea; C2 – Y condylar fracture through trochlea with comminution of supracondylar area; C3 – comminuted articular fracture.

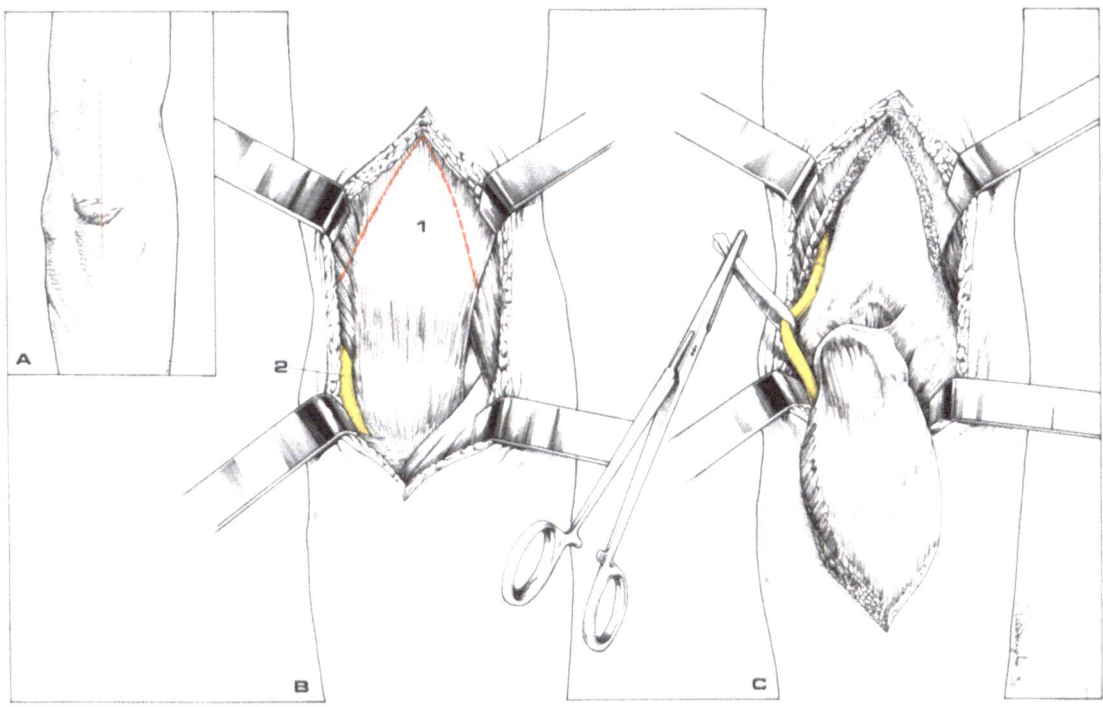

Fig. 2. - Exposure of the distal third of the humerus and the elbow: A) vertical dorsal incision; B) inverted V-shaped incision of the triceps; C) isolation of the ulnar nerve (2) and detachment of the tricipital flap (1).

eral side of the joint and the anterior and posterior sides of the distal epiphysis.

Extensive exposure on the anterior side of the humerus should be avoided in order to prevent ossification of the anterior brachialis.

Internal fixation techniques

In epitrochlear detachment, as in condylar and trochlear fractures, fixation is done with either 4 mm cancellous or malleolar screws depending upon the size of the fragment.

If the fragment is small, the perforation should start from the fracture surface in order to avoid cleavage. In transverse or comminuted supracondylar fractures, surgery is indicated primarily in the presence of displaced fragments that cannot be reduced.

Usually, a 1/3 tubular plate is placed on the lateral side, and its screws are inserted in traction if the fracture is oblique.

Occasionally, a shorter second 1/3 tubular plate is placed on the posteromedial side to increase stability.

Internal fixation is strongly indicated in condylar fractures through the trochlea, as it is the only way to reconstruct the articular surface. The operation is usually very difficult both in the reduction stage, which is like putting together the pieces of a mosaic, and in the fixation stage.

To be stable, the fixation should always start from the trochlea, keeping its anatomical width in mind. This structure is fixed with either a transversally-placed 4 mm cancellous or malleolar screw, which is then attached to the lateral side of the diaphysis with a 1/3 tubular plate.

Application of a second, shorter 1/3 tubular plate on the posteromedial side is often necessary.

The small fragments can be fixed with either biodegradable Kirschner wires or 2.7 mm cortical screws.

In comminuted fractures a temporary fixation with Kirschner wires may be useful, but they must be placed so as not to hinder the introduction of the plate.

If a metaphyseal bone defect remains, an

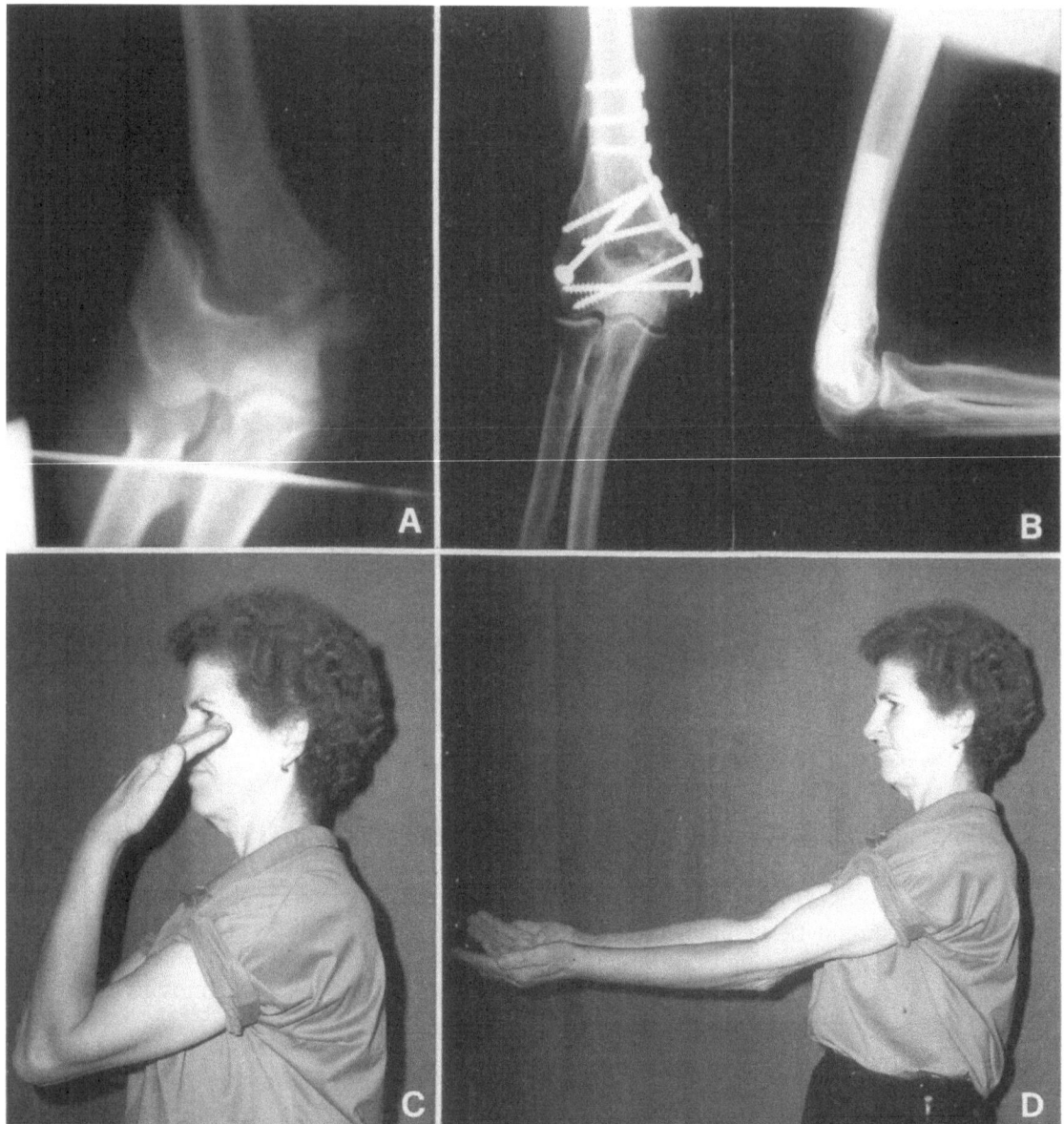

Fig. 3. - G.P., age 57 (A2 fracture): A) Preoperative radiograph with the limb in skeletal traction; B) radiograph 3 years after surgery reveals para-articular calcifications; C,D) clinical examination after 3 years shows slight limitation of range of motion (flexion normal, extension -20 degrees).

autogenous corticocancellous graft may be necessary. The graft can be taken from the olecranon, or it can be made up of the smallest fragments at the fracture site.

At the end of the operation the elbow is passively flexed and extended in order to test the stability of the implant and plan the postoperative management accordingly. No fixation device should occupy the coronoid or olecranon fossae at any time, lest it hinder flexion and extension.

POSTOPERATIVE MANAGEMENT

If the fixation proves stable, active mobilization consisting of flexion and extension can begin on the second day, after removal of the drainage fluid.

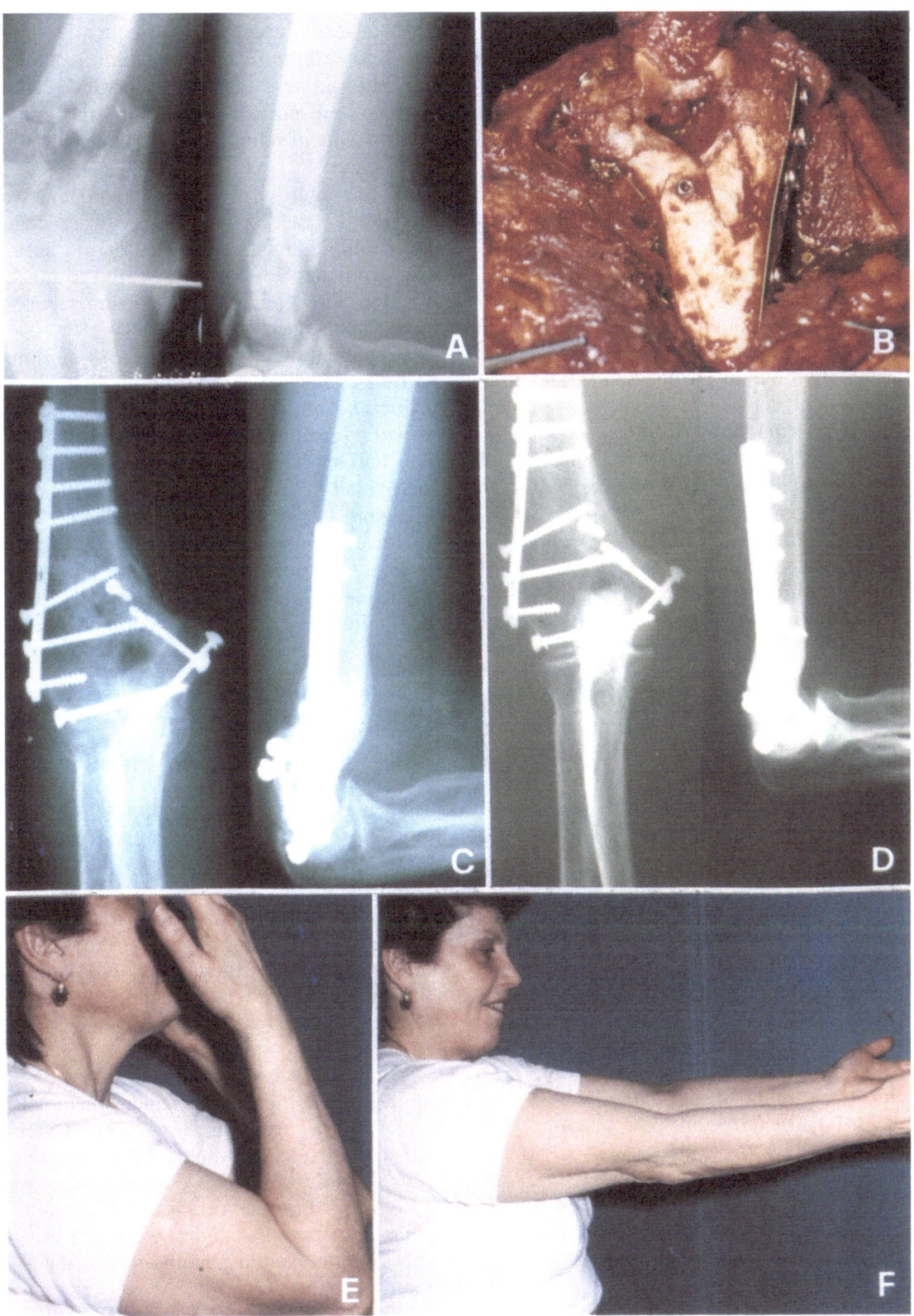

Fig. 4. - C.A., age 57 (C3 fracture): A) Preoperative radiograph with limb in skeletal traction; B) completed fixation; C,D) radiographs both 5 months and 5 years after surgery show formation of callus; E,F) clinical examination 5 years after surgery shows excellent functional recovery with only slight limitation of flexion (-20 degrees).

For at least 20 days, any type of passive mobilization that could cause para-articular ossifications with resulting stiffness should be avoided. The patients should therefore alternate posterior cast immobilization with gradual, active, independent mobilization.

The average period of partial immobilization is 20 days.

PATIENTS

Thirty-two patients, 23 males and 9 females, were treated using the above method at the Divisione di Ortopedia e Traumatologia of the Ospedale Civile at Sassuolo (Modena) from 1982 to 1986.

Referring to the Müller classification, we were able to distinguish the following fracture types:
- A1 fracture: 2 cases
- A2 fracture: 2 cases
- A3 fracture: 3 cases
- B1 fracture: 1 case
- B2 fracture: 1 case
- B3 fracture: 1 case
- C1 fracture: 6 cases
- C2 fracture: 7 cases, 2 of which were open, 1 accompanied by humeral shaft fracture, and 1 by olecranon fracture
- C3 fracture: 9 cases

RESULTS

Postoperative complications included 3 cases of neurologic deficit, 2 involving the radial nerve and 1 the ulnar nerve. All 3 cases healed spontaneously. There was also one case of pseudarthrosis caused by a technical error in the fixation (instability of device).

Twenty-one of the 32 patients were present at the follow-up examination (3 A fractures, 1 B fracture, and 17 C fractures). The average follow-up period was 3½ years (range 6 months - 6.2 years). None of the patients had limited pronation or supination, significant pain in the joint (except the patient with pseudoarthrosis), or neurologic deficit over the long-term.

In all cases except 3 (subsequently subjected to arthrolysis), radiographic examination showed an evident joint line and restoration of the normal anatomy of the joint. Five patients developed para-articular ossifications.

In the interest of clinical homogeneity, only the 17 cases of C fracture were considered in the functional evaluation of the results, studying with particular care the range of active elbow flexion and extension according to Kapandji (3).

No patient recovered full range of motion: the best result had a 15-degree limitation of flexion and no limitation of extension, while the worst result had a flexion deficit of 25 degrees and an extension deficit of 30 degrees. The overall average was a 15-degree flexion deficit and a 21-degree extension deficit.

However, all patients recovered at least a 90-degree portion of the total range of flexion and extension and, most importantly, this portion included the most functionally useful sectors of movement.

CONCLUSIONS

In light of our results, already partially analyzed in a previous publication (5), the validity of AO internal fixation in the treatment of fractures of the distal humerus in the adult seems evident.

The AO method, if performed correctly, makes stable fixation possible even in severely comminuted fractures. Consequently, it allows anatomical reconstruction of the distal epiphysis and restoration of normal joint anatomy.

A stable fixation makes early joint mobilization possible, thereby shortening functional recovery time. The results are significantly better than those attained with either conservative treatment or fixation with Kirschner wires only.

Both the functional results and the time to healing clearly justify surgical treatment using stable fixation even in fractures where the alternative is arthroplasty.

REFERENCES

1) DECOULX P., DUCLOUX M., HESPEEL J., DECOULX J.: Les fractures de l'extremité inférieure de l'humérus chez l'adulte. *Rev. Chir. Orthop.* 1980; Supp. II: **66**.

2) GHEZZI L.M.: *Le fratture dell'estremità distale dell'omero nell'adulto.* Atti XXV Convegno Nazionale Club Italiano A.O., Paternò, Taormina, 27, 14-16 settembre 1984.

3) KAPANDJI I.A.: *Fisiologia articolare.* Soc. Ed. Demi, Roma, 1974.

4) LECESTRE P.: Les fractures de l'extremité inférieure de l'humérus chez l'adulte. *Rev. Chir. Orthop.* 1980; **66**.

5) LUPPINO T., FIOCCHI R., SALSI A., STEFANINI T.: L'osteosintesi solida mediante tecnica A.O. nelle fratture comminute intraarticolari distali dell'omero. *G.I.O.T.* 1989; **15**(2): 183-188.

6) MÜLLER M.E., ALLGOWER M., SCHNEIDER R., WILLENEGGER M.: *Manuale dell'osteosintesi. Tecniche raccomandate dall'A.O.* Piccin Ed., Padova, 1981.

7) ZINGHI G.F., SABETTA E., DONATI D., BUNGARO P.: Le fratture dell'estremità inferiore dell'omero nell'adulto. *G.I.O.T.* 1988; **14**(2): 215-224.

Fractures of the proximal ulna

U. Passaretti - M. Misasi

Fractures of the proximal ulna include both olecranon and coronoid fractures and, more precisely, are meta-epiphyseal fractures of the ulna.

Relatively rare among the fractures of the upper limb, they are more common in adults than in children or the elderly.

Percentage-wise, fractures of the olecranon are more common than fractures of the coronoid.

The anatomical region in question consists of the proximal humeroulnar and radioulnar joints, the different components of which ensure their stability. For example, the first mechanism of arrest, and therefore protection, during both hyperflexion and hypertension of the ulna is the depth of the coronoid and olecranon fossae, which causes the apophysis to come to a halt against the bone surface in case of extreme elbow movement.

At full flexion the coronoid apophysis can reach the bottom of the fossa only when the tension of the extensor muscles is neutralized and the resistance of the posterior marginal fibers of the lateral ligaments is overcome. Likewise, the extension of the ulna is arrested by the resistance of the flexor muscles and the tension produced by the anterior marginal bundles of the lateral ligaments.

Nevertheless, despite the inherent protective bony structures (crest of the semilunar notch, concave portion of the trochlea, olecranon, and coronoid apophysis), longitudinal dislocation is fairly common.

As a matter of fact, in case of severe trauma (a fall on the outstretched hand, for example) the top of the olecranon smashes into the olecranon fossa, causing posterior dislocation.

Rarer are dislocations that occur only after the rupture of one of the two strong lateral ligaments; these are almost always accompanied by posterior dislocation because of the simultaneous laceration of the capsule.

Another factor that can facilitate dislocation is the position of the elbow in 45-degree flexion, since in that position neither the coronoid nor the olecranon are inside their fossae and are therefore vulnerable.

The orbicular ligament together with the strong lateral ligaments (stiff reinforcing bundles that radiate from the distal edges of the epicondyles to the edges of the semilunar notch inside the fibrous layer of the capsule) constitute the stabilizing component of the proximal radioulnar joint.

The orbicular ligament detaches anteriorly and posteriorly from the edge of the radial notch of the ulna and effectively reinforces even the lateral side of the capsule. Therefore, all these capsuloligamentous structures plus the particular conformation of the bony elements give the proximal humeroulnar and radioulnar joints remarkable stability, which in adults can be overcome only by severe trauma.

FRACTURE OF THE OLECRANON

These fractures occur mainly in young adults, more rarely in the elderly, and very seldom in children. Since they are articular lesions, even minimal shifting of the reduction can lead to arthritis. The insertion of the triceps on the tip of the olecranon makes accurate reduction using simple orthopedic treatment impossible.

The mechanism of injury in olecranon fractures can be either direct or indirect.

1) Indirect mechanism
In most cases this consists of strong contractions of the triceps during forced flexion

of the forearm against the trochlea. The modality consisting of forearm extension is rarer; in that case the olecranon is held in the olecranon fossa by the action of the elbow ligaments.

2) Direct mechanism

Both occupational and motor vehicle accidents have made this type of trauma more common. Because of the force of the direct trauma, severe exposure, contusions, and skin lacerations are also inflicted.

Fractures of the olecranon can be:
a) isolated
b) multiple
c) associated with other lesions

a) **Isolated fractures** were divided by Merle d'Aubigué into three categories:

Type I: fractures of the tip of the olecranon, the only periarticular fractures. Shifting is variable and depends on the contraction of the triceps.

Type II: fractures of the middle portion. These are the most common. They are different from fractures of the base because they leave a piece of coronoid surface intact and preserve the stability of the elbow. The displacement of the fragments can be serious or not depending upon the integrity of the fibrous structures that insheath the posterior fascia of the olecranon. When these remain intact, the fragments are only minimally displaced; if they are damaged, however, the upper fragment is lifted up by the triceps and then slides posteriorly. The fracture site is then located under the skin.

Type III: fracture of the base. These are unstable fractures that involve the distal and horizontal portions of the semilunar notch. Significant displacement of the fragments is rare because they are not subject to strong muscular traction.

b) **Multiple fractures** are relatively common and usually the result of direct trauma. Treatment requires precise indications, but they vary from case to case. The fractures are categorized as follows:

— *double fracture*: fracture of the middle portion accompanied by fracture of the base; presence of a *middle fragment*;

— *comminuted fracture*: comminution of fragments. The coronoid apophysis usually remains intact, ensuring stability;

— *olecranon-coronoid fracture*: typically unstable primarily because of coronoid fracture.

c) **Fractures associated with other lesions** include:

— fracture of the proximal ulna with dislocation of the radial head. This combination is improperly considered a Monteggia fracture-dislocation;

— transolecranon elbow dislocations: al-

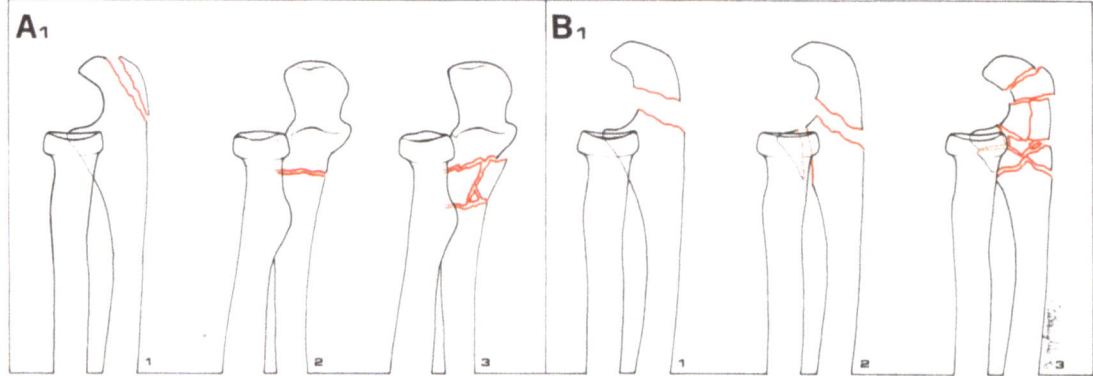

Fig. 1. - Schematic drawing of the Müller classification of fractures of the proximal ulna. A1: periarticular fractures subdivided into fractures of the tuberosity (1), and simple (2) and multiple (3) metaphyseal fractures. B1: articular fractures subdivided into mid-olecranon fractures (1), olecranon-coronoid fractures (2), and comminuted epi-metaphyseal fractures.

ways caused by severe trauma and often open, they result in radioulnar instability. The radius and ulna are rarely torn apart, since as long as the orbicular ligament is undamaged the radioulnar joint remains intact.

Bigat and Thomine recognize two clinical types:

Type I: oblique fracture of the base of the olecranon with no damage to the ligamentous insertions, which preserve the humerus-olecranon congruity.

Type II: comminuted fractures (severe, direct trauma, fracture is often open) of the middle portion of the olecranon; congruity of humerus and olecranon is destroyed.

Along with this classification should be mentioned the one proposed by Professor Müller in his book dedicated to the AO fracture classification.

Müller submits that a fracture classification using common nomenclature is indispensable for the evaluation of various potential treatments. To adequately document a fracture, the orthopedist must not only consider the fracture line visible on the AP and lateral radiographs, but also all the other factors that determine the severity of the fracture, such as the complexity of the therapeutic problems, the complications observed in similar cases, and the risk of permanent disability.

The fracture designation must be simple and easily memorized. Müller divides the skeleton into 9 segments and the fractures into 3 main categories, called *A-B-C*, each of which is in turn divided into three subgroups.

Fractures of the proximal ulna are categorized as follows:

A1: periarticular fractures subdivided into three groups:

1) fractures of the tuberosity

2) isolated metaphyseal fractures

3) multiple metaphyseal fractures

B1: articular fractures also subdivided into three groups:

1) mid-olecranon

2) olecranon-coronoid

3) comminuted epi-metaphyseal.

Though this modern classification proposed by Müller, which is useful above all for facilitating the entry of case data into a computer, should be kept in mind, we prefer the more practical classification system previously described.

Treatment

For the above reasons, treatment of these fractures requires not only accurate reduction but also stabilization. Simple cast immobilization is indicated only for fractures with no or minimal displacement, that is, for fractures which should remain stable even after casting (which should be done with elbow flexed to 90 degrees and forearm in zero position). Immobilization should not last more than 3

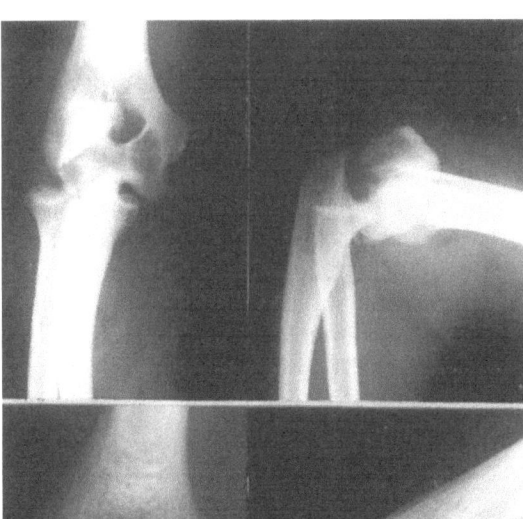
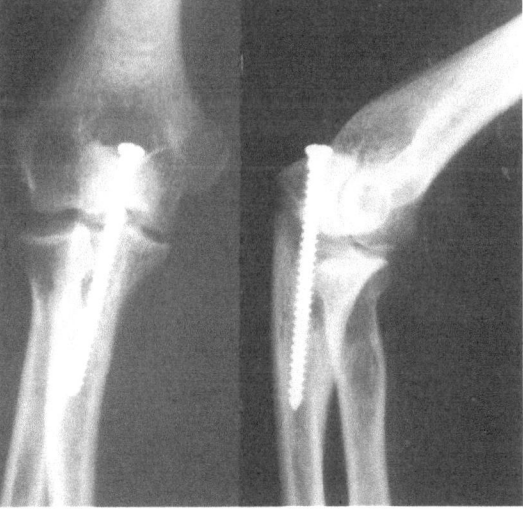

Fig. 2. - In mid-olecranon fractures the displacement of the fragments can be more or less evident depending upon the integrity of the fibrous structures that insheath the posterior fascia of the bone. Use of a screw ensures stable fixation of the fragments.

weeks due to the need for early active reeducation (important in all articular fractures).

Surgical treatment is adopted in all other cases because of the severity of the lesions. The choice of internal fixation device varies according to the type of fracture.

Incorrect indications and/or poor execution of surgery can result in serious limitations in overall function of the entire limb, with pain and decreased work capacity in addition to visible aesthetic damage.

Elective internal fixation can be done using a variety of methods and devices, such as encirclage, screws (cortical and cancellous), plates and screws, combinations of different devices, and olecranectomy.

Encirclage

It is and it was the most frequently used fixation device, but its adoption is justified in only a few types of fracture, such as the Merle d'Aubigné types I and II.

Simple encirclage is in fact insufficient in elbow flexion because of the strong diastasic action of the triceps on the proximal fragment. Fixation should therefore be readied with a single or double figure-8 encirclage.

In oblique fractures, which are less stable, the encirclage fixation can be strengthened

with two traction Kirschner wires.

This reduction is more stable and thus the period of immobilization is reduced to 15 days in a foam-rubber splint with the joint flexed at 45 degrees.

Screws

Both cortical and cancellous screws may be used. The former are indicated for oblique epi-metaphyseal fractures in which there is often a large diaphyseal fragment, thus especially for type III fractures. In type II fractures, however, a large cancellous screw should be inserted perpendicularly into the fragment and situated in the center of the medullary canal.

Plate and screw fixation

This device is used in complex epi-metaphyseal fractures with 2 or more fragments, also known as type III fractures. These fractures often cause secondary arthritis because of the frequent presence of a "decalage" of the anterior articular surface.

Stabilization of the various fragments makes early mobilization possible, which is essential for good functional results.

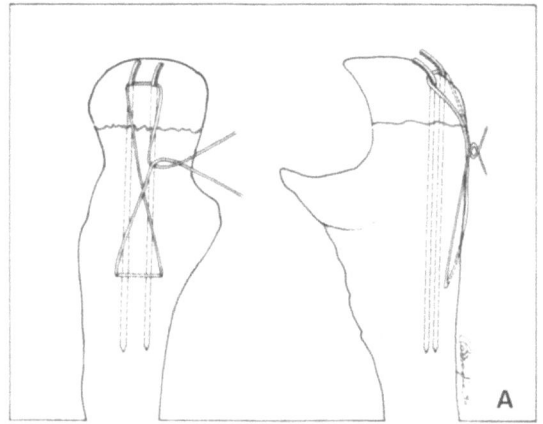 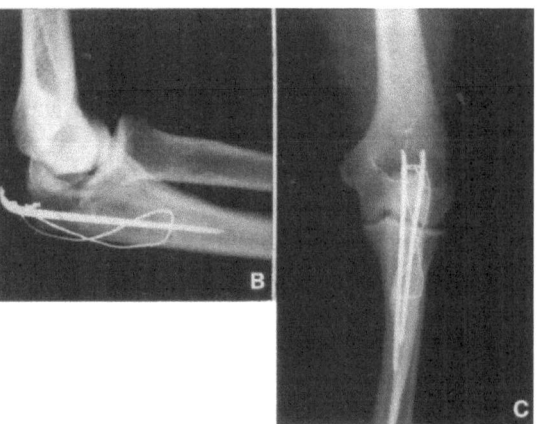

Fig. 3. - A) Schematic drawing of dynamic internal fixation performed by Weber et al.; it is called haubanage in French and Zuggurtungsosteosynthese in German. The combination of Kirschner wires and figure-8 encirclage transform the diastasic force of the triceps into a compression force at the fracture site. B,C) Example of a fracture treated by this method. Active flexion and extension are allowed after two weeks of elbow immobilization in a foam-rubber splint.

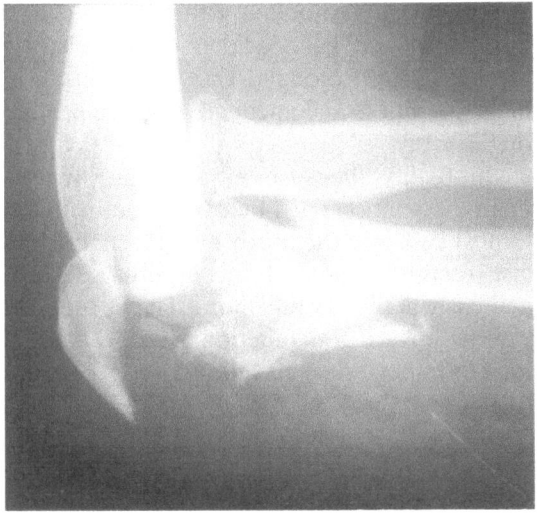

Fig. 4. - Olecranon fracture with transolecranon dislocation of both forearm bones (Bigat-Thomine fracture type II). Caused by severe trauma, often open, and accompanied by comminution of the semilunar notch, treatment of these lesions is always surgical and always immediate, dynamic internal fixation being strongly indicated.

Combinations of different internal fixation devices

The most frequently used combinations are simple or figure-8 encirclage with screws and/or mid-medullary nails. These combinations are necessary because of the anatomic variability of the fractures; different choices must be made according to skin exposure, comminution, and the frequent presence of fractures and dislocations of other joint components.

The choice of internal fixation device therefore depends on the personal preference of the surgeon, but must be made with the goal of allowing the earliest active mobility possible without immobilizing the joint in an orthesis or cast for a long period of time.

Olecranectomy

This procedure is indicated only for severely comminuted, often open fractures which cannot be fixed any other way.

However, it only produces good results if the tip of the coronoid is intact and if it is still possible to reinsert the triceps tendon so that elbow stability is preserved.

It is adopted more frequently in inveterate or incorrectly treated fractures accompanied by secondary pseudoarthrosis. Olecranectomy is justified in these cases, allowing an even earlier postoperative mobilization. The operation is performed using a subperiosteal approach; reinsertion of the triceps tendon is unnecessary.

FRACTURES OF THE CORONOID PROCESS

Pure coronoid fractures are uncommon; they are usually combined with posterior dislocation or proximal meta-epiphyseal elbow fractures. While they may be a result of indirect trauma with the elbow either hyperextended or flexed, they are more often caused by direct trauma, when the end of the elbow in flexion is hit very hard and an *olecranon-coronoid fracture* is provoked.

Either a tomography or thorough multiview radiographs are essential, especially when almost asymptomatic fractures, such as chip fractures of the tip of the coronoid, are suspected.

Pure coronoid fractures may involve the tip or the base.

1) In *fractures of the tip of the coronoid*, a small fragment is usually detached and may, in rare cases, even become an intraarticular loose body. In this instance surgical removal may be indicated. In all other cases, treatment consists of immobilization for 15 days without therapeutic massages in the subsequent rehabilitation phase because of the risk of calcifications in the anterior brachialis muscle.

2) In *fractures of the coronoid base*, the detached fragment is bigger and includes both the coronoid and a portion of the semilunar notch. It is therefore an articular fracture with humeroulnar incongruity. When the coronoid fragment is large, the action of the anterior brachialis muscle pushes it upward causing either dislocation or subluxation and therefore instability. This is easy to reduce but difficult to contain.

For this reason internal fixation is necessary. A cortical screw placed horizontal to the coronoid process and inserted from back to front is enough to ensure stable fixation of the fragment.

CONCLUSIONS

Fractures of the proximal ulna, although rare, can result in permanent *aesthetic* and *functional* problems, and even disability.

The reason for this must be sought in diagnostic errors (such as failure to recognize coronoid tip fractures on the x-ray) as well as incorrect choice of treatment.

Incorrect treatment, both insufficient and excessive, is the main risk. For example, an unstable and imprecise internal fixation can lead to painful radioulnar arthritis with severe joint stiffness. These syndromes can also be provoked by prolonged cast immobilization in an attempt to see adequate fracture healing on the x-ray.

In reality, because of articular involvement the fixation must be carried out with the utmost care and the following objectives: precise reconstruction of the articular surface and early active mobilization. This is the only way to ensure the functional recovery of a joint as important as the elbow.

REFERENCES

1) ALLIEU Y., VIDAL J.: Fractures de l'extrémité supérieure des deux os de l'avant-bras. *Encycl. Med. Chir.*, Paris (Appareil Locomoteur) 5, 14042 B-10, 1977.

2) ANDRÉ S., MICHELUTTI D., TOMENO B.: Les fractures de l'olecrane. *Rev. Chir. Orthop.* 1983; **69**: 629, 636.

3) BIGA N.: *Fractures de l'olecrane avec luxation en avant des deux os de l'avant-bras ou luxation transolécraniennes. A propos de 11 cas.* Thèse, Rouen, 1972.

4) BOITZY A.: L'ostheosynthèse par hauban. *Rev. Chir. Orthop.* 1983; **69**: 348.

5) JUDET R., LACOSTE A.: Traitement des fractures de l'olecrane par ligature extraosseuse aux orins (technique du bouchon de champagne). *Actualité de chirurgie orthopédique de l'hospital R. Poincaré* 1968; **VI**: 32-40.

6) MÜLLER M.E.: *Classificazione A.O. delle fratture.* Springer Verlag, Berlin, 1987.

7) MÜLLER M.E., ALLGOWER M., WILLENEGGER H.: *Technique of internal fixation of fractures.* Springer Verlag, Berlin, Heidelberg, New York, 1965.

Fractures of the proximal radius in adults

G. Guida - G. Iolascon - G. Marrone - A. Toro - A. Siano

Fractures of the proximal radius are a subject of considerable current interest because of the uncertainty surrounding some of the therapeutic problems. Several of these concerns, such as the indications for various treatments according to the type of lesion as well as the effects of resection of the radial head on both elbow stability and the distal radioulnar joint, are still controversial: a review of the literature still shows considerable difference of opinion.

Furthermore, the incidence of fractures of the proximal radius is certainly underestimated. They may go unobserved due to very mild symptoms or a negative initial radiographic examination. Only a more comprehensive examination including radiographs in various degrees of pronation and supination can reveal these fractures.

In 1954 Mason proposed his classification of radial head fractures that is now the standard, dividing them into three categories:

Type I: undisplaced fracture
Type II: fracture with displaced fragment
Type III: comminuted fracture.

This classification seems incomplete after a review of both other studies and our own patients. It does not cover fractures of the radial neck (Fig. 2), which occur in a significant number of adults (about 18% of our patients), nor does it consider the size of the fragment in fracture types I and II.

We would therefore like to propose a new classification system that takes these elements into consideration: an integration of the Mason (17), Radin *et al.* (24), Bakalim (3), and Arner, Ekengren, and Von Schreeb (2) classifications (Fig. 3).

The type I fractures (undisplaced) are divided into three categories according to the size of the fragment. If it involves up to 1/3 of the surface of the radial head, it is called type IA (Fig. 4); 1/2 of the surface, IB (Fig. 5); and 2/3 of the surface, IC (Fig. 6).

The type II fractures (displaced) are also divided into three categories - IIA (Fig. 7), IIB (Fig. 8), and IIC (Fig. 9) - according to the size of the fragment.

Comminuted fractures are designated as type III (Fig. 10).

Type IV fractures consist of undisplaced radial neck fractures (Fig. 11), while type V refers to displaced radial neck fractures (Fig. 12).

As we will demonstrate shortly, this classification is useful for determining therapeutic indications.

MATERIALS AND METHODS

We reviewed 151 patients, 79 males (52.3%) and 72 females (47.7%), who were 44.2 years old on average (range 18-74).

Fifty-one percent of the cases were affected on the left side, and 49% on the right.

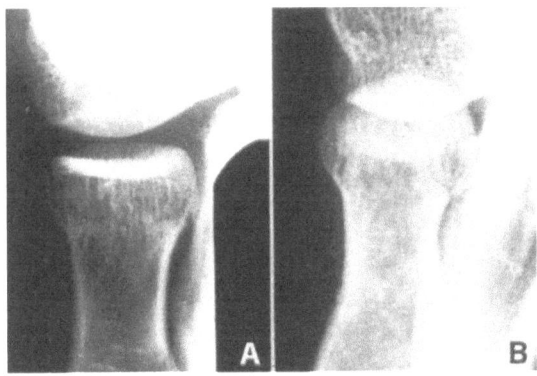

Fig. 1. - X-rays taken in different degrees of forearm pronation and supination reveal (B) a fracture that cannot be seen with (A) standard radiographs.

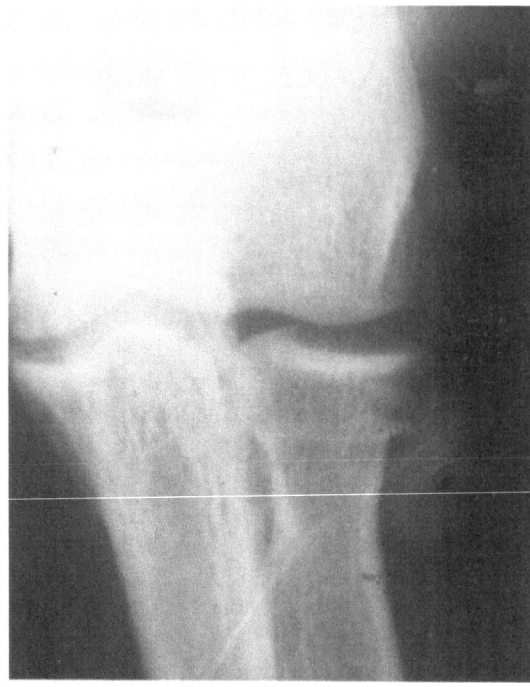

Fig. 2. - Fracture of the radial neck in an adult.

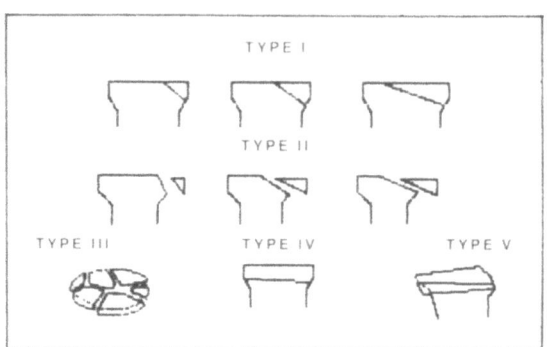

Fig. 3. - Proposed classification system for fractures of the proximal radius.

Table 1

Type of fracture	No. of patients	Subcategories
I	22 (14.6%)	IA = 6 IB = 12 IC = 4
II	63 (41.7%)	IIA = 27 IIB = 27 IIC = 9
III	39 (25.8%)	
IV	15 (10%)	
V	12 (7.9%)	

The distribution according to the type of fracture was as follows (Table 1):

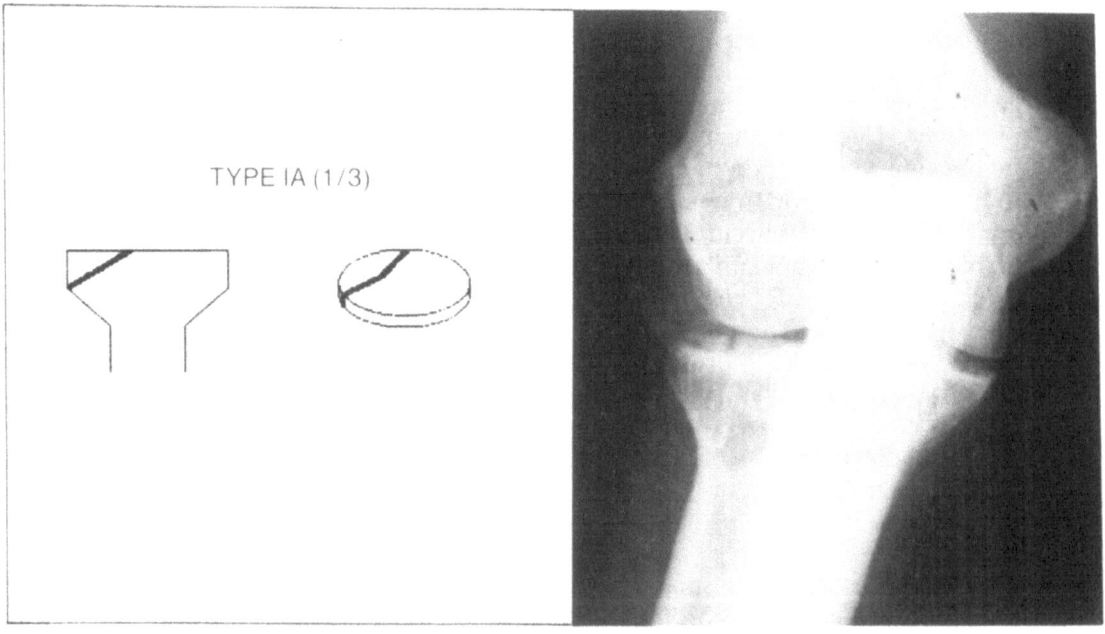

Fig. 4. - Type IA fracture: the undisplaced fragment involves about 1/3 of the surface of the radial head.

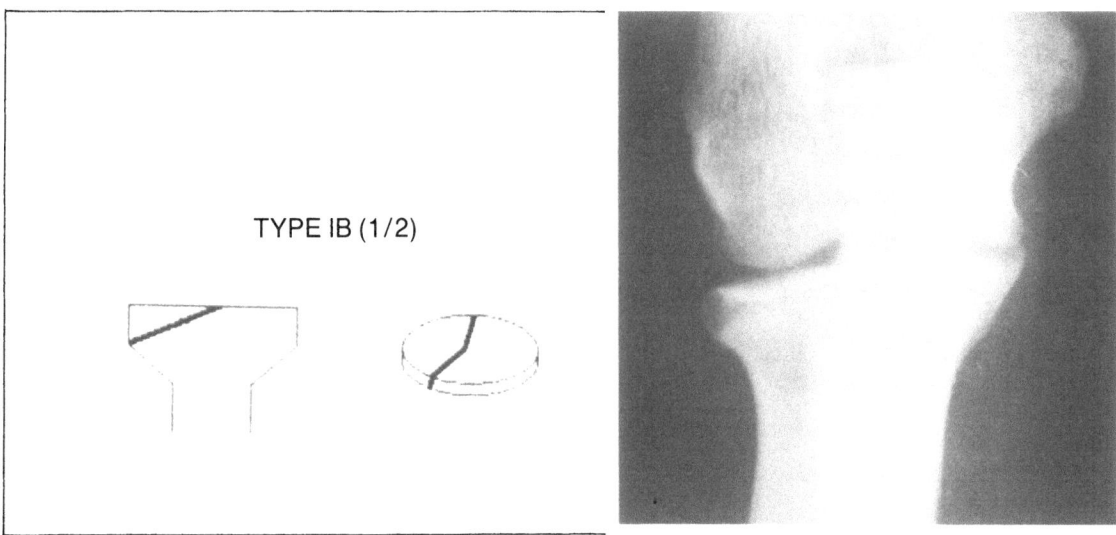

Fig. 5. - Type IB fracture: the undisplaced fragment involves about 1/2 of the radial head.

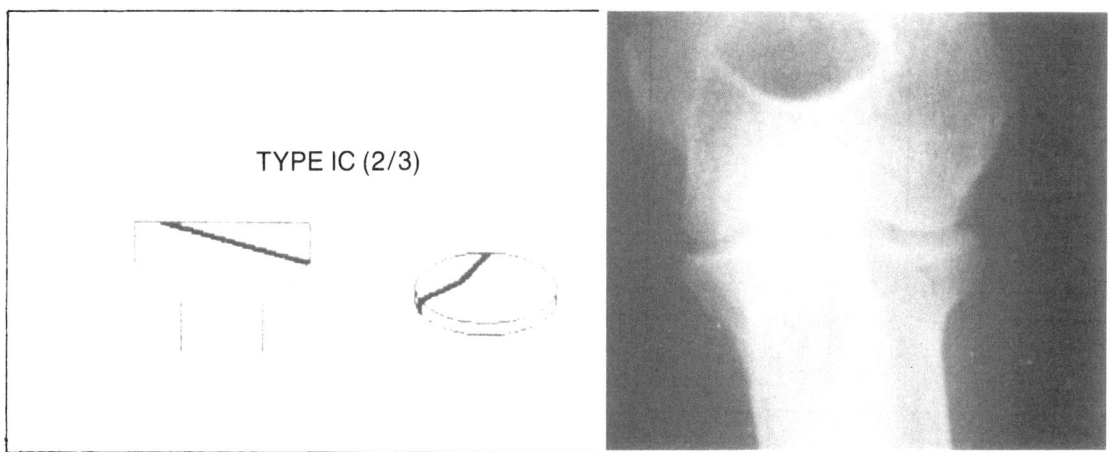

Fig. 6. - Type IC fracture: the undisplaced fragment involves 2/3 of the radial head.

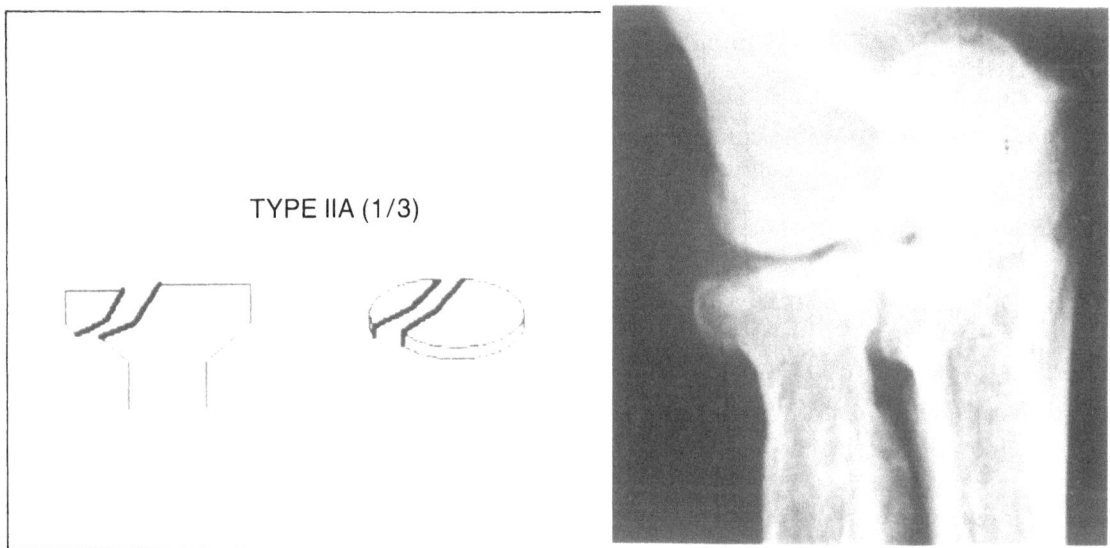

Fig. 7. - Type IIA fracture: the displaced fragment involves about 1/3 of the radial head.

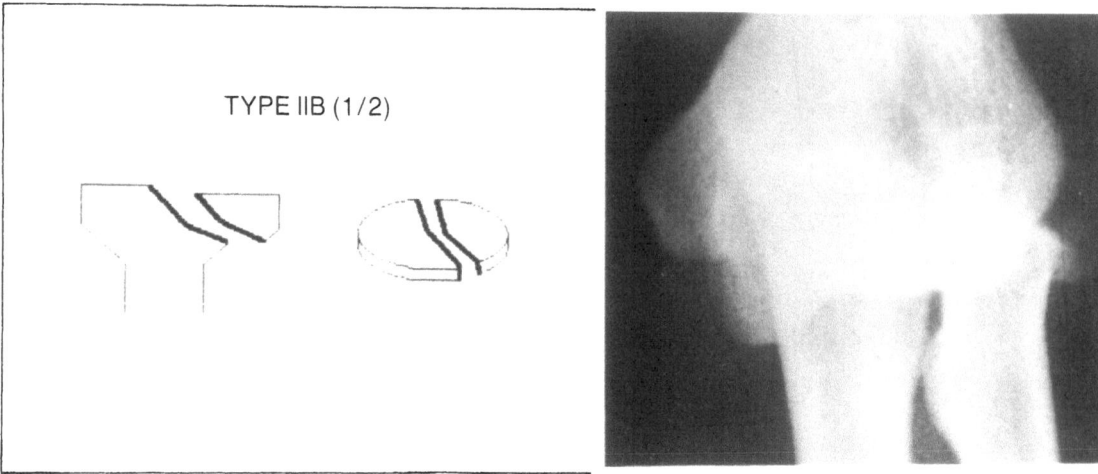

Fig. 8. - Type IIB fracture: the displaced fragment involves about 1/2 of the radial head.

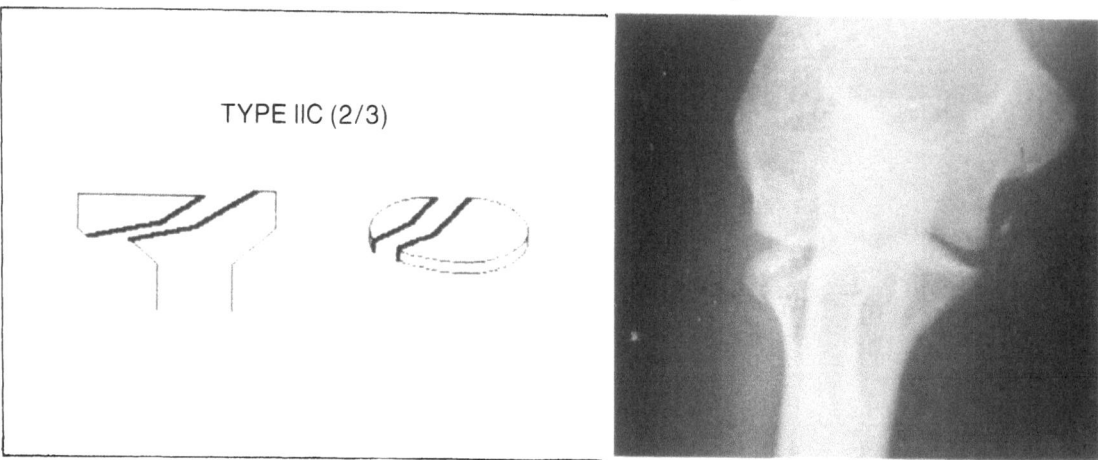

Fig. 9. - Type IIC fracture: the displaced fragment involves about 2/3 of the radial head.

RADIAL HEAD FRACTURES ASSOCIATED WITH OTHER LESIONS

There are many possible combinations of fractures and capsuloligamentous lesions.

Possible fracture sites are:
- proximal ulna
- medial epicondyle
- lateral epicondyle
- distal radius
- scaphoid.

The capsuloligamentous lesions consist of:
- elbow displacement
- lesion of the ulnar collateral ligament
- lesion of the distal radioulnar joint.

In our study, 50 patients (33%) had other lesions in addition to the radial head fracture (Figs. 13-14):
- 13 elbow dislocations
- 9 distal radioulnar joint subluxations
- 35 fractures of the proximal ulna
- 3 fractures of the distal radius
- 1 scaphoid fracture.

Some patients had more than one associated lesion.

TREATMENT

Since the severity of the lesion varies considerably according to whether the radial head fracture is isolated or associated with

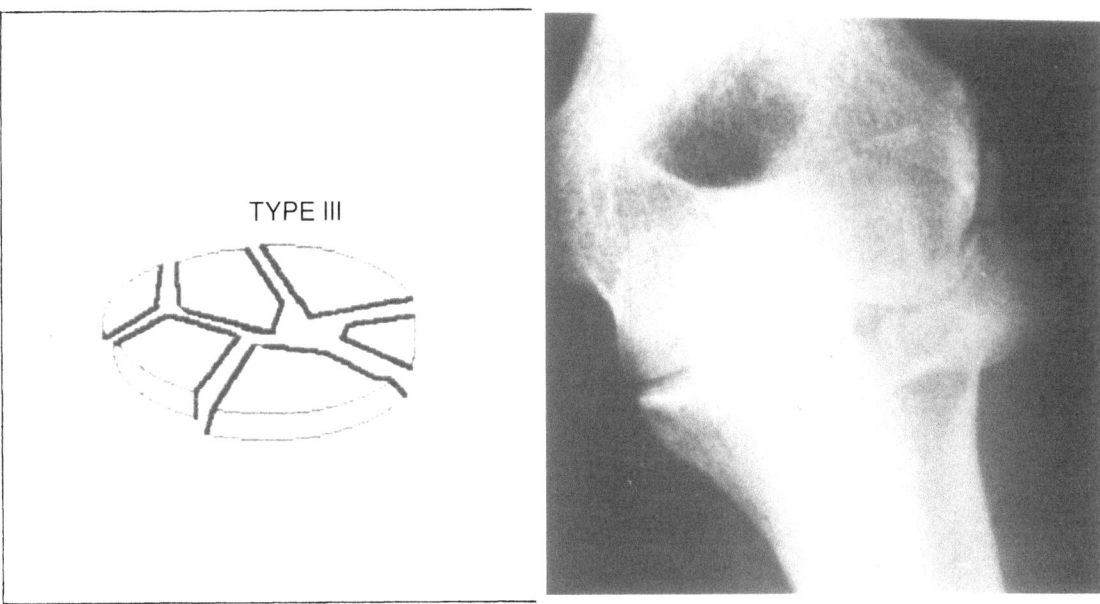

Fig. 10. - Type III fracture: comminuted.

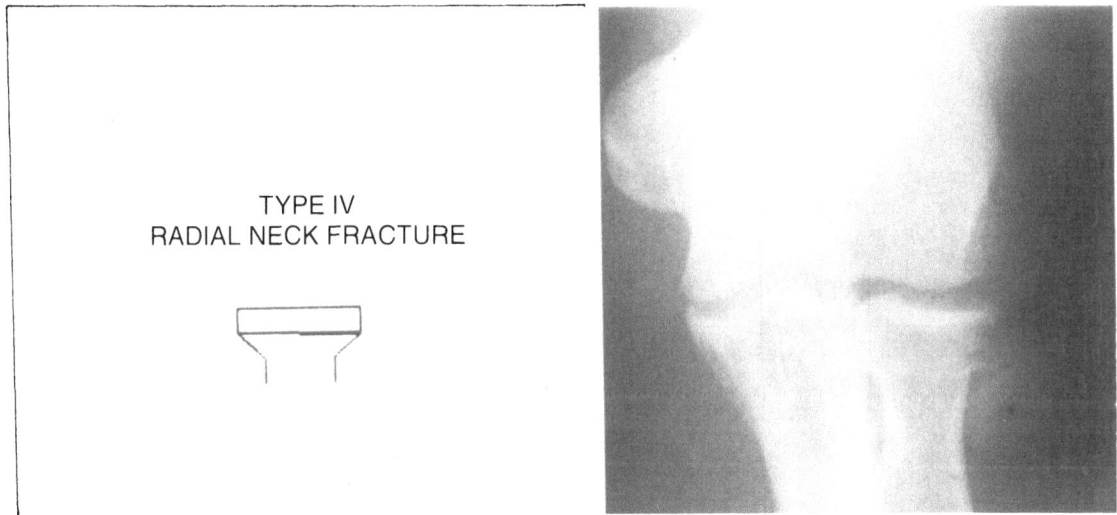

Fig. 11. - Type IV fracture: undisplaced radial neck fracture.

other lesions, we divided the treatments and the results they yielded into two groups.

In isolated fractures the treatment consisted of cast immobilization for all of the type I fractures, for 42 of 45 type II fractures, for 9 of 21 type III fractures, and for 10 radial neck fractures (types IV and V).

Resection was not once employed in type I or type IV fractures, yet was used in 3 type II fractures, 12 of 21 type III fractures, and 3 of 9 type V fractures (Table 2):

In fractures combined with other lesions, resection was performed in 17 of 50 cases along with treatment of the associated lesion, internal fixation, or reduction of the dislocation.

RESULTS

The results were evaluated according to the Radin *et al.* criteria and designated as good, fair, or poor.

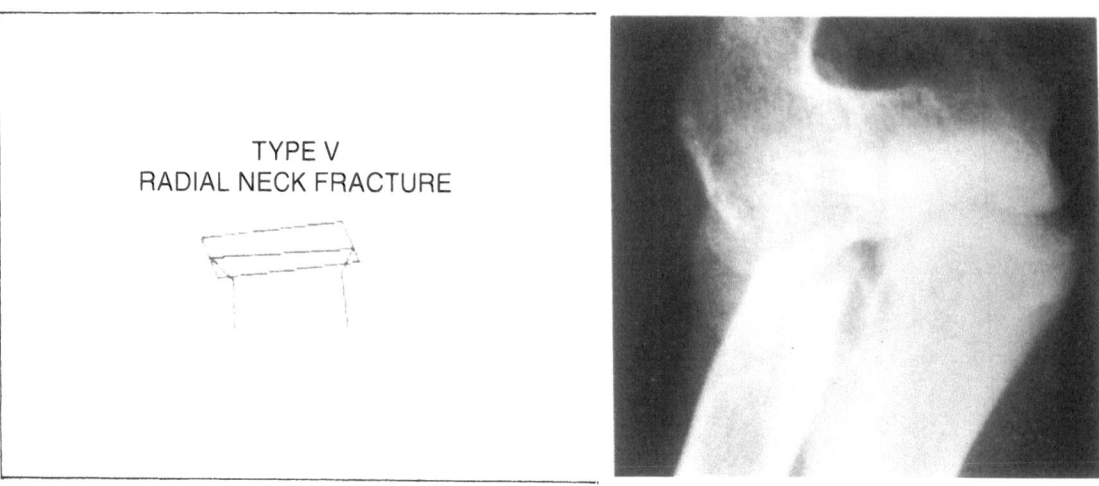

Fig. 12 - Type V fracture: displaced radial neck fracture.

Table 2
ISOLATED FRACTURES OF THE PROXIMAL RADIUS.
TREATMENT ACCORDING TO TYPE OF FRACTURE

	I			II			III	IV	V
	A	B	C	A	B	C			
Cast	6	12	4	18	21	3	9	4	6
Resection	–	–	–	2	–	1	12	–	3

Table 3
ISOLATED FRACTURES OF THE PROXIMAL RADIUS.
RESULTS ACCORDING TO CHOICE OF TREATMENT

TYPE I FRACTURES						
Conservative treatment				**Resection**		
				Total		Total
	A	B	C		A B C	
Good	6	11	3	20	– – –	
Fair	–	1	1	2	– – –	
Poor	–	–	–	–	– – –	

Table 4
ISOLATED FRACTURES OF THE PROXIMAL RADIUS.
RESULTS ACCORDING TO CHOICE OF TREATMENT

TYPE II FRACTURES						
Conservative treatment				**Resection**		
				Total		Total
	A	B	C		A B C	
Good	16	16	1	33	1 – 1	2
Fair	2	3	1	6	1 – –	1
Poor	–	2	1	3	– – –	–

Good: joint motion deficit of less than 10%, no pain; fair: joint motion deficit of less than 30% and /or moderate pain; poor: joint motion deficit of more than 30% and/or acute pain.

The results for the isolated fractures were as follows: type I fractures (Table 3) all good after non-operative treatment; type II fractures (Table 4) relatively good — 3 poor, 7 fair, and 35 good results.

In type III fractures, non-operative treatment yielded the same results as resection of the radial head; it also produced good results in fractures of the radial neck (Table 5).

The fractures combined with other lesions provide interesting evidence: the results in cases treated with radial head resection (for the most part serious lesions) are even slightly inferior to the results of treatment without resection (Table 6).

DISCUSSION

A review of the literature reveals that most authors recommend non-operative treatment for type I fractures and radial head resection for type III fractures. Opinions differ as to the best treatment for type II fractures.

We will now go through the various types of fractures:

1) *Undisplaced fractures (type I):*

Table 5

ISOLATED FRACTURES OF THE PROXIMAL RADIUS.
RESULTS ACCORDING TO CHOICE OF TREATMENT

TYPE III FRACTURES		
	Conservative treatment	Resection
Good	6	7
Fair	2	3
Poor	1	2
TYPE IV FRACTURES		
	Conservative treatment	Resection
Good	3	–
Fair	1	–
Poor	–	–
TYPE V FRACTURES		
	Conservative treatment	Resection
Good	4	1
Fair	1	1
Poor	1	1

Table 6

FRACTURES OF THE PROXIMAL RADIUS COMBINED
WITH OTHER LESIONS. RESULTS ACCORDING TO
CHOICE OF TREATMENT

Without resection of the radial head							
	II			III	IV	V	Total
	A	B	C				
Good	4	3	1	1	8	1	18
Fair	3	2	1	1	2	1	10
Poor	–	1	1	1	1	1	5
With resection of the radial head							
	II			III	IV	V	Total
	A	B	C				
Good	–	–	1	4	–	–	5
Fair	–	–	1	4	–	–	5
Poor	–	–	–	7	–	–	7

Most authors report good results after non-operative treatment. Some (1, 14, 16) boast better results with early mobilization, which can cause secondary displacement, as reported by Radin *et al.* (24) and Bakalim (3), if the fragment involves over 1/3 of the surface of the radial head. Based on both these findings and the results of our own study, we believe that 3 weeks of immobilization in either a plaster cast or an elbow splint that allows forearm pronation and supination is the treatment of choice for type IA fractures. For types 1B and 1C, however, more rigorous therapy is needed: 3 weeks of immobilization

in a long-arm cast that does not allow pronation and supination. Our results with the above treatments were consistently good.

2) *Displaced fractures (type II)*:

The division of this group into three categories according to the size of the displaced fragment is especially useful. When the fragment involves less than 1/3 of the radial head surface (IIA), non-operative treatment is strongly indicated, yielding good results as shown by our data. We had satisfactory results with non-operative treatment even in the IIB and IIC fracture groups, as did other authors (1, 3, 5, 10, 24) who achieved equally good or better results with non-operative treatment as with resection of the radial head.

3) *Comminuted fractures (type III)*:

According to most authors, surgery is indicated for these fractures. Nonetheless, a series of studies (1, 2, 4, 5, 6, 7, 10, 29) obtained good or fair results with non-operative treatment in an equal or higher (1) percentage of cases.

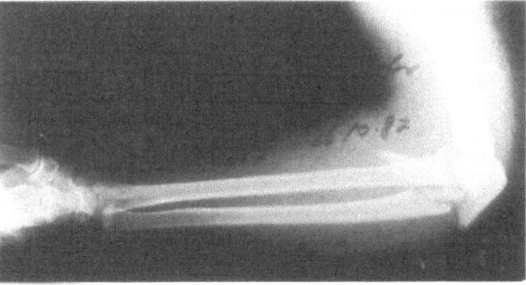

Fig. 13. - Type III fracture combined with subluxation of the distal radioulnar joint.

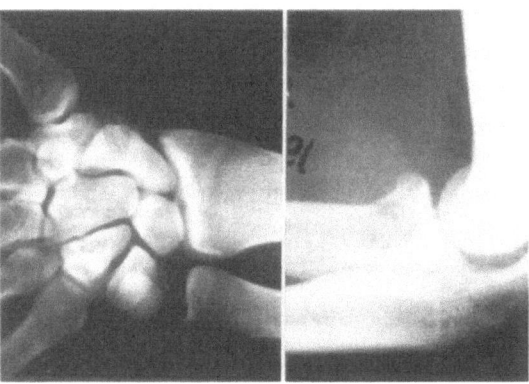

Fig. 14. - Type IB fracture combined with scaphoid fracture.

We had good or fair results in 80% of the cases of type III, type IIB, and type IIC fractures treated with resection of the radial head.

It should be noted, however, that the patients who were not treated with resection of the radial head because of problems of stability caused by other concomitant lesions (elbow dislocation or fracture of the proximal ulna) obtained equally satisfactory results, considering that their lesions were much more severe.

We believe that the statement "comminution of the fracture and severe displacement of the fragment (in type II) are formal indications for resection of the radial head" must be rethought, since conservative treatment yields equally good results. Moreover, resection of the head can bring on problems such as elbow instability, reduced limb strength, valgus deformity, ossification, long-term arthritic changes in the elbow, and subluxation of the radioulnar joint. Even though these complications do not usually compromise the long-term outcome, as shown in this and other studies, they do add to the already existing problems and are one more reason to attempt conservative treatment. We believe that the

only absolute indication for surgery is the presence of an intraarticular loose body, as Miller, Drennan, and Maylahn (15) have already stated.

4) *Radial head fractures combined with other lesions*:

In cases of radial head fracture associated with elbow dislocation or fracture of the proximal ulna, the associated lesion is the more serious of the two and thus has therapeutic priority.

Therefore, after reduction of the dislocation or reduction and internal fixation of the ulnar fracture, further treatment is restricted to removal of loose bodies or resection in cases of comminuted or type V fractures.

If necessary, resection can be performed after stability is regained. This option after non-operative treatment, as demonstrated by Broberg and Morrey (5), may improve elbow function and reduce pain to such an extent that good and excellent results are achieved in 80% of the cases. Delayed resection may also be useful in cases of fracture of the proximal radius where conservative treatment has failed.

REFERENCES

1) ADLER J.B., SHAFTAN G.W.: Radial head fractures, is excision necessary? *J. Trauma* 1964; **4**: 115-136.
2) ARNER O., EKENGREN K., VON SCHREEB T.: Fractures of the head and neck of the radius. *Acta Chir. Scand.* 1957; **112**: 115-134.
3) BAKALIM G.: Fractures of radial head and their treatment. *Acta Orthop. Scand.* 1970; **41**: 320-331.
4) BOHLER L.: *Treatment of fractures*. Grune and Stratton, New York, 1956.
5) BROBERG M.A., MORREY B.F.: Results of delayed excision of the radial head after fracture. *J. Bone Jt Surg.* 1986; 669-674.
6) BUSH L.F., MC LAIN E.J.: Operative treatment of fractures of the elbow in adults. *Am. Acad. Orthop. Surgeons* 1959; **16**: 265-277.
7) CHARNLEY J.: *Fractures of the head of the radius. Closed treatment of common fractures*. E. and S. Livingstone, Edinburgh 1963.
8) COLEMAN D.A., BLAIR W.F., SHURR D.: Resection of the radial head for fracture of the radial head. *J. Bone Jt Surg.* 1987; **69-A**, 385-392.
9) ESSEX-LOPRESTI P.: Fractures of the radial head with distal radio-ulnar dislocation. *J. Bone Jt Surg.* 1951; **33-B**: 244-247.

10) GOLDBERG I., PEYLAN J., YOSIPOVITCH Z.: Late results of excision of the radial head for an isolated closed fracture. *J. Bone Jt Surg.* 1985; **45-A**: 675-679.
11) HIDAKA SHIGEI, GUSTILO R.B.: Refracture of bones of the forearm after plate removal. *J. Bone Jt Surg.* 1984; **66-A**: 1241-1243.
12) HOTCHKISS R.N., WEILAND A.J.: Valgus stability of the elbow. *J. Orthop. Res.* 1987; **5**: 372-377.
13) HUDSON D.A., DE BEER J. DE V.: Isolated traumatic dislocation of the radial head in children. *J. Bone Jt surg.* 1988; **69-B**: 378-381.
14) JOHNSTON G.W.: A follow-up of one-hundred cases of fracture of the head of the radius with a review of the literature. *Ulster Med. J.* 1962; **31**: 51-56.
15) KLAUD MILLER G., DRENNAN D.B., MAYLAHN D.J.: Treatment of displaced segmental radial head fractures. *J. Bone Jt Surg.* 1981; **63-A**: 712-717.
16) MASON J.A., SHUTKIN N.M.: Immediate active motion treatment of fractures of the head and neck of the radius. *Surg. Gynec. Obstet.* 1943; **76**, 731-737.
17) MASON M.L.: Some observations on fractures of the head of the radius with a review of one-

hundred cases. *Br. J. Surg.* 1954; **42**: 123-132.

18) McDougall A., White J.: Subluxation of the inferior radio-ulnar joint complicating fracture of the radial head. *J. Bone Jt Surg.* 1957; **39-B**: 279-287.

19) Mackay I., Fitzgerald B., Miller J.H.: Silastic replacement of the head of the radius in trauma. *J. Bone Jt Surg.* 1979; **61-B**: 494-497.

20) Morrey B.F., An K.N.: Functional anatomy of the ligaments of the elbow. *Clin. Orthop. Rel. Res.* 1985; **201**: 84-90.

21) Morrey B.F., An K.N., Stormont T.J.: Force trasmission through the radial head. *J. Bone Jt Surg.* 1988; **70-A**: 250-256.

22) Morrey B.F., Askew L., Chao E.Y.: Silastic prosthetic replacement for the radial head. *J. Bone Jt Surg.* 1981; **63-A**: 454-458.

23) Morrey B.F., Chao E.Y., Hui F.C.: Biomechanical study of the elbow following excision of the radial head. *J. Bone Jt Surg.* 1979; **61-A**: 63-68.

24) Radin E.L., Riseborough E.J.: Fractures of the radial head. *J. Bone Jt Surg.* 1966; **48-A**: 1055-1064.

25) Rymaszewski L.A., Mackay I., Amis A.A., Miller J.H.: Long-term effects of excision of the radial head in rheumatoid arthritis. *J. Bone Jt Surg.* 1984; **66-B**: 109-113.

26) Smith F.M.: *Surgery of the elbow.* Springfield, Illinois, Thomas, 1954.

27) Swanson A.B., Jaeger S.H., La Rochelle D.: Comminuted fractures of the radial head. *J. Bone Jt Surg.* 1981; **63-A**: 1039-1049.

28) Taylor T.K.F., O'Connor B.T.: The effect upon the inferior radio-ulnar joint of excision of the head of the radius in adults. *J. Bone Jt Surg.* 1964; **46-B**: 83-88.

29) Wade P.A.: *Surgical treatment of trauma.* Grune and Stratton, 1960.

30) Weseley M.S., Barenfeld P.A., Eisenstein L.A.: Closed treatment of isolated radial head fractures. *J. Trauma* 1983; **23**: 36-39.

Treatment of pure elbow dislocation: long-term results

V. Patella - B. Moretti - V. Pesce - G. Lo Bianco - S. Chirianni

In the field of elbow traumatology the incidence of pure dislocation varies, depending on the study, from 10% to 30% and is considered to have a relatively good prognosis.

To understand the pathogenesis of dislocation, we must consider both the external dislocating forces and the intrinsic bonds that oppose these forces. The joint components and the capsuloligamentous structures provide this internal resistance by virtue of their shape. These structures passively reinforce the joint in conjunction with the active stabilizing forces produced by the muscular structures. However, it is important to remember that the fully extended elbow joint, with the forearm supinated, may have a physiologic valgus angulation of up to 25 degrees; this condition is important for the conveyance of the external forces along preferential weight-bearing axes.

Of all the various classification systems that have been proposed (Bohler, Vigliani *et al.*, Messina *et al.*, etc.), this study uses the one devised by Smith (1972), which distinguishes between dislocation of both radius and ulna (posterior, posterolateral, posteromedial, and anterior), isolated dislocation of the radius, isolated dislocation of the ulna, and divergent dislocation of radius and ulna.

Pure posterior dislocation is usually a result of indirect trauma such as a fall on the palm of the hand with elbow extended and forearm supinated; the dislocating force tends to be transmitted dorsal to the transverse axis of the elbow and may cause anterior capsuloligamentous damage, more specifically tears on the anterior side of the collateral ligaments and sometimes on the insertion of the anterior brachialis and anconeus muscles.

In posterolateral and posteromedial dislocation, the indirect mechanism of injury is the dorsolateral or dorsomedial transmission of force upon the slightly flexed elbow, forcing it into an unnatural valgus or varus angulation. Pure lateral and medial dislocations, however, may be provoked by either direct trauma to the proximal third of the forearm with shoulder and elbow fixed or a forward fall with the arm under the body, forcing the elbow into an abnormal valgus or varus angulation.

Anterior dislocation can be triggered either directly by trauma to the olecranon with elbow flexed or indirectly by a forward fall with the forearm under the body, forcing it first into an unnatural valgus angulation (medial capsuloligamentous lesion) and then flexing and rotating it. Finally, isolated dislocation of the radial head is brought about by hyperextension of the forearm on the arm causing tearing of both the joint capsule and the orbicular ligament.

We reviewed 285 patients treated for pure elbow dislocation at the 1ª Clinica Ortopedica dell'Università di Bari from 1950 to 1988. The patients were 32 years old on the average (range 4-76), and 110 (38.8%) had been less than 15 years old at the moment of trauma; 177 (62%) were male, and neither the right nor the left side was prevalently affected. The lesion was acute in 269 cases, inveterate in 16 (more than two weeks), and open in two.

The dislocation was posterior in 59% of the cases, posterolateral in 36%, isolated radial in 3%, and anterior or posteromedial in 1%.

The trauma was a fall in 60% of the cases, a sports injury in 35%, and a motor vehicle accident in the other 5%.

Primary treatment consisted of closed reduction and cast immobilization in 259 cases (96.3%); the other 10 lesions (3.7%) required open reduction and immobilization in a long-

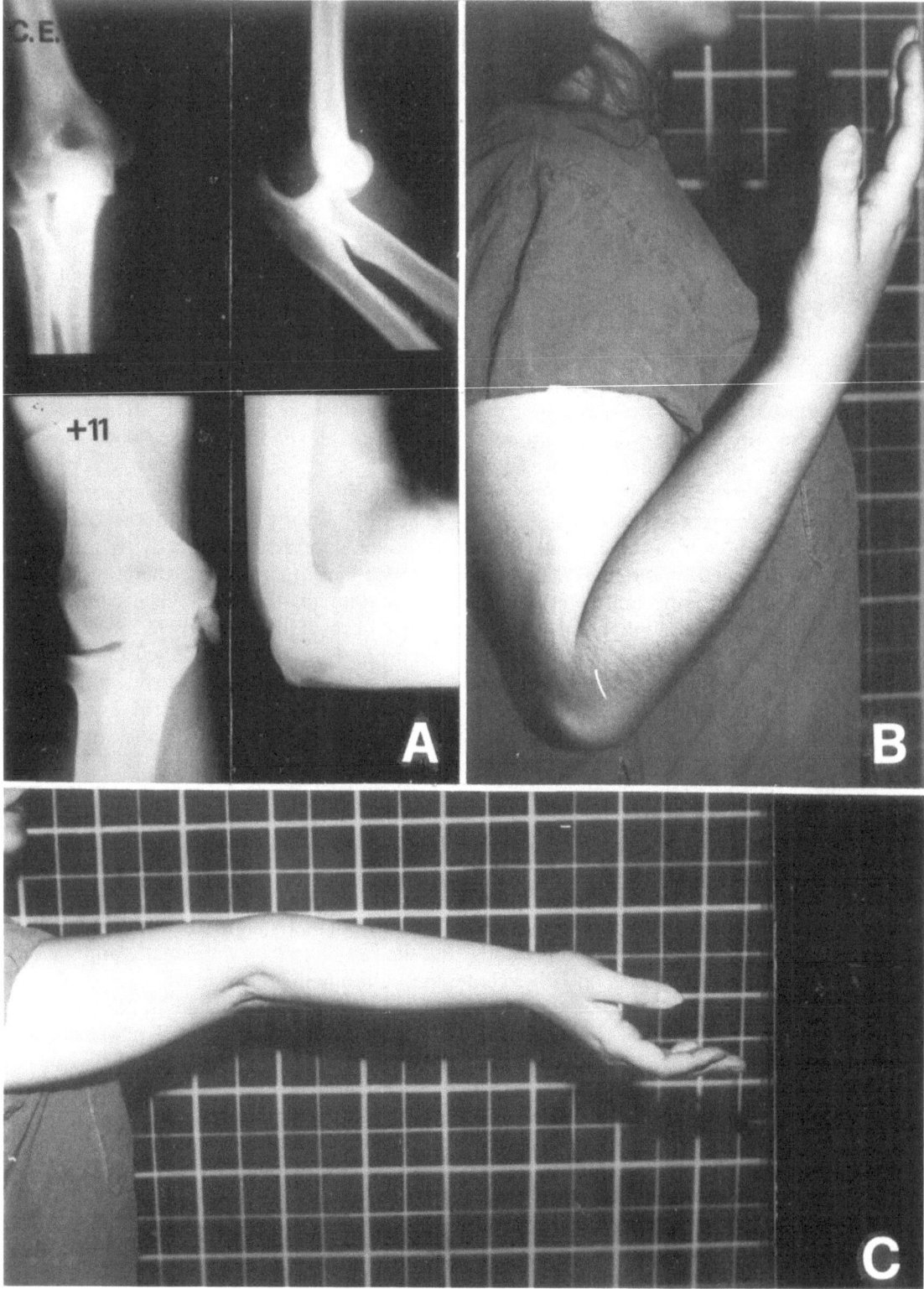

Fig. 1. - A) Radiograph of posterior dislocation before and 11 years after injury; B,C) despite calcifications of the ulnar collateral ligament, the patient shows full functional recovery.

arm cast for an average of 20 days (range 3-38). Just after the trauma 10 patients had peripheral nervous lack, ulnar nerve paresis in all cases and additional median nerve paresis in 4 cases, which gradually subsided. No late vascular complications were observed either after surgery or after immobilization.

Seventy-one patients (25%) were reviewed clinically and radiographically after an average of 11 years (range 1-18). The clinical criteria were pain, joint function, residual instability, and stabilized neurovascular lack; the clinical results were classified as excellent, good, fair, or poor.

An excellent result was achieved in 25 patients (36%), 95% of whom were under 15 years of age. These cases showed almost no pain or joint instability and had full functional recovery with no vascular lack (Fig. 1 A-C).

Thirty-three patients (46%) were classified as good. Their clinical features were slight pain, which was felt for the most part in the morning and during changes in the weather, joint motion limitation of less than 20 degrees (loss of flexion and/or extension), slight instability that is mostly subjective and felt only during physical exertion, and no neurovascular lack.

Thirteen patients (18%) were classified as fair. They had instability and moderate pain during physical exertion, especially when the dominant limb was injured; even in the absence of neurovascular lack, except for occasional paresis of the median or ulnar nerve dermatome, there was limitation of joint motion up to 40 degrees (Fig. 2 A-C).

In this study there were no decidedly poor results, defined as presence of acute and persistent pain (even at night), severe instability with possible redislocation, functional limitation of more than 40 degrees, and stabilized neurovascular lack.

The radiographic criteria were heterotopic ossifications, joint instability, and signs of arthritic degeneration.

Calcifications or periarticular ossifications, which were frequently located along the collateral ligaments and near the anterior capsuloligamentous area, were observed in 41% of the patients. Another 31% showed joint instability, which was revealed by the valgus stress test with the elbow fully ex-

tended and the gravity stress test with elbow extended, hand holding a 1.5 kg weight, and the distal and middle thirds of the humerus supported. The radiographic signs of medial laxity were mild in all cases, and there was no correlation between them and the instability during physical exertion reported by the patients (Fig. 3 A-B).

Degenerative arthritis, present in 45% of the cases, featured subchondral sclerosis, narrowing of the joint space, and osteophyte production; however, radiographic findings and clinical features did not always agree, except for a few cases with radiographic signs of sclerosis and osteophytosis who also had slight functional limitation.

Fourteen inveterate dislocations were reviewed after the same average follow-up period as the acute dislocations. Three cases were treated with closed reduction and cast immobilization, while 11 underwent open reduction and then cast immobilization for an average of 4 weeks.

The clinical result was defined as good in two patients and fair in the remaining 12, one of whom had stabilized ulnar nerve paralysis. Radiographic signs of degenerative arthritis and periarticular ossifications were present in all cases, while the incidence of residual joint instability was almost the same as in acute dislocation.

The conclusions that can be drawn from this study are as follows:

1) the best results were achieved in patients under 15 years of age;

2) there was a direct correlation between the extent of the functional lack and the length of the period of immobilization; the "ideal" period of immobilization is 10-15 days;

3) recurrence of pain, whether due to prolonged physical exertion or changes in the weather, whether constant, occurring mostly at night, or occurring first thing in the morning, was related to the length of the period of immobilization in all cases. The pain may be a consequence of chondral lesions, which cannot be diagnosed radiographically, caused by dislocation and/or reduction;

4) prolonged immobilization does not prevent residual instability;

5) physical therapy is essential for reduc-

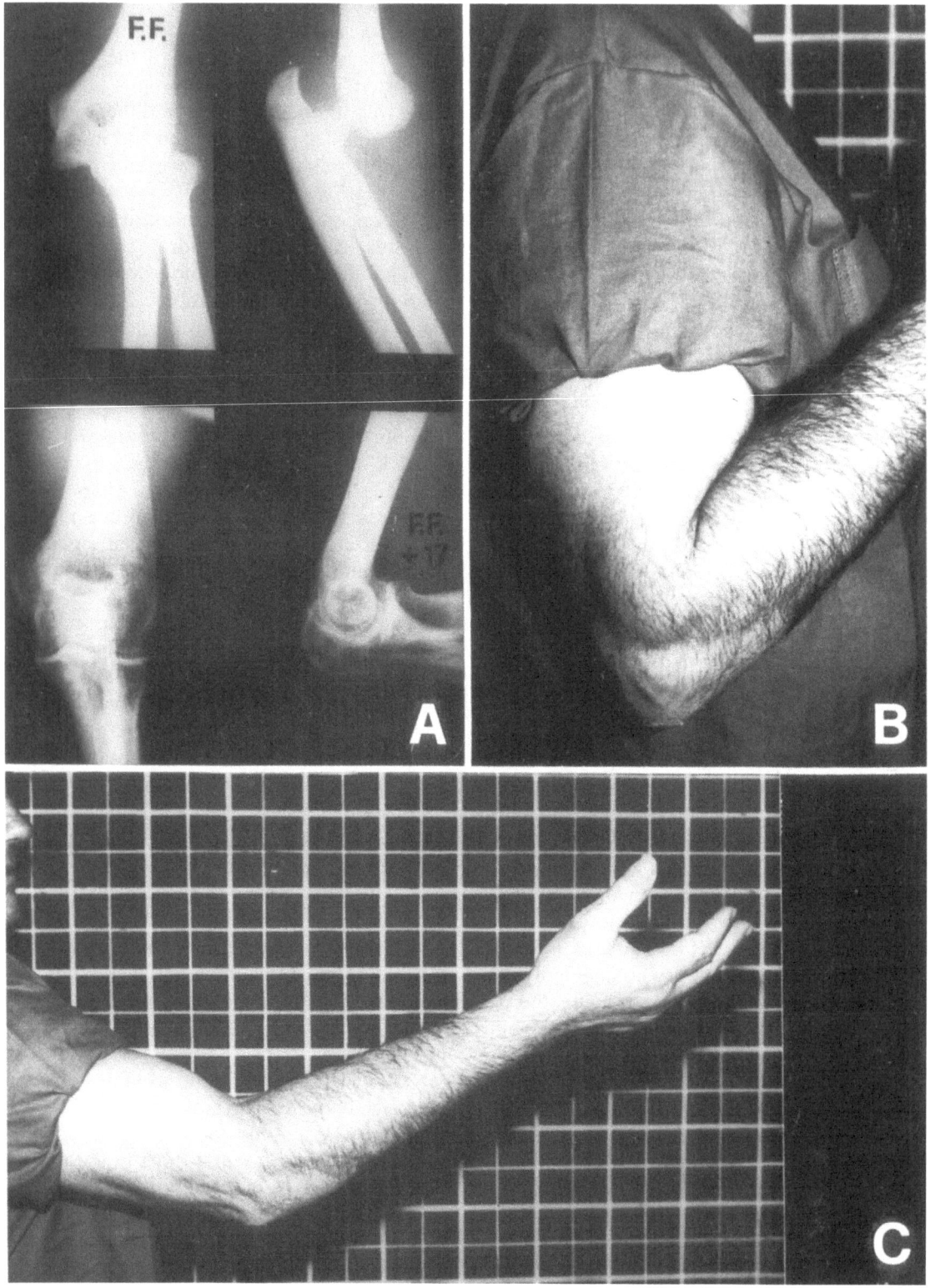

Fig. 2. - A) Radiograph of posterolateral dislocation before and 17 years after injury reveals signs of arthritic degeneration; B,C) clinically, elbow extension is limited (fair result).

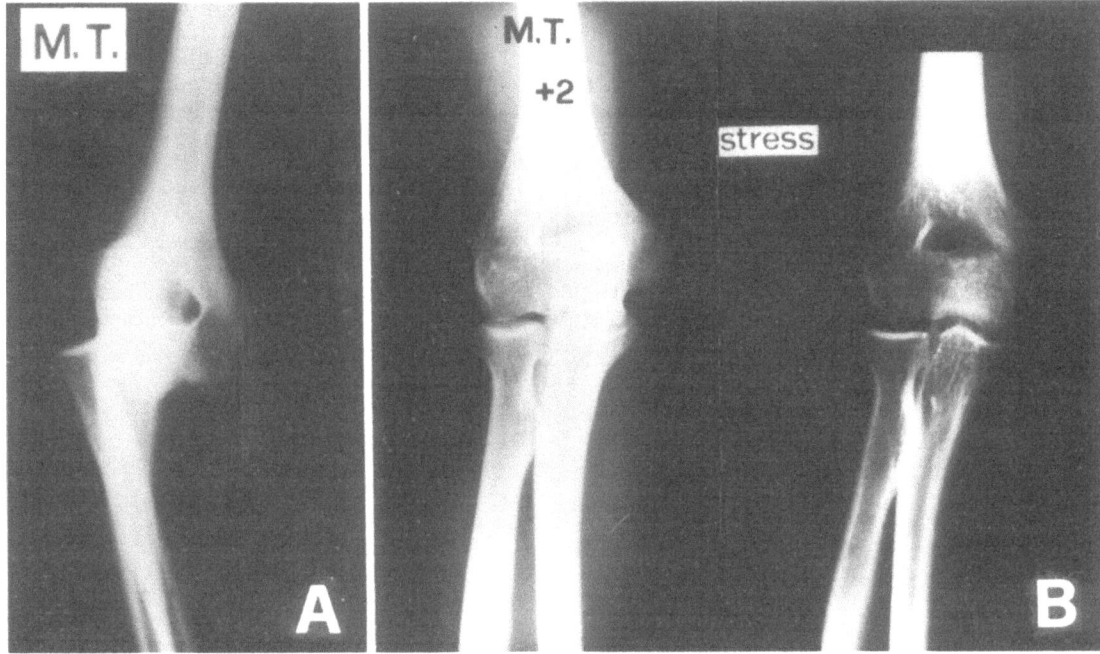

Fig. 3 - A) Radiographic view of posterolateral dislocation two years after trauma; B) the valgus stress test shows moderate laxity and opening of the medial joint space.

ing calcification (probably through rapid restoration of muscle tone and trophism, tissue elasticity, and local circulation), loosening the articular and periarticular scars, and promoting healing of the chondral and articular lesions that contribute to residual pain;

6) negative results in inveterate disloca-

tions are caused by and proportional to the permanence of the dislocation and the length of the period of immobilization; both open and closed reduction, which are more extensive procedures in these lesions than in acute lesions, can cause further articular, capsuloligamentous, and vascular damage.

REFERENCES

1) CROVA M., ROSSI P., DETTONI A., SABATINO C.: La lussazione del gomito. Revisione di 100 casi. *Minerva Ortop. e Traumatol.* 1988; **39** (11): 845.

2) DICKSON R.A.: Reversed dynamic slings. A new concept in the treatment of post-traumatic elbow flexion contractures. *Injury* 1976; **8**: 35.

3) DURIG M., MULLER W., RUEDI T.P., GAUER E.F.: The operative treatment of elbow dislocation in the adult. *J. Bone Jt Surg.* 1979; **61-A**: 239.

4) GIANCECCHI F., CAVAZZUTI A., TARTAGLIA I., CARRETTI P., ROTINI R.: Lussazioni e fratture-lussazioni di gomito (studio di 48 casi controllati a distanza). *Chir. Org. Mov.* 1982-1983; **68**: IV-VI.

5) GLYNN J.J., NIEBAUER J.J.: Flexion and extension contracture of the elbow. Surgical

management. *Clin. Orthop.* 1976; **117**: 289.

6) JOHANSSON O.: Capsular and ligament injuries of the elbow joint: a clinical and arthrographic study. *Acta Chir. Scand.* 1962; Suppl., **287**: 159.

7) JOSEFSSON P.O., JOHNELL O., GENTZ C.F.: Long-term sequelae of simple dislocation of the elbow. *J. Bone Jt Surg.* 1984; **66-A**: 927.

8) JOSEFSSON P.O., NILSSON B.E.: Incidence of elbow dislocation. *Acta Orthop. Scand.* 1986; **57**: 537.

9) MARTINI M., HALLAJ N., DAOUD A., DESCAMPS L.: Les luxations traumatiques récentes du coude. A propos de 94 observations. *Acta Orthop. Belg.* 1978; **44**.

10) MEHLOFF L.T., NOBLE P.C., BENNETT J.B., TULLOS H.S.: Simple dislocation of the elbow in the adult. *J. Bone Jt Surg.* 1988; **70-A**: 244.

11) MORREY B.F., AN K.N.: Articular and ligamentous contributions to the stability of the elbow joint. *Am. J. Sports Med.* 1983; **11**: 315.

12) MOUTERDE P., LORTAT-JACOB A., KENESI C.: Luxation postérieure du coude. Etude expérimentale. *Acta Orthop. Belg.* 1975; **41**: 505.

13) PROTZMAN R.R.: Dislocation of the elbow. *J. Bone Jt Surg.* 1978; **60-A**: 539.

14) SALTER R.B., SIMMONDS D.F., MALCOLM B.W., RUMBLE E.J., MACMICHAEL D., CLEMENTS N.D.: The biological effect of continuous passive motion on the healing of full thickness defects in articular cartilage. An experimental investigation in the rabbit. *J. Bone Jt Surg.* 1980; **62-A**: 1232.

15) SCHWAB G.H., BENNETT J.B., WOODS G.W.: Biomechanics of elbow instability: the role of the medial collateral ligament. *Clin. Orthop.* 1980; **146**: 42.

16) URBANIAK J.R., HANSEN P.E., BEISSINGER S.F., AITKEN M.S.: Correction of post-traumatic flexion contracture of the elbow by anterior capsulotomy. *J. Bone Jt Surg.* 1985; **67-A**: 1160.

17) VIGLIANI F., ATTUBATO M.: La nostra esperienza nel trattamento delle lussazioni di gomito. *Arch. Putti* 1959; **11**: 354.

Fracture-dislocation of the elbow: evaluation of long-term results

V. Patella - B. Moretti - V. Pesce - G. Lo Bianco - S. Chirianni

We have intentionally separated the discussion of pure dislocation of the elbow from that of fracture-dislocation, since the latter presents different problems of etiology, treatment, and results.

The mechanism of injury is practically the same as that of pure dislocations, even if, in the cases complicated by fractures and/or joint lesions, the intensity of the trauma is greater. Another explanation for these complications is the physiologic valgus angulation of the elbow (0-25°) which, at the moment of trauma, directs the damaging centripetal force as well as the position of the elbow, the same direction of the force that causes the shifting of the joint components and the violent defensive muscle contraction which is proportionate to the extent of the dislocation.

Various classification systems for fracture-dislocation of the elbow have been proposed (Bohler, Biebl, Watson-Jones, Merle d'Aubigné, etc.); this study uses the classification put forth by Vigliani and Attubato, which is simple yet covers the wide variety of pathological forms, emphasizing the priority of either the dislocation or the fracture, depending on the lesion.

As for the shifting of the joint components, however, we have adopted the classic division described in the previous chapter.

When we refer to dislocation-fracture, we mean that the dislocation is the principal lesion and the fracture or epiphyseal detachment may be considered an epiphenomenon, especially in less severe cases. Included in this category are dislocations combined with small avulsion fractures, small articular fractures, and undisplaced, stable fractures of one or more joint components. The fractures and joint lesions do not usually complicate treatment of the dislocation in these cases, even though it is sometimes impossible to reduce the diastasic bone fragments, especially in avulsion fractures.

We define fracture-dislocation, on the other hand, as dislocation of the joint components complicated by a joint fracture at least as important as the capsuloligamentous lesion. Included in this category are dislocations with an either simple or comminuted displaced epiphyseal fracture or a comminuted fracture of more than one epiphysis. In these cases treatment should aim not only to restore the normal anatomical relationships between the joint components, but also to reduce the associated fractures in order to stabilize the reduction of the dislocation.

This study comprises 118 patients treated for elbow dislocation complicated by fracture from 1950 to 1988 at the 1ª Clinica Ortopedica dell'Università di Bari. Seventy-eight of these (66%) were male; the average age was 29 (range 2-73), and 35.2% of the patients (42) had been under 15 years old at the time of trauma.

Neither the left nor the right side was significantly prevalent; none of the fractures were open, and 110 lesions were considered acute while the remaining 8 were inveterate. The associated fractures affected the following structures in order of frequency: the radial head (31%), the medial epicondyle (22%), the lateral condyle (17%), the olecranon (11%), the lateral epicondyle (10%), the coronoid process (4%), the trochlea (4%), and the distal humeral epiphysis (1%).

The trauma was a fall in 55% of the cases, a sports injury in 20%, and a motor vehicle accident in 25%; comparing this to the corresponding data on pure elbow dislocations, we found that motor vehicle accidents were much more likely to cause fracture-dislocations, which are more severe and have a poorer prognosis.

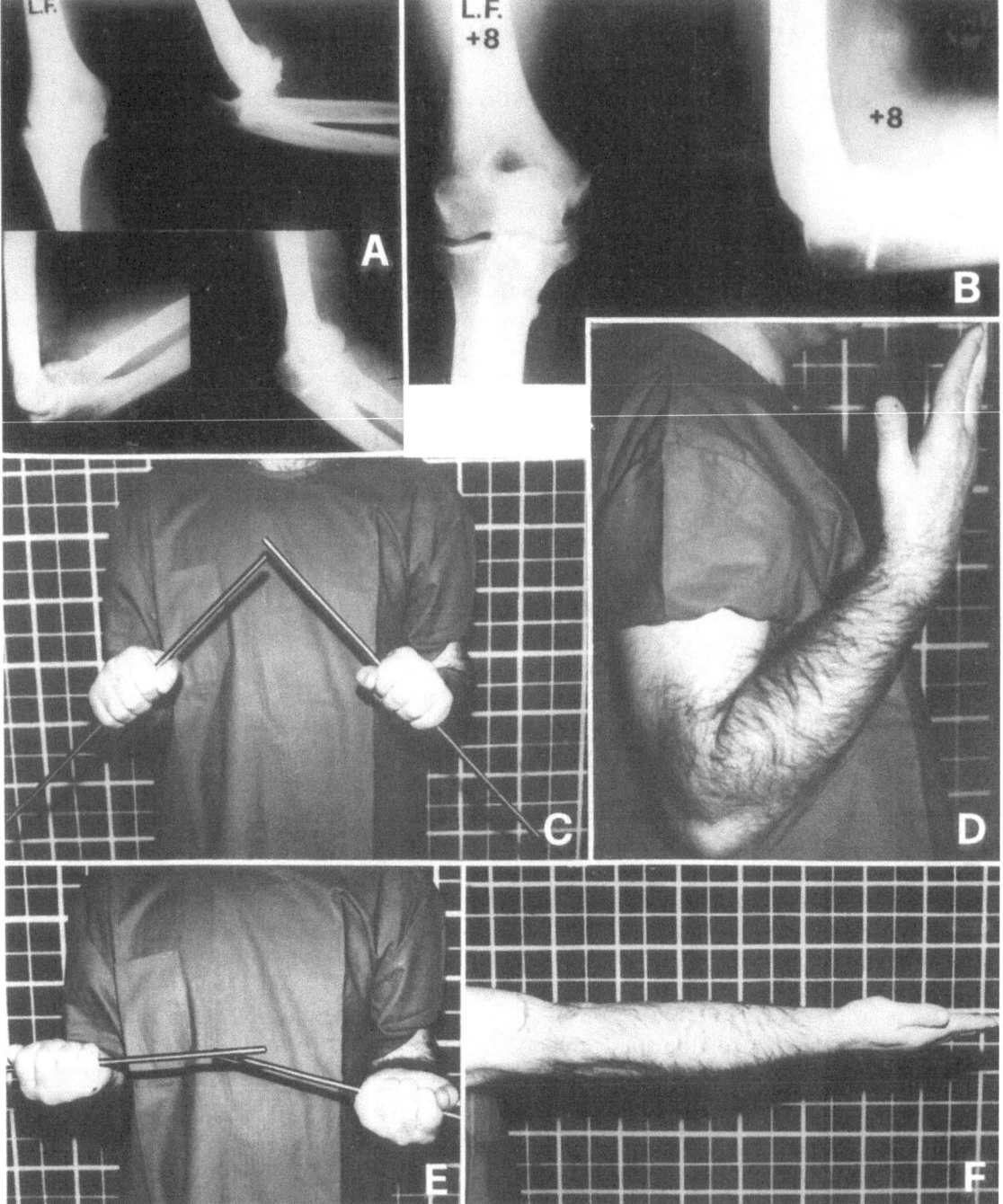

Fig. 1. - A) Radiograph of posterior dislocation of the elbow with fracture of the coronoid process both before and 8 years after treatment of the dislocation and screw fixation of the fracture; B) note the arthritic degeneration with marginal osteophytosis; C-F) clinical view of the same case shows an excellent result with total functional recovery.

The treatment consisted of closed reduction followed by cast immobilization in 57% (67) of the cases, while open reduction followed by cast immobilization lasting an average of 28 days (range 7-70) was adopted in the other 43% (51). There was a greater tendency towards open reduction and a higher average period of immobilization than re-

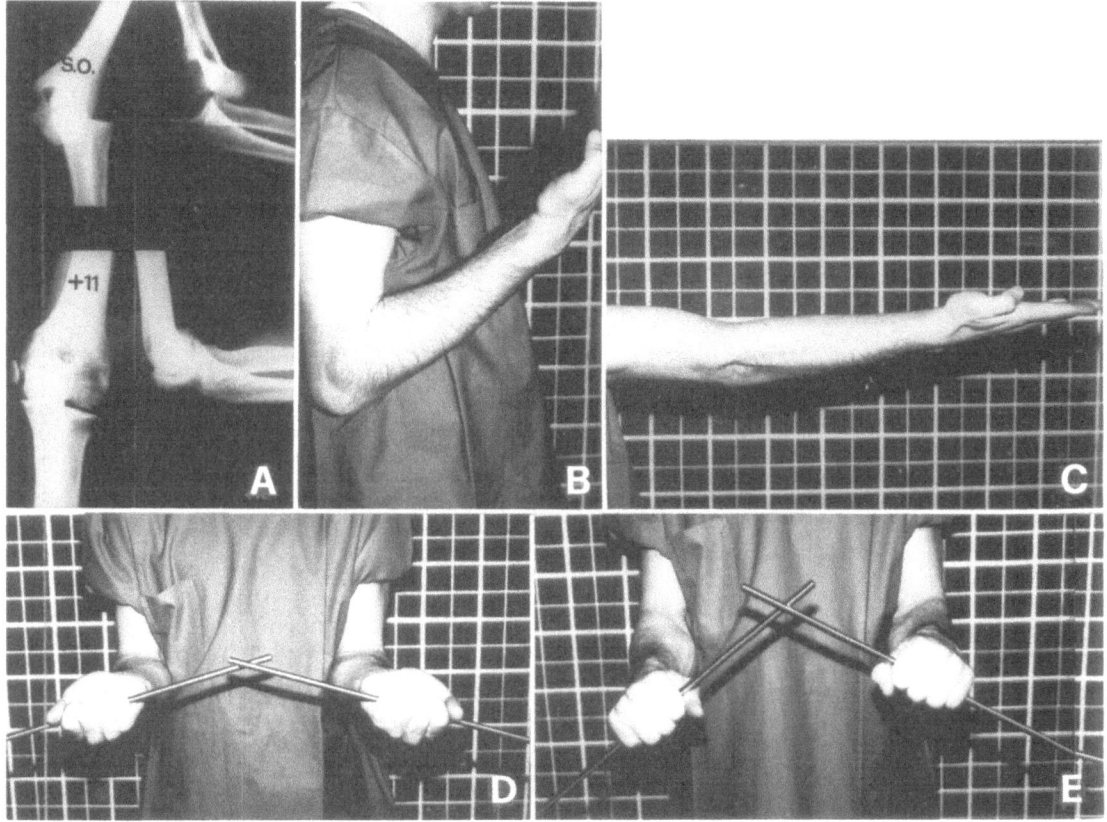

Fig, 2. - A) Radiograph of posterolateral dislocation of the elbow with fracture-diastasis of the medial epicondyle both before and 11 years after trauma; pseudoarthrosis and signs of arthritic degeneration do not compromise the functional outcome (B-E), which is good.

ported in the study of pure elbow dislocations.

We observed five cases of immediate and three cases of late peripheral nervous lack; the latter involved the radial nerve and appeared after surgery, while four of the former involved the ulnar nerve; the remaining case showed paresis of both the radial and ulnar nerves. This last patient had developed an anterior compartment syndrome immediately after the trauma, but it subsequently subsided almost completely and left no significant scars.

Forty-two patients (35.6%) were clinically and radiographically reviewed after an average of 12.6 years (range 1-27). Even though we were able to review only a relatively small number of patients, the length of the follow-up period allows us to draw several conclusions.

The clinical and radiographic evaluation was the same as was performed in the cases of pure elbow dislocation. The clinical features evaluated were pain, joint function, joint instability, and residual neurovascular lack. The results were excellent in 6 cases (14%), good in 24 (57%), and fair in the remaining 12 (29%). What has already been said regarding the patients with problems following pure elbow dislocation can help to explain the above categories. The radiographic evaluation, on the other hand, revealed heterotopic ossifications in 70% of the cases, joint instability (positive valgus stress test) in 35.7%, signs of degenerative arthritis in 65%, and accurate fracture reduction. As pointed out in the study of pure elbow dislocation (*see* previous chapter), the clinical and radiographic results do not always correspond, except in cases of severe joint degeneration or severe alteration of the geometric constants of the

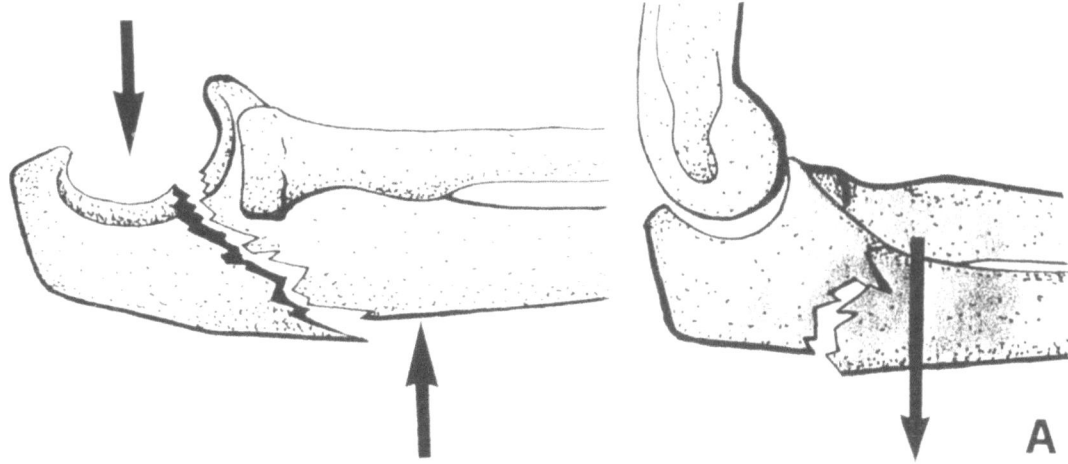

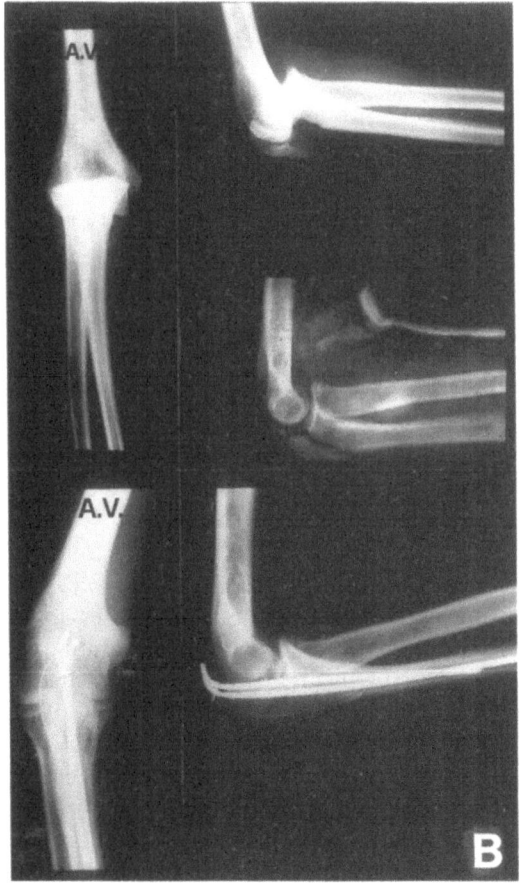

Fig. 3. - A) Drawing illustrating the location of the olecranon fracture in simple anterior radioulnar fracture-dislocation (*left*) and simple posterior elbow fracture-dislocation (*right*). B) X-ray of a simple anterior fracture-dislocation of the elbow treated first with closed reduction of the dislocation and then with internal fixation of the olecranon using the Weber technique and wires due to instability.

joint components due to inaccurate reduction (Figs. 1-2).

We will now discuss the 4 most common types of lesion found in this study: anterior or posterior radioulnar fracture-dislocation, dislocation with coronoid fracture-diastasis, dislocation with radial head fracture, and dislocation with epitrochlear fracture-diastasis.

Fracture-dislocation of the proximal radius and ulna does not disturb the normal relationship between the two bones, which usually remain solidly attached to one another.

We differentiated the lesions with anterior dislocation (AFD) from those with posterior dislocation (PFD) and then further divided both groups according to the type of fracture, simple or comminuted. In simple AFD the mechanism of injury is direct trauma to the slightly flexed elbow, causing fracture and diastasis of the olecranon up to the coronoid. In simple PFD, on the other hand, the mechanism of injury is indirect trauma from a fall on the hand with the elbow flexed and the forearm supinated; in these cases the fracture line is usually located at the base of the olecranon and coronoid (Fig. 3A).

We prescribed surgical treatment for these simple lesions (AFD and PFD): open reduction of the radial head to ensure joint stability and internal fixation of the olecranon using the Weber technique and either screws or wires (Fig. 3B).

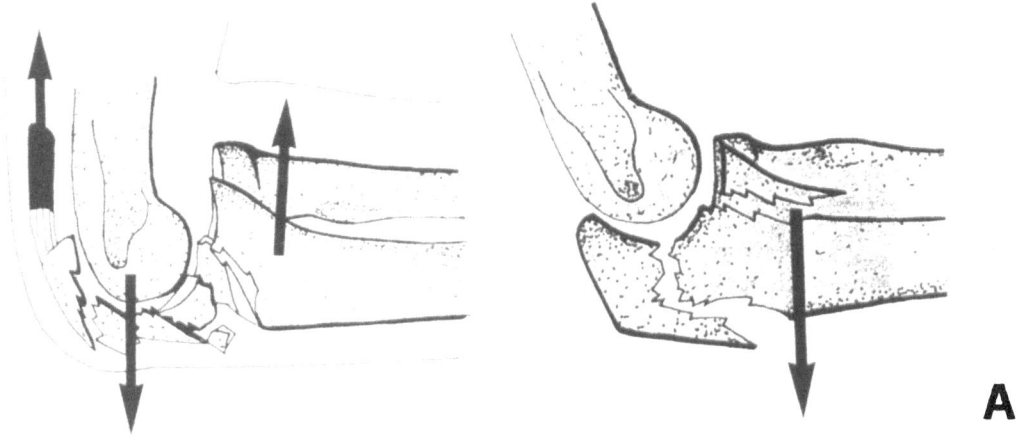

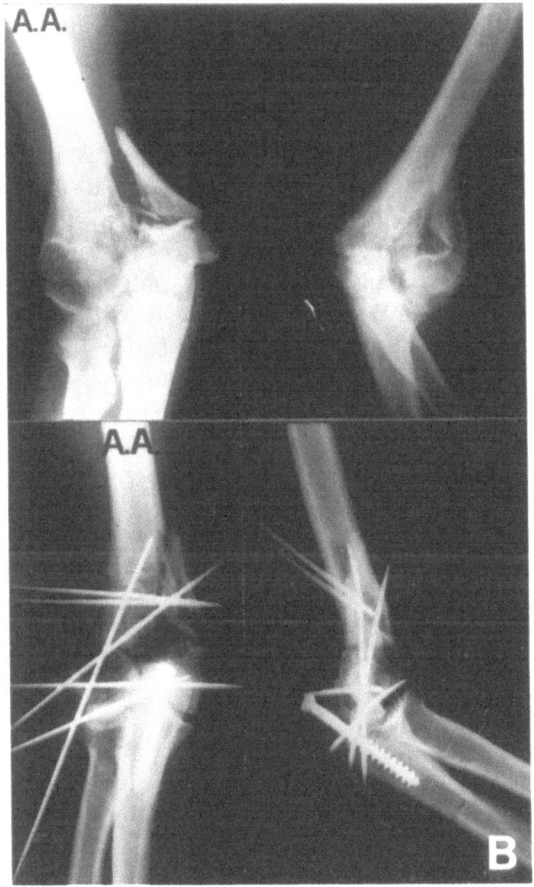

Fig. 4. - A) Drawing showing the location of the olecranon fracture in comminuted anterior radioulnar fracture-dislocation (left) and comminuted posterior elbow fracture-dislocation (right). B) X-ray of olecranon-distal humerus fracture with anterior subluxation treated surgically, using a posterior transolecranal approach for minimal interfragmentary fixation.

direct, inflicted by a fall on the hand with elbow flexed and forearm supinated. Three main fragments - olecranal, coronoid, and metaphyseal - can usually be identified (Fig. 4A). The other element in the pathogenesis of this lesion, the first being axial compression caused by the fall described above, is direct anteroposterior trauma to the forearm combined with muscle tension, resulting in displacement of the fragments and joint dislocation. The olecranal fragment tends to shift in a posterior and proximal direction, while the coronoid fragment usually heads anteromedially; the metaphyseal fragment remains attached to the radial head and is displaced posteriorly with respect to the lateral humeral condyle.

The comminuted fractures were treated non-operatively with closed reduction and cast immobilization when there was only slight displacement of fragments and when the reduction of the dislocation ensured good reconstruction of the articular surfaces. Surgical treatment consisted of minimal internal fixation of the fragments (Fig. 4B), with the possibility of subsequent olecranectomy or temporary stabilization with transarticular Kirschner wires. Transarticular external fixa-

Comminuted AFD is usually caused by direct trauma to the flexed elbow, thus the pretension of the triceps explains the evident displacement of the larger olecranal fragment. In comminuted PFD, on the other hand, the trauma responsible for the lesion is usually in-tion on the elbow joint was used in only a few cases. A posterior surgical approach was used for the fixation of comminuted fractures of the olecranon and the distal humerus, while a lateral approach was used for fixation of the coronoid when this was necessary. The average period of immobilization after conservative treatment was about 40 days, compared to only 20 days after surgical treatment. The long-term clinical results of both surgical and conservative treatment were more or less the same, especially in the most severely comminuted fractures.

In dislocation with coronoid fracture we observed a constant traction mechanism in the following types of fracture (in order of frequency): posterior, posterolateral, and anterior. In these cases conservative treatment, consisting of immobilization in a long-arm cast with elbow flexed, was reserved for small fractures with mild displacement, while surgical treatment using screws or the pull-out technique was adopted for fractures of the entire coronoid with severe displacement (Fig. 1).

Radial head fracture commonly accompanies posterolateral dislocation, occurring less frequently with pure posterior dislocation. Conservative treatment was used in undisplaced fractures, while single-fragment fractures with displacement were treated with reconstructive surgery consisting of internal fixation with either metal or biodegradable nails. Finally, ablative surgery was reserved for comminuted radial head fractures with evident displacement in patients over 15 years of age. In our experience the results of ablative surgery have featured immediate valgus instability of the joint, yet this has mostly subsided over time and has been followed by good functional recovery with only slight instability. In almost all these cases, there was radiographic evidence of joint degeneration that did not, however, correspond to severe functional limitation.

Finally, fracture of the medial epicondyle occurred most frequently in posterior and posterolateral dislocation of the elbow. This lesion usually consisted of fracture-diastasis of the apophysis due to forced valgus angulation of the elbow and generally occurred before the age of 16-18.

In the follow-up examination, signs of stabilized ulnar nerve damage were present in 13.8% of the patients; this complication almost always arose after injury.

Open reduction and internal fixation with screws or nails was adopted only in cases classified as Watson-Jones type III or IV. The peripheral neurologic complications were treated with neurolysis and anteposition of the ulnar nerve only in cases with severe clinical defects and neuroelectric signs of significant nerve and muscle damage.

REFERENCES

1) ALEFRAM P.A., BAUER C.H.: Epidemiology of fractures of the forearm. A biomechanical investigation of bone strength. *J. Bone Jt Surg.* 1962; **44-A**.

2) COSCO F., SPECCHIA L., POLI G.: Valutazione dei risultati a distanza del trattamento della frattura-lussazione congiunta di gomito. *Chir. Org. Mov.* 1987; **72**: 49.

3) DONATI D.: La lussazione traumatica del gomito associata a frattura del condilo esterno. Descrizione di un caso. *Chir. Org. Mov.* 1986; **71**.

4) GIANCECCHI F., CAVAZZUTI A., TARTAGLIA I.: Lussazioni e fratture-lussazioni di gomito. *Chir. Org. Mov.* 1983; **68**: 653.

5) KAPLAN S.S., RECKLING F.W.: Fracture separation of the lower humeral epiphysis with medial displacement. *J. Bone Jt Surg.* 1971; **53-A**.

6) KEON-COHEN B.T.: Fracture at the elbow. *J. Bone Jt Surg.* 1966; **48-A**.

7) MALCAPI C., GIANNANGELI F.: Le fratture-lussazioni del gomito. *Min. Ortop.* 1973; **24**: 133.

8) MAROTTE J.H., SAMUEL P., LORD G., BLANCHARD J.P., GUILLAMON J.L.: La fracture luxation conjointe de l'extremité supérieure des deux os de l'avant-bras. *Rev. Chir. Orthop.* 1982; **68**: 103.

The Monteggia lesion

A. Vaccari - A. Montorsi - F. Boselli - A. Folloni - C. Cordella

INTRODUCTION

The Monteggia lesion is named after Giovanni Battista Monteggia, who first reported it in 1814 (13). He defined it as a traumatic lesion featuring a fracture of the proximal ulna and an anterior dislocation of the proximal epiphysis of the radius. In later years this theory was modified by other authors. In 1855, Malgaigne reported that fracture of the ulna at any level can be accompanied by proximal dislocation of the radius (12), an idea that Hamilton had already expressed in 1850 (8). These reports convinced many that the Monteggia fracture-dislocation, as had been described by the author, could not be considered an isolated lesion but rather a group of traumatic lesions that, according to Bado (1967), "have in common dislocation of the humeroradioulnar joint combined with ulnar fracture (2)."

CLASSIFICATION

After Monteggia's original concept of 1814 was modified through the broadening of the definition and the introduction of other variations of the lesion, several classifications were proposed.

The **Watson-Jones classification** was the most widely used system for many years (17), and is based on the site of dislocation of the radial head. The three main categories of lesions are as follows:

Type 1: typical Monteggia lesion, or Watson-Jones extension fracture combined with anterior dislocation of the radial head (Fig. 1).

Type 2: reverse Monteggia lesion, or Watson-Jones flexion fracture with posterior dislocation of the radial head (Fig. 2).

Type 3: Monteggia lesion with lateral dislocation of the radial head (Fig. 3).

In 1959 **Bado** proposed a more precise classification, distinguishing 4 types of lesions (1):

Type 1: ulnar shaft fracture at any level with anterior angulation combined with anterior dislocation of the radial head. It is the most common variation (about 60% of cases) (Fig. 4).

Type 2: proximal metaphyseal ulnar frac-

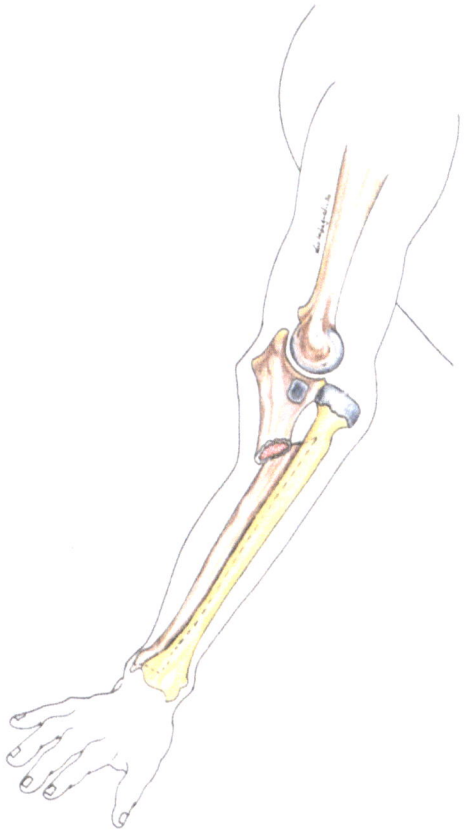

Fig. 1. - Monteggia lesion, or Watson-Jones extension fracture combined with anterior dislocation of the radial head.

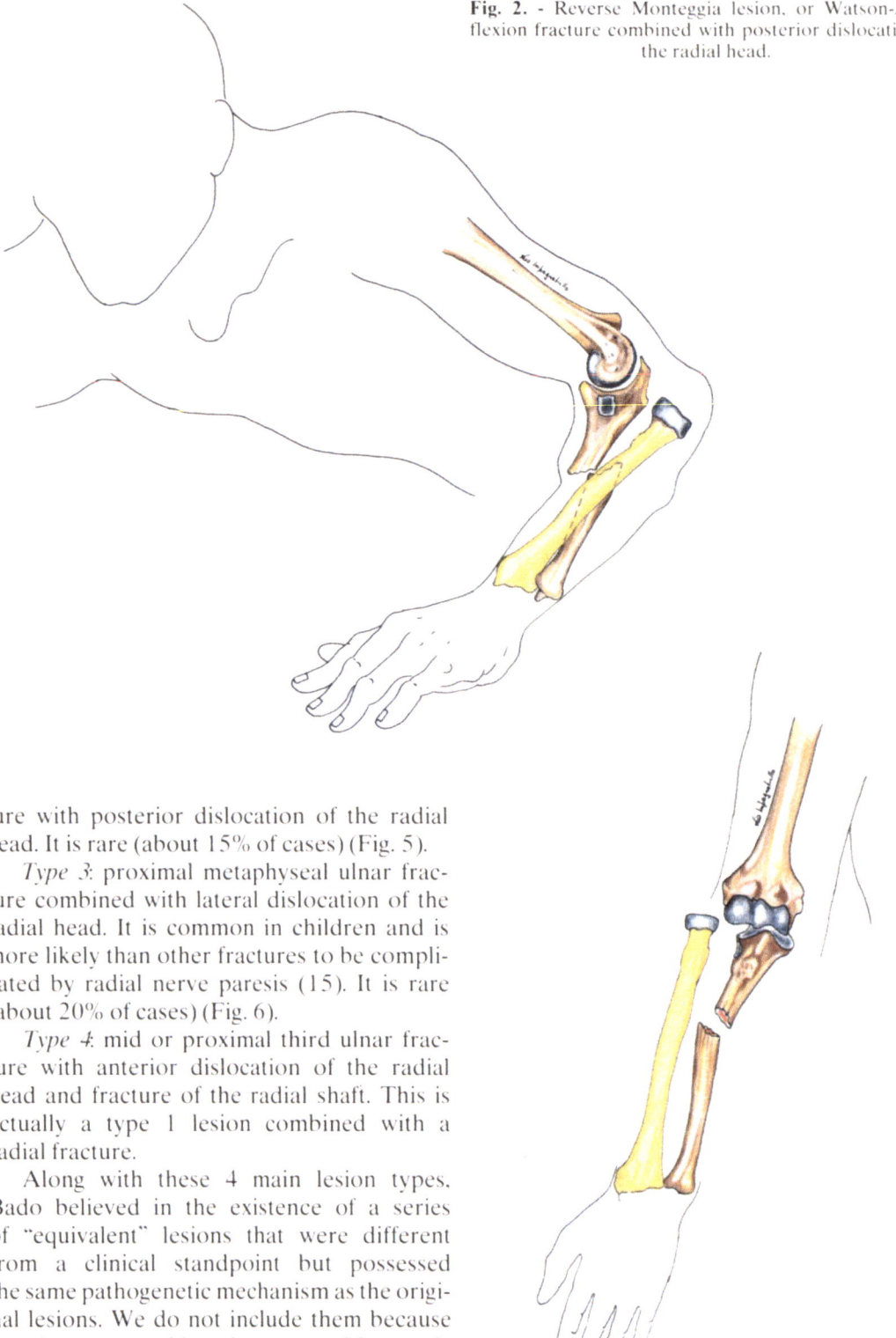

Fig. 2. - Reverse Monteggia lesion, or Watson-Jones flexion fracture combined with posterior dislocation of the radial head.

ture with posterior dislocation of the radial head. It is rare (about 15% of cases) (Fig. 5).

Type 3: proximal metaphyseal ulnar fracture combined with lateral dislocation of the radial head. It is common in children and is more likely than other fractures to be complicated by radial nerve paresis (15). It is rare (about 20% of cases) (Fig. 6).

Type 4: mid or proximal third ulnar fracture with anterior dislocation of the radial head and fracture of the radial shaft. This is actually a type 1 lesion combined with a radial fracture.

Along with these 4 main lesion types, Bado believed in the existence of a series of "equivalent" lesions that were different from a clinical standpoint but possessed the same pathogenetic mechanism as the original lesions. We do not include them because we do not consider them true Monteggia lesions.

Although the Bado classification is an improvement over the earlier Watson-Jones

Fig. 3. - Type 3 Watson-Jones fracture with lateral dislocation of the radial head.

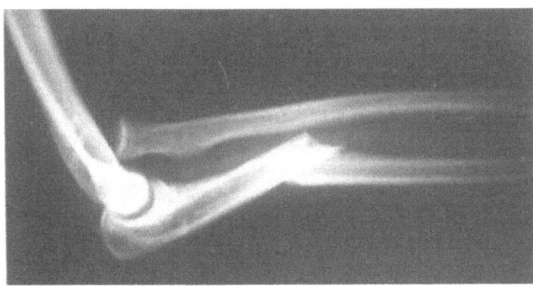

Fig. 4. - Monteggia fracture-dislocation (Bado type 1 or Trillat group 1).

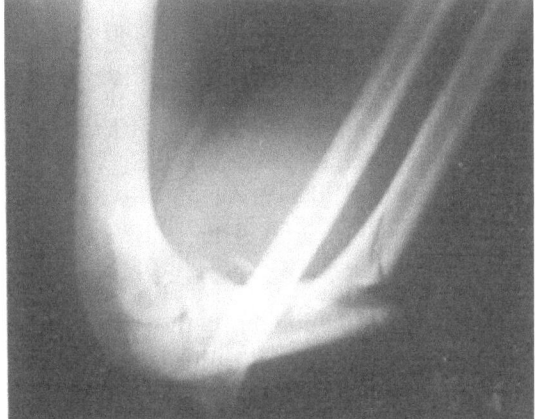

Fig. 5. - Monteggia fracture-dislocation (Bado type 2 or Trillat group 1).

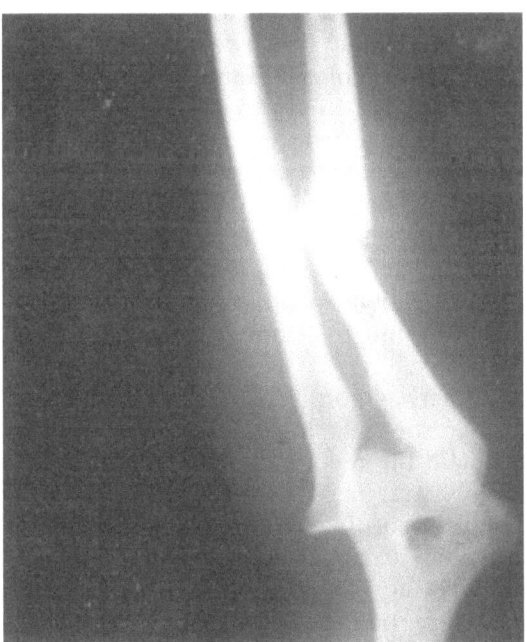

Fig. 6. - Monteggia fracture-dislocation (Bado type 3 or Trillat group 1).

system because it is based on the site of the fracture as well as the type of dislocation, it was further modified by Trillat *et al.* in 1969 (15). These authors argued that the Bado classification did not cover a lesion that they believed to be very common, that is, a meta-epiphyseal fracture in the adult combined with posterior or anterior dislocation of the radial head. This is not covered in the Bado type 3 category because the dislocation is not lateral and the lesion is typical in the adult. According to Trillat, a Monteggia lesion in which the ulnar fracture is at a proximal or midshaft level is not related to a lesion in which the ulnar fracture is at the level of the olecranon, even if the type of radial head dislocation is the same in both cases. In fact, the first instance involves a forearm fracture and the second an elbow fracture, so the differences are not only clinical but also therapeutic and prognostic. Based on these facts, Trillat *et al.* proposed their own classification system, consisting of 3 categories:

Group 1: includes all lesions consisting of ulnar shaft fractures at any level combined with anterior, posterior, or lateral dislocation. The ulnar fracture may be single, multiple, or comminuted. They may occur in both children and adults and their mechanism is trauma to the forearm.

Group 2: includes meta-epiphyseal ulnar fractures with anterior, posterior, or lateral radial head dislocation. The general appearance of the fracture may vary as in group 1.

The etiology and pathogenesis of these lesions is related to trauma to the elbow rather than the forearm.

Group 3: includes group 1 and 2 lesions that are accompanied by a lesion of either the humerus, the radius, or the wrist.

Therefore, the Trillat classification concentrates on the site of the ulnar fracture and the possible associated fracture and/or other lesions. No special emphasis is given to direction of the dislocation of the radial head.

ETIOLOGY AND PATHOGENESIS

The etiology and pathogenesis of these lesions is usually indirect trauma to the forearm. In the Bado type 1 lesion, the cause is forced rotation (6). In a forward fall, while the hand is hyperextended and the forearm is pronated, the trunk rotates laterally and transmits lateral rotation of the limb to the hand resting firmly on the ground. This further pronates the forearm, which was already fully pronated at impact. The proximal ulna is thus fractured, while the radius is forced into full pronation and crosses the mid-proximal ulna. Then the proximal ulna, acting as a fulcrum, pushes the radius and dislocates its head anteriorly. In the Bado type 2 lesion, the mechanism is a direct, rotatory force that supinates the forearm. Type 3 is caused by direct trauma to the medial side of the elbow, with or without rotation (1). The radial head is dislocated laterally away from the ulna, causing rupture of the oblique cord and Denucé quadrate ligaments, the interosseous membrane, and the capsule of the proximal radioulnar joint (16).

DIAGNOSIS

Diagnosis is generally quite easy, provided that the orthopedist collects the data relative to the trauma from the patient's medical history, performs a thorough clinical examination, and requests both lateral and AP radiographs. The main clinical features are pain and severe functional limitation of the elbow, as well as the characteristic deformity. Forearm and hand are locked in pronation. Active movement is impossible while passive mobilization is limited by pain. If the fracture is compound, the wound is located either anteriorly or posteriorly depending upon the type of lesion. The radiologic exam is essential: there can be no doubt about the diagnosis when the radial head dislocation and the ulnar fracture are observed on the two projections. In instances of isolated ulnar fracture, an x-ray of the elbow must be taken in order to observe the condition of the humeroradioulnar joint and exclude a possible Monteggia lesion. Finally, it is important not to underestimate the possibility of additional fractures to nearby structures such as the distal humerus and the wrist.

TREATMENT

Treatment of Monteggia fracture-dislocations is different in children and adults.

Treatment in children

Conservative orthopedic treatment is usually adopted. Almost all authors agree that this yields good results if executed within the first few hours after trauma (5, 7, 10, 11, 14).

Reduction of the radial head and realignment of the ulna are usually achieved quite easily if the proper methods are used. The patient is put under general anesthesia and the surgeon reduces the fracture with the elbow flexed to 90 degrees and the forearm fully supinated. Immediate application of counter-traction above the elbow is necessary. After reduction, the arm is immobilized in a cast maintaining both the traction on the forearm and the position of the limb: elbow flexed and forearm slightly supinated. Maintaining this position is usually not difficult if the fracture has been reduced correctly. Subsequent displacement of the ulna may occur, however, in which case a second attempt at closed reduction should be made only within the first two weeks after the trauma. A radiologic exam should always be done after 7-10 days to check the status of the reduction, which, according to some authors (14), is acceptable if the fracture is angled no more than 10 degrees in either the sagittal plane (lateral x-ray) or the horizontal plane (AP x-ray). The period of cast immobilization varies from 5 to 7 weeks, then thorough elbow rehabilitation is necessary.

Other authors have observed that the transverse metaphyseal fractures tend to maintain the reduction, while the more distal oblique ones tend toward subsequent displacement. In these cases an intramedullary nail (percutaneous Kirschner wire) may be necessary. Surgical intervention is rarely necessary because of irreducibility of the dislocation: in this instance reconstruction of the lacerated orbicular ligament may be indicated.

Treatment in adults

Treatment in the adult is more difficult and controversial compared to treatment in the child. When a Monteggia lesion is present, closed reduction is indicated in any case because it often achieves immediate reduction of the radial head with resulting reduction of the ulnar fracture. Nevertheless, a review of the literature reveals that conservative treatment in the adult usually yields an unsatisfactory result compared to that achieved in the child (3, 4, 15). All this is explained by the high incidence of pseudoarthrosis. The key to the treatment of these lesions is the healing of the ulnar fracture, which seems more difficult in a Monteggia lesion than in an isolated fracture because of the associated instability of the elbow provoked by the dislocation and the ligamentous lesion. The two conditions

that form the basis of the etiology and pathogenesis of pseudoarthrosis are then created: the biological condition (ulnar fracture, healing of which is notoriously difficult in the adult) and the mechanical condition (micromotion of the fracture site due to proximal instability). Therefore, the purpose of surgery is to remove these conditions and promote healing, usually easier at the metaphyseal level, with fixation devices that reduce and stabilize the fracture and, if necessary, repair or reconstruction of the torn orbicular ligament.

Some authors think both of these operative stages are always indicated and should be performed at the same time (3). Others prefer to first stabilize the ulna with intramedullary nails or screws and to perform surgery on the radial head only when it is unstable or irreducible (15). In this instance the most com-

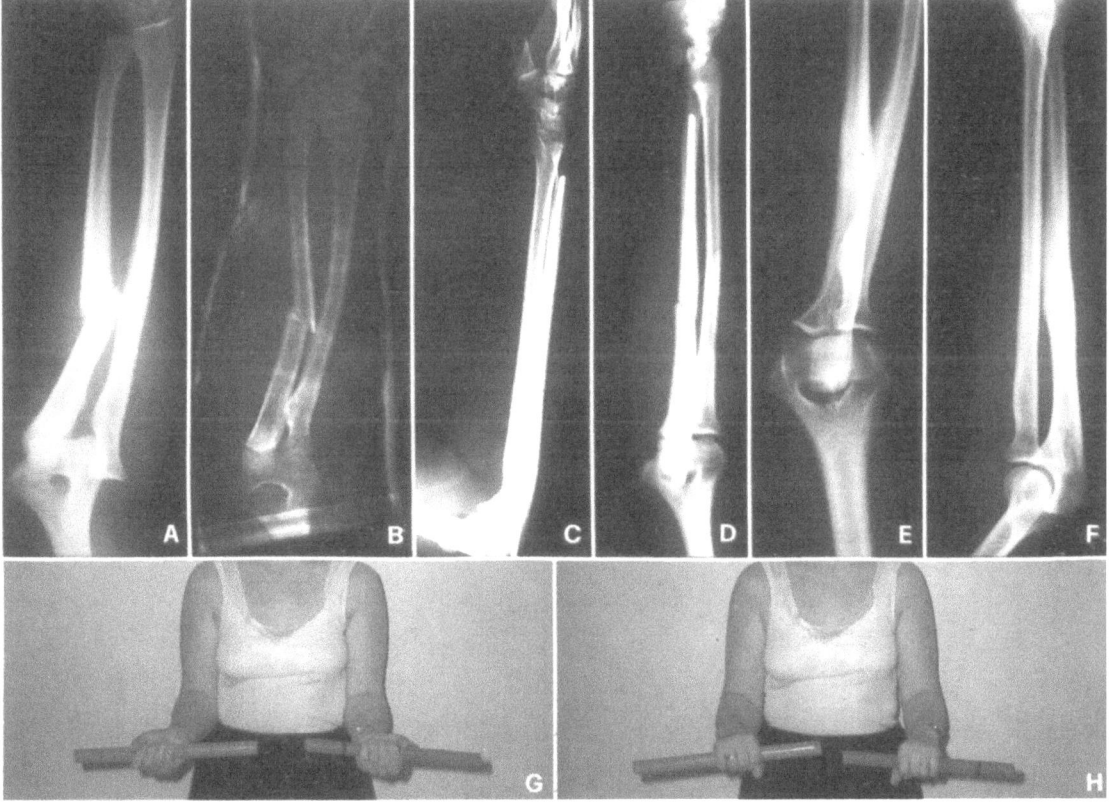

Fig. 7. - O.L., patient 12: A) Radiograph of Monteggia fracture-dislocation (Bado type 3 or Trillat group 1). B) Radiograph after reduction and casting: ulnar angulation is greater than 10 degrees in the horizontal plane. C,D) Radiograph after internal fixation of ulna with Rush nails. E,F) Follow-up radiograph shows good fracture healing and no angulation. G,H) The clinical examination shows no limitation of pronation or supination.

mon approach is Ollier's, which requires an incision from the end of the ulna, 4-5 cm below the elbow joint, extending proximally along the edge of the triceps tendon. The muscles that insert on the ulna are moved toward the radial portion of the incision. Using this approach, both procedures can be done through only one incision. Other authors perform both internal fixation of the ulna, with either intramedullary nails or plates, as well as open reduction of the radial head stabilized with Kirschner wires (4).

We prefer closed reduction of the dislocation and internal fixation of the ulna, choosing the fixation devices according to the site of the lesion. If the fracture is metaphyseal or meta-epiphyseal, percutaneous Kirschner wires may be used (Fig. 9). If the lesion is either lower or diaphyseal, we prefer Rush nails or plates and screws (Figs. 7-8). If the radial head is still unstable after the ulnar reduction (this can be checked with fluoroscopic imaging), we perform a temporary percutaneous stabilization of the bone with a transcondylar-radial Kirschner wire. Only in very rare cases of irreducibility of the dislocation after ulnar fixation do we recommend surgical reduction of the radial head and reconstruction of the orbicular ligament. The period of cast immobilization varies from 6 weeks to 3 months, even if the fixation is stable, in order to promote good capsuloligamentous scarring.

MATERIALS AND METHODS

From January 1979 to March 1989, 16 patients (9 males and 7 females) who were

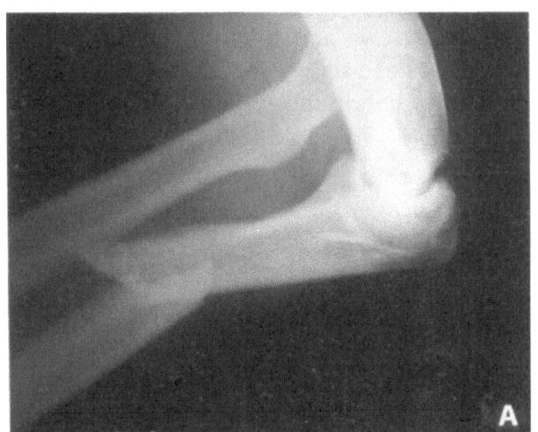

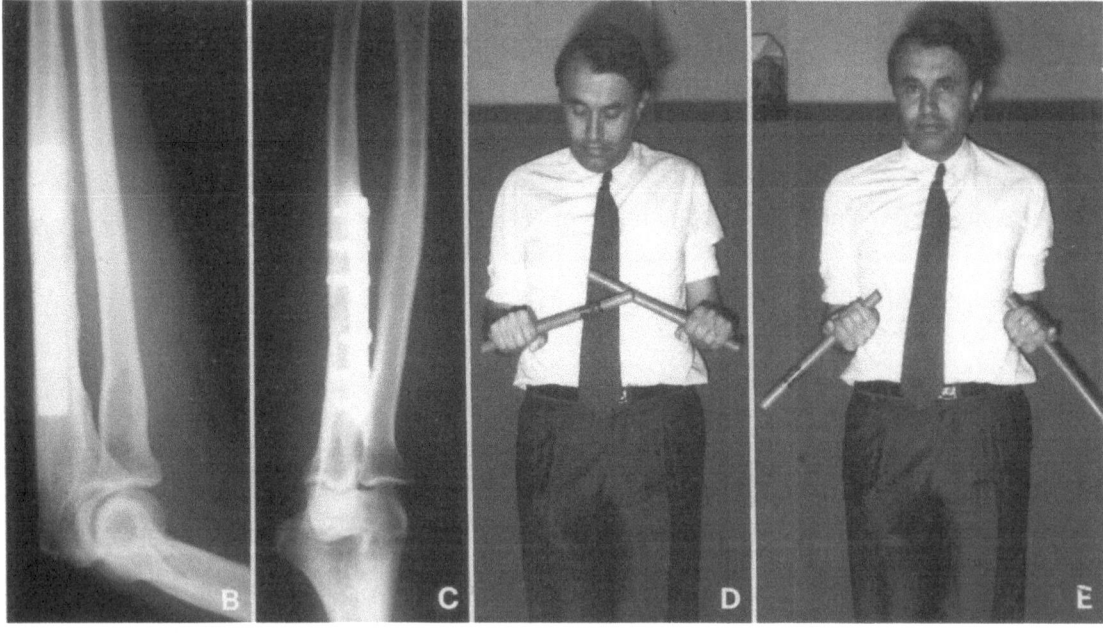

Fig. 8. - K.J., patient 2: A) Monteggia lesion (Bado type 1 or Trillat group 1). B,C) Follow-up radiograph shows healing and no angular deviation. D,E) The clinical examination shows an excellent outcome.

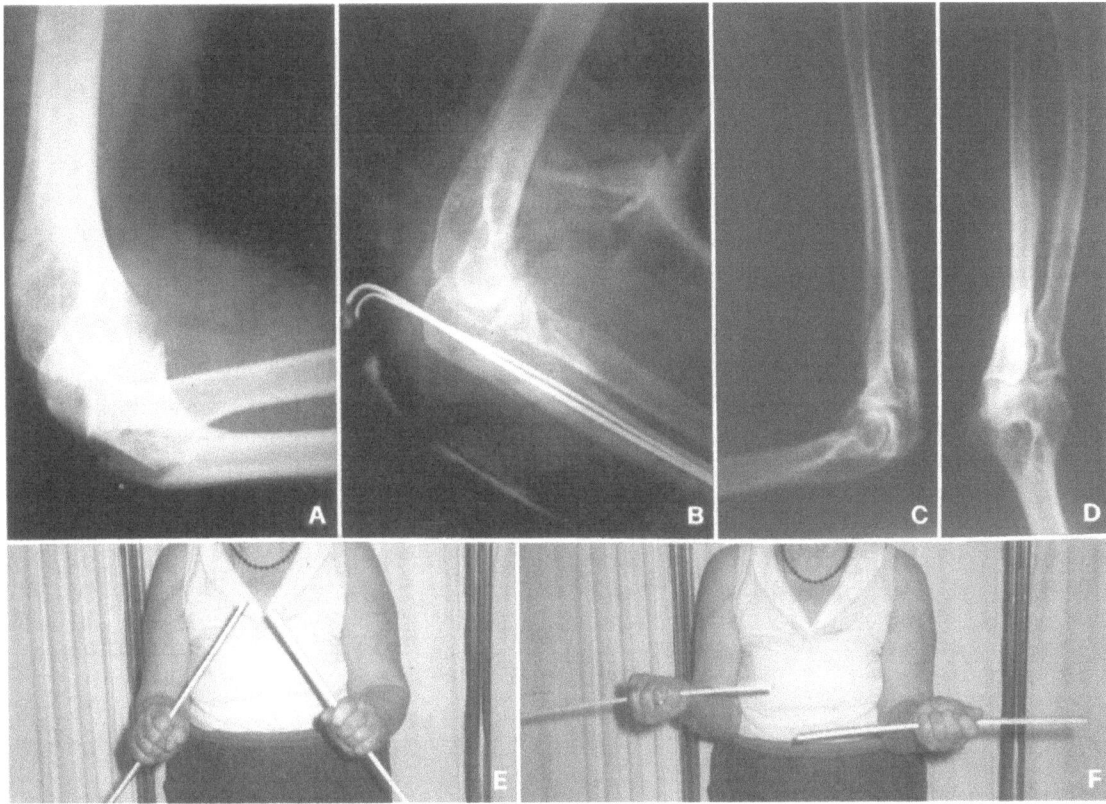

Fig. 9 - F.I., patient 8: A) Monteggia fracture-dislocation (Bado type 2 or Trillat group 2). B) Radiologic view after reduction, percutaneous fixation with two Kirschner wires, and casting. C, D) Follow-up x-ray shows perfect healing and restoration of anatomical alignment. E,F) The clinical exam shows an excellent outcome.

35.5 years old on average (range 5-72) were treated for Monteggia lesion. The left elbow was affected in 9 cases and the right in 7. The breakdown of our patients according to the Bado classification is as follows: type 1, 6 cases; type 2, 8 cases; type 3, 2 cases, and type 4, no cases. According to the Trillat classification, on the other hand, there were type 1, 8 cases; type 2, 8 cases; and type 3, no cases. In 11 cases the fixation device used was the intramedullary nail (Rush, Kirschner, Steinmann), in 2 cases an A.O. plate, and in 1 case a Hoffmann external fixation device. Closed reduction was performed in the child patient. Only one patient did not undergo ulnar fixation. Surgical repair of the orbicular ligament was performed twice. The radial head was removed in 3 cases. All patients (except the one treated with external fixation) underwent cast immobilization (Table 1).

RESULTS

All cases were reviewed after a follow-up period ranging from 6 months to 10 years. The clinical criteria regarded joint function (flexion and extension of the elbow, pronation and supination of the forearm), and the radiologic criteria (using two views) were ulnar fracture healing, presence of periarticular calcifications, the ulnar axis, and the relationship of the radial head to the other structures. Both pain (absent, occasional, during exertion, constant) and resumption of previous activity (total, partial, or completely lacking) were evaluated. The results were evaluated using a point system explained in

Table 1

Case	Age	Sex	Side	Ulnar fixation	Radial head stabilization	Radial head resection	Cast
1. T.F.	21	M	L	Steinmann nail	Dynamic	No	Yes
2. K.J.	35	M	L	Plate	No	No	Yes
3. P.E.	25	M	L	Rush	No	Yes	Yes
4. D.M.	36	M	L	Rush	No	No	Yes
5. C.G.	22	M	R	Kirschner	Dynamic	No	Yes
6. B.E.	5	F	R	Orthopaedic	No	No	Yes
7. G.M.	72	F	L	Plate	No	Yes	Yes
8. F.I.	75	F	R	Percutaneous Kirschner	No	No	Yes
9. G.R.	18	M	L	External fixation	No	Yes	No
10. F.E.	25	M	R	Rush	No	No	Yes
11. M.M.	17	F	R	Kirschner	No	No	Yes
12. O.L.	43	F	R	Rush	No	No	Yes
13. L.N.	69	F	L	Percutaneous Kirschner	No	No	Yes
14. G.L.	35	M	L	Kirschner	No	No	Yes
15. P.G.	30	M	R	No	Kirsch.	Yes	Yes
16. B.G.	40	F	L	Rush and graft	No	No	Yes

Table 2

Flexion-extension	Up to 145° Up to 100° Up to 50° Less than 50°	Score = 4 Score = 3 Score = 2 Score = 0
Pronation	Up to 85° Up to 60° Up to 30° Less than 30°	Score = 4 Score = 3 Score = 2 Score = 0
Supination	Up to 90° Up to 60° Up to 30° Less than 30°	Score = 4 Score = 3 Score = 2 Score = 0
Healing	YES NO	Score = 4 Score = 0
Calcification	YES NO	Score = 0 Score = 4
Radial head	In place Dislocated	Score = 4 Score = 0
Pain	Absent Occasional During exertion Constant	Score = 4 Score = 3 Score = 2 Score = 0
Resumption of activity	Total Partial Completely lacking	Score = 4 Score = 2 Score = 0
Outcome	Poor Fair Good Excellent	Score = 0-20 Score = 21-27 Score = 27-30 Score = 31-33

Table 2, and were as follows: 7 excellent, 5 good, 1 fair, and 3 poor.

DISCUSSION

Some conclusions can be drawn in light of the results. A tendency toward surgical treatment is usually correct in adult patients, yet inadequate treatment should be avoided. One of the unsatisfactory results was almost certainly due to incorrect treatment: the fracture had been correctly stabilized with a plate, but the radial head had been resected causing elbow destabilization and pseudoarthrosis. After surgery using a nail without a graft, hypertrophic nonunion occurred (patient 7).

In another poor result, the dislocation had been reduced and the radial head had been stabilized with a transhumero-radial Kirschner wire, but cast immobilization was used instead of surgical fixation of the ulnar fracture. This allowed the micromotion of the fracture site that broke the Kirschner wire. The fracture was subsequently fixed and the radial head resected. The result was unsatisfactory because in addition to elbow instability there was dislocation of the distal ulnar epiphysis (patient 15). The third poor result was also treated with radial head resection and intramedullary nailing of the ulna. Removal of the radial head again played an important role in the outcome (patient 3).

This study, unlike others, counts only one child patient. This is due to the fact that we included only patients who were actually admitted to the hospital, and not those who were treated on an out-patient basis. There were no cases of infection and no vascular or nervous complications.

CONCLUSIONS

The Monteggia fracture-dislocation is in itself benign if treated correctly. The goal of treatment should be an ulnar fixation that promotes fracture healing: rigid fixation of the shaft and dynamic fixation of the proximal metaphysis. Surgery of the radial head is usually unnecessary, and should not be used in any case as primary treatment. Failure is always due to incorrect treatment.

REFERENCES

1) BADO J.L.: *The Monteggia lesion*. Thomas, Springfield 1959.
2) BADO J.L.: The Monteggia lesion. *Clin. Orthop.* 1967; **50**: 71-86.
3) BOYD H.B., BOALS J.C.: The Monteggia lesion: a review of 159 cases. *Clin. Orthop.* 1969; **66**: 94-100.
4) BRUCE H.E., HARVEY J.P., WILSON J.C.: Monteggia fractures. *J. Bone Jt Surg.* 1974; **56-A**: 1563-76.
5) DUBUC J.E., ROMBOUTS J.J., VINCENT A.: Les luxations de l'extrémité proximale du radius chez l'enfant. *Acta Orthop. Belg.* 1984; **50** (6): 815-836.
6) EVANS E.M.: Pronation injuries of forearm with special reference to anterior Monteggia fracture. *J. Bone Jt Surg.* 1949; **31-B**: 578.
7) FOWLES J.V., SLIMAN N., KASSAB M.T.: The Monteggia lesion in children. *J. Bone Jt Surg.* 1983; **65-A** (9): 1276.
8) HAMILTON, 1850. Quoted by Bado J.L. (1)
9) HOLST-NIELSEN F., JENSEN V.: Tardy posterior interosseous nerve palsy as a result of an unreduced radial head dislocation in Monteggia fractures: a report of two cases. *J. Hand Surg.* 1984; **9** (4): 572-575.
10) KALAMCHI A., WILMINGTON, DELAWARE: Monteggia fracture-dislocation in children: late treatment in two cases. *J. Bone Jt Surg.* 1986; **68-A** (4): 615-619.
11) LEFTS M., LOCHT R., WIENS J.: Monteggia fracture-dislocations in children. *J. Bone Jt Surg.* 1985; **67-B** (5): 724-727.
12) MALGAIGNE, 1855. Quoted by Bado J.L. (1).
13) MONTEGGIA G.B.: *Istituzioni chirurgiche*. Milano, 1814.
14) PAPAVASILIOU V.A., NENOPOULOS S.P.: Monteggia-type elbow fractures in childhood. *Clin. Orthop. Rel. Res.* 1988; **233**: 230-233.
15) TRILLAT A., MARSAN C., LAPEYRE B.: Classification et traitement des fractures de Monteggia: à propos de 36 observations. *Rev. Chir. Orthop.* 1969; **55** (7): 639-658.
16) VERNERET C., LANGLAIS J., POULIQUEN J.C., RIGAULT P.: Luxations anciennes post-traumatiques de la tête radiale chez l'enfant. *Rev. Chir. Orthop.* 1989; **75**: 77-89.
17) WATSON-JONES R.: *Fractures and joint injuries*. Williams and Wilkins, Baltimore, 1955, 4ª ed., vol. 2, 572-581.

Neurovascular complications in the post-traumatic elbow

A. Landi - O. Soragni - G.L. Sacchetti - R. Cavana - G. Caserta

INTRODUCTION

The elbow joint is surrounded by vascular and nervous structures that are vulnerable to direct trauma as well as a consequence of articular and periarticular traumatic syndromes. The density of these structures contributes to the high incidence of iatrogenic lesions, mostly involving the three main nerves (median, ulnar, and radial), caused by application or removal of metal fixation devices.

Neurovascular complications generally arise in infancy, and late nerve compression syndromes are the result of altered growth patterns (cubitus varus and valgus) caused by epiphyseal trauma that is either not diagnosed or incorrectly treated.

Vascular complications

Treatment of vascular lesions has been modified over the years.

During World War II, when damaged arteries were systematically ligated, amputation was necessary in 56% of the patients with proximal lesions of the deep brachial artery, 26% of the patients with distal lesions and 39% of the patients whose radial and ulnar arteries were ligated simultaneously (1).

Emergency treatment of vascular lesions, first performed during the Korean War, radically changed the prognosis, as none of the 80 cases later required amputation (40). It should be noted that of the 65 vascular lesions reported in the University of Louisville study, only two were caused by elbow fracture-dislocation (1).

Vascular complications in the elbow are most commonly caused by supracondylar extension fractures (15). Lipscomb reports the experience of the Mayo Clinic and Founda-

tion (15) of 11 cases of brachial artery lesion in 108 supracondylar extension fractures, and Spear (31), analyzing a previous study, reports 4 complete lacerations of the artery.

Therefore, a case of acute vascular complications with typical symptoms – pallor, no peripheral pulse, pain and distal anesthesia – should be treated with reduction to prevent elbow flexion; the limb should then be put in skeletal traction and kept under close observation. The signs of impending Volkmann's contracture that would make vessel exploration advisable are acute edema, preventing adequate collateral circulation, and lack of improvement in the condition of the peripheral circulatory system. Whitesides et al. (39), Eaton and Green (4), and Mubarak and Carrol (23) proved that Volkmann's contracture is often caused by an undiagnosed compartment syndrome that may exist apart from severe arterial lesion. For the purposes of classification, however, it is important to categorize Volkmann's contracture according to Holden's etiologic criteria (11) that we have modified (14).

Type 1 is the result of lesion of a main arterial branch proximal to the site of muscle ischemia. This type can be subdivided into three categories: in *1a*, a lesion that threatens the viability of the limb, provokes muscle necrosis yet spares the overlying skin; *1b*, however, is the result of a revascularization syndrome; which leads to an unexpected and inadequately treated compartment syndrome; *1c* is due to damage or compression of the vascular pedicle of a muscle provided with only a single vascular supply.

Type 2 is the result of direct trauma to the various compartments or indirect trauma to the structures inside these compartments. This type is comprised of two subcategories: *2a* when the compartment syndrome affects a healthy structure, and *2b* when the syndrome is aggravated by other systemic factors such as CO poisoning, hemophilia, etc. (14). Today, the lower incidence of Volkmann's contracture is attributable to better monitoring techniques such as direct evaluation of the compartmental pressure (23, 29) and the study of muscular energy metabolism using magnetic resonance spectroscopy of P31 (10). Since Volkmann's contracture is in most cases a consequence of an inadequately treated compartment syndrome, subjective clinical features such as pallor, pain when muscles are stretched in the compartment, and absence of pulse alone are not completely reliable for diagnosis, but should be confirmed if possible with imaging studies.

The easiest way to monitor the development of a compartment syndrome is to measure the pressure in the volar compartments of the forearm (39). Heppenstall (10) reports that fasciotomy is not indicated due to the fact that the compartmental pressure remained at more than 30 mm/Hg for over 8 hours (21, 22), but rather by the difference between the average arterial pressure and the compartmental pressure (ΔP).

As a matter of fact, when spectroscopy and compartmental measurements were done in men (10), at least 3 cases with intra-compartmental pressure around 60 mm/Hg yet $\Delta P \geq 40$ mm/Hg had normal metabolic profiles of the muscles. These cases were taken under observation and the problems eventually disappeared spontaneously. When they do not, however, volar fasciotomy is recommended once the brachial artery, which may be bruised, completely lacerated, or pinched by the fracture, has been examined (Fig. 1). Sometimes adventitiectomy is sufficient, and occasionally resuturing or grafting is necessary.

The good results reported in the past achieved with fascio-cutaneous decompression (15) and ligature of the lacerated ends of the artery were attributed to the disappearance of the peripheral reflex spasm according to Lériche's theory. In most cases the cure of the vascular symptoms is probably related to the direct benefits of fasciotomy and the indirect benefits of fascio-cutaneous

decompression on the collateral circulatory system.

We agree with Watson-Jones (38) that an impending Volkmann's syndrome in no case justifies open reduction of the fracture.

Neurologic complications

On this subject, we believe the experience of R. Watson-Jones (37), which was presented in July of 1929 at the convention of the American Orthopedic Society in Liverpool, to be particularly relevant even today. The subject of his report was primary neurologic lesions in the elbow, and it was based on 5000 cases of joint fracture.

Based on the A.O. classification, reported by Randelli, elbow fractures are divided into the categories of articular and periarticular. Under the periarticular category, neural lesions associated with supracondylar and epitrochlear fractures are described.

Under the articular category, the complications are associated with epiphyseal trauma or fractures of the trochlea and capitulum. For the forearm side of the elbow joint, the most common neural complications associated with the Monteggia lesion, radial head fracture, and olecranon fracture are reported.

DISLOCATION OF THE ELBOW

Elbow dislocation can happen at any age. It accounts for 6% of all traumatic lesions of the elbow in children. The bones of the forearm are usually dislocated in a posterior, posterolateral, or posteromedial direction, and the brachialis muscle is torn away from the coronoid process (37).

The mechanism of injury is usually a fall on the outstretched hand with arm abducted, forearm pronated, and elbow slightly flexed (30). In the 97 cases of elbow dislocation reported by Watson-Jones (37), the direction of the dislocation and the type of neural complication are recorded quite precisely. In 2 of 32 cases of pure posterior dislocation, there was only one instance of radial nerve palsy, which disappeared shortly after reduction.

Only 1 of 29 cases of posterolateral dislo-

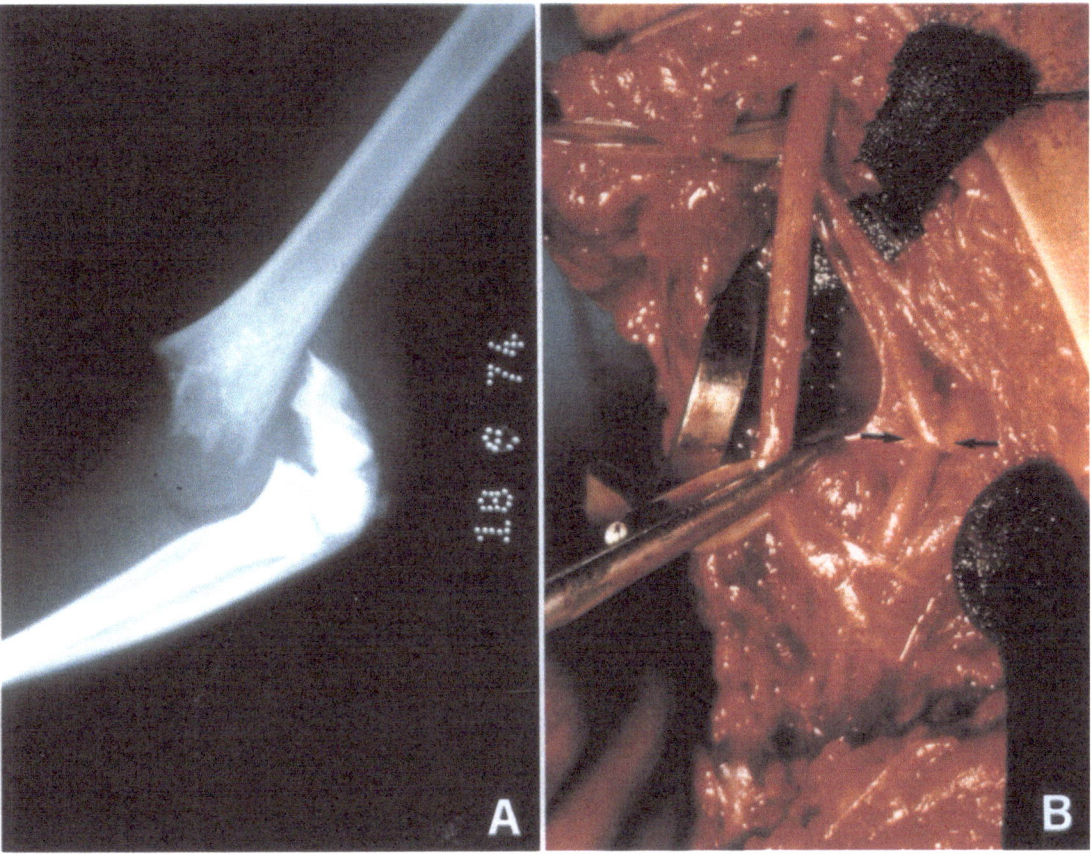

Fig. 1. - P.M., male aged 9: Supracondylar fracture of the right elbow (A). Peripheral ischemic syndrome: emergency exploration reveals the brachial artery pinched (arrow) by the fracture (B). Fasciotomy is performed on the forearm, adventitiectomy on the artery, and Kirschner wire fixation on the fracture. The outcome features severe elbow stiffness that leaves arthroplasty as the only option.

cation showed temporary paralysis of the median nerve. The ulnar nerve is the most commonly affected neurologic structure (12 of 16 of the cases of pure lateral elbow dislocation). That the ulnar nerve is never involved in posterolateral dislocation can be explained by the fact that the roof of the epitrochlear-olecranal groove is torn and the nerve, sliding backwards, can achieve full mobility and therefore escape traction.

In pure lateral dislocation, on the other hand, the integrity of the groove allows traction on the nerve and thus paralysis.

As for Italian authors, Traina (SERTOT, Bologna 1989: personal communication) studied 20 cases of elbow dislocation in children and reported 2 partial radial nerve deficits and 2 ulnar nerve deficits, all temporary ex-

cept for one case in which the ulnar nerve had to be anteposed.

DISLOCATION OF THE ELBOW WITH FRACTURE OF THE EPITROCHLEA

According to Watson-Jones (37), 25% of elbow dislocations are accompanied by epitrochlear fracture. The epitrochlea ossifies at about 18 years old, and up to this age the epiphyseal line is an area of minor resistance. Therefore, lacking the medial restraint, the median nerve can become entrapped inside the joint either during or following incorrect reduction maneuvers.

The rarity of median nerve injury following elbow dislocation is proven by the existence of only 19 cases reported in literature (Table 1) (29). One of the striking features is the young age of these patients (average age 8.2) as well as the relatively long delay (average 7.8 months) before diagnosis and treatment. Nerve entrapment usually occurs in the joint (16 cases), in the epitrochlear callus in case of fracture (2 cases), or in the scar tissue (1 case). There are 3 different modalities of entrapment (6, 9) (Table 2):

1) in posterolateral dislocation, a rupture of the medial portion of the capsule with detachment of the epitrochlear muscles at their insertion points (A)

2) entrapment of the nerve in the callus of an epitrochlear fracture (B)

3) hooking of the nerve, which is folded over and pinched in the joint during incorrect reduction (C); this is one of the rare cases in which epitrochlear fracture is not present.

Table 1

MEDIAN NERVE ENTRAPMENT FOLLOWING ELBOW DISLOCATION

Author	Age	Type of paralysis	Delay before diagnosis and treatment	Joint motion deficit	Location	Arthro-tomy	Treatment	Result	
								Joint motion	Functional recovery
J. Bonvallet 1977	7	Total	5 months	N.R.	Joint	NO	None	N.R.	Unsatisfactory
E.S. Gurdjian 1945	7	Total	5 1/2 months	N.R.	Joint	YES	Neurolysis	N.R.	Good
H.M. Smathers 1945	41	Total	N.R.	N.R.	Scar tissue	NO	Neurolysis	N.R.	Good
L. Mannerfelt 1968	9	Partial	7 days		Joint	YES	Neurolysis	Normal	Excellent
R. Steiger et alii 1969	11	Partial	4 months	Normal	Epitrochlear callus	NO	Neurolysis	Normal	Excellent
	8		10 months	N.R.	Joint	YES	Neurolysis	N.R.	Unsatisfactory
P. Fourrier et alii 1977	11	Partial	21 months	20° flex. 20° ext.	Joint	YES	Neurolysis	Normal	Excellent
J. Hallet 1981	9	Total	2 years	15°	Joint	YES	Neurolysis	N.R.	Unsatisfactory
J.W. Pritchett 1984	8	Total	8 weeks	Normal	Epitrochlear callus	NO	Neurolysis	Normal	Excellent
E.W. Floyd III et alii 1987	13	Total	1 day	20° flex. (gen. anaesth.)	Joint	NO	Neurolysis	Normal	Excellent
	10	Total	1 day	90° flex.	Joint	NO	Neurolysis	Normal	Good
D. Pritchard et alii 1973	12	Partial	8 months	N.R.	Joint	YES	End to end suture	Normal	Excellent
N.A. Rana et alii 1974	8	Total	1 year	N.R.	Joint	YES	End to end suture	N.R.	Excellent
I. Matev 1976		Total	3 months	40° ext.	Joint	NO	End to end suture	Slightly limited	Excellent
	10	Total	1 year	Normal	Joint	NO	End to end suture	N.R.	Insufficient follow-up
N.E. Green 1983	7	Total	4 months	45° ext.	Joint	NO	End to end suture	N.R.	Excellent
H. Ayala 1983	9	Total	3 months	N.R.	Joint	NO	End to end suture	N.R.	Good
	11	Partial	15 months	N.R.	Joint	NO	5 cm resection and graft	N.R.	Good
G. Sacchetti et alii 1989	7	Total	1 year	Normal	Joint	NO	4 cm resection and graft	N.R.	Excellent

The symptoms, especially at the onset, are not uniform. Pain is often absent (18) and paralysis incomplete. A precise neurological examination covering both motor and sensory elements is difficult in children, and, when a simple neuropraxic lesion is suspected, a decision to refrain from exploration is legitimate (28). After 3 weeks an EMG can provide objective information about the type of nerve damage. Three months after dislocation a cortical depression can be seen on the distal humeral metaphysis on the ulnar side and is interpreted as a sign of interruption of the local periosteal reaction due to the abnormal position of the nerve. A streak is also evident at the densest margins distal to the cortical depression, which corresponds to the course of the posteriorly dislocated nerve (18). The neurologic lesion is caused by a combination of traction and friction, and recovery of the nerve, after it is replaced in its anatomical position, is quite rapid.

MRI is the only useful scanning technique in this phase, since it is capable of showing the nerve entrapped in the joint. In late exploration, if the nerve is completely paralyzed, nerve resection and neurorrhaphy by means of either an end to end suture or a graft are indicated.

Good results are possible if the suture is made within 2 months after trauma according to both Merle D'Aubigné (19) and our own experience (29) (Fig. 2).

ELBOW DISLOCATION WITH ENTRAPMENT OF THE EPITROCHLEAR FRAGMENT IN THE JOINT

In children, fracture-dislocation of the epitrochlea usually occurs due to the traction of the flexor muscles when the elbow is dislocated laterally. During reduction, the avulsed epiphysis can easily become entrapped in the joint space (Table 3). In all 5 cases of pure lateral dislocation with the epitrochlear fragment in the joint reported by Watson-Jones, the ulnar nerve was affected. Therefore, in a case of complex elbow trauma when the epitrochlea cannot be seen on the standard x-ray, there is a good chance that the epitrochlear fragment is inside the joint space, providing further grounds for surgery. As a matter of fact, if the bone fragment is not removed there could be permanent consequences such as limited range of motion and subsequent arthritic changes. Furthermore, the compressed ulnar nerve could be irreparably damaged. For these reasons, reduction and fixation of the epitrochlea as well as

Table 2

A

B

C

decompression of the nerve must be performed immediately; otherwise there is no other option but anteposition of the nerve. One of our patients who was treated one month after trauma and reviewed 10 years later achieved a good functional result yet showed grasp weakness as well as deficit of the third palmar interosseous muscle (Fig. 3).

SUPRACONDYLAR FRACTURES

In the 87 cases reported by Watson-Jones (37), both the displacement of the fragments and the type of immediate or late paralysis it caused are described in detail.

This study suggests that primary involvement of the ulnar nerve is very rare (4 cases), possibly because severe anterolateral displacement also occurs very seldom.

This study shows no primary involvement of the median nerve, while according to D.M. Brooks (Modena, 1976: personal communication), Jones (12), and our own experience, it can be affected by extension fracture.

We agree with D.M. Brooks that paralysis most frequently strikes the anterior interos-

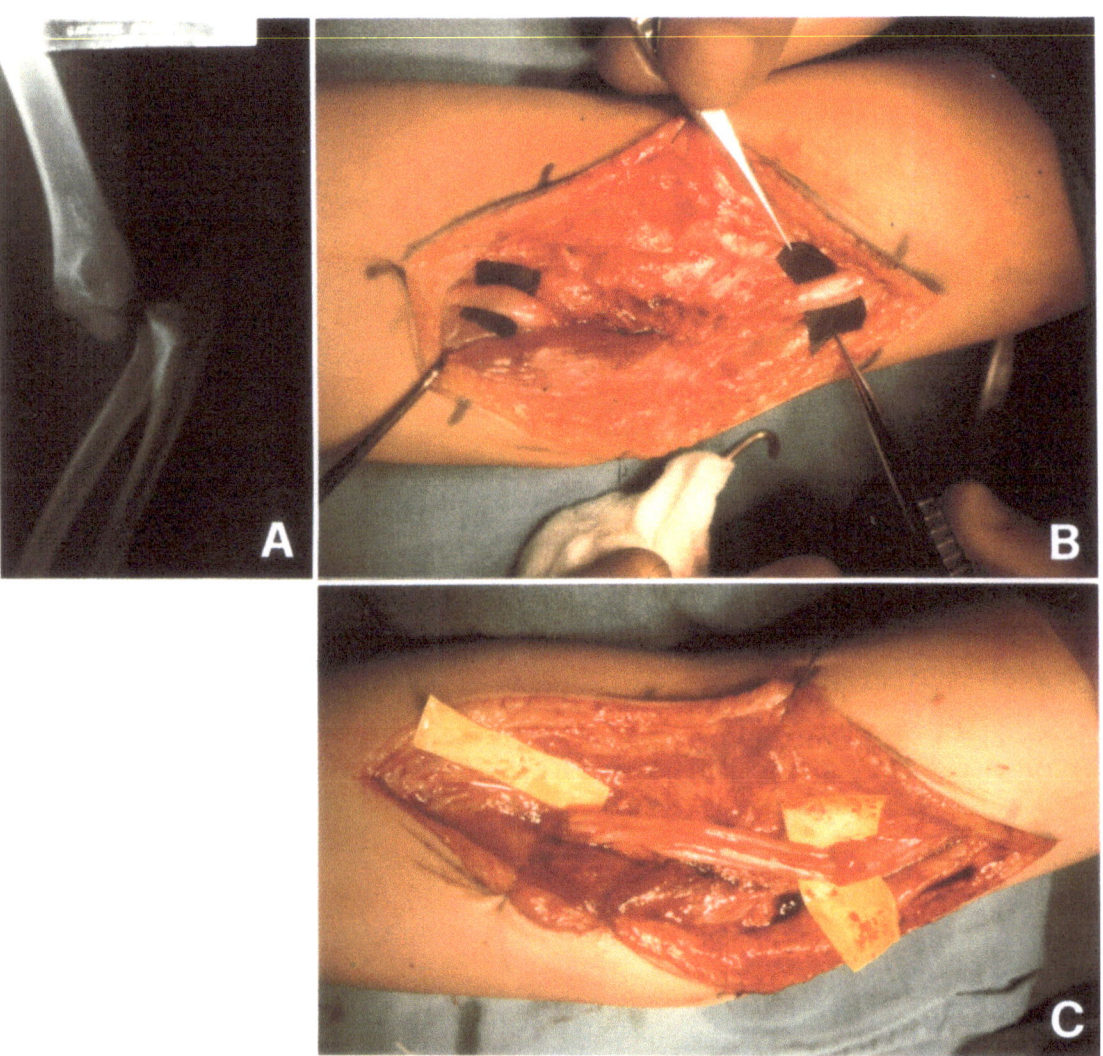

Fig. 2. - G.A., male aged 7: Posterolateral dislocation of the right elbow (A). The dislocation is reduced with the patient under general anesthesia in another hospital. After 8 months of persistent sensory and motor problems due to high paralysis of the median nerve, the antecubital fossa is explored. The median nerve appears to be entrapped in the joint (B). The loose ends are resectioned and sutured with sural nerve grafts (C). After 1 year the nerve shows complete recovery of motor and sensory functions.

seous nerve. Spinner (34) argues that the lesion is a result of traction on the nerve in the proximal forearm rather than a direct supracondylar contusion.

As for the radial nerve, Watson-Jones (37) reports two cases of temporary paralysis accompanying posterolateral displacement of the distal fragment. Our experience regards 3 cases of total paralysis of this nerve that, later examined, was shown to be completely severed in two patients (7 and 8 years old) and intact in the third patient (10 years old). Internal neurolysis in the third patient produced only partial recovery.

Of the 51 cases of humeral fracture reported by Postacchini (25), 11 were accompanied by supracondylar fracture. The paralysis disappeared spontaneously in 10 cases, persisting in only one patient. Therefore, the possibility that the radial nerve may be completely torn as a result of a supracondylar fracture should be considered, even if there have been only 4 reported cases.

Martin (17) recently reported another case in which the proximal segment of the nerve was retracted into the arm, necessitating the use of long sural nerve grafts. In spite of this, a good functional result was achieved.

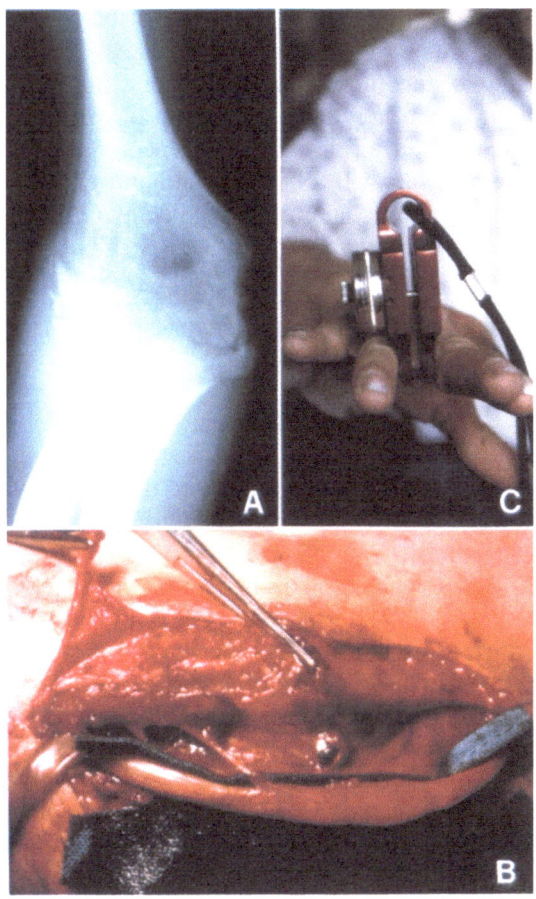

Fig. 3. - V.D., male aged 14: Epitrochlear right fracture of the elbow. Displaced fragment inside the joint and entrapment of ulnar nerve resulting in total paralysis (A). Removal of the epitrochlear fragment from the joint, fixation with a screw, and neurolysis of the ulnar nerve (B). Long-term result features deficit of the third palmar interosseous muscle (C).

Table 3

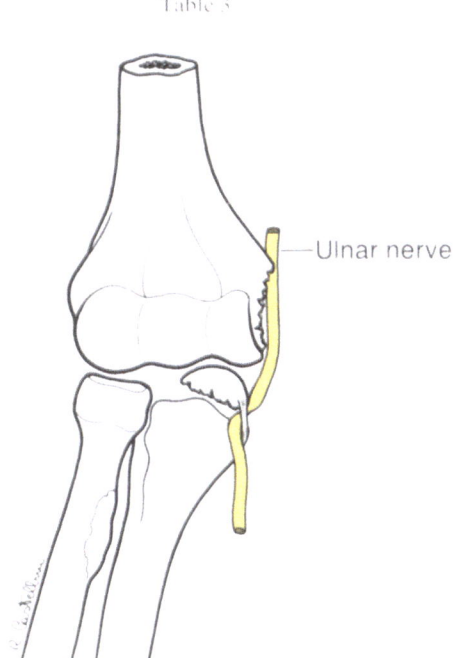

Ulnar nerve

EPIPHYSEAL TRAUMA OF THE TROCHLEA

Supracondylar fractures are rarely complicated by delay or angular deviation in the growth of the distal humerus, and when this does occur the cause is either segmental damage or compression of the underlying epiphysis. A type V Salter-Harris fracture of the trochlea becomes apparent in adulthood as a cubitus varus and is accompanied by local compression of the ulnar nerve. In teenage patients corrective osteotomy is the usually suggested treatment, but when nerve compression is diagnosed in an adult, only the neurologic complication is treated by the surgeon, as the range of motion is usually normal. The angled course of the nerve makes simple decompression insufficient; anteposition of the nerve itself is necessary. In these cases Sahito (Tel Aviv, 1989: personal communication - IFSSH) recommends medial neurolysis in conjunction with deep anteposition of the nerve.

EPIPHYSEAL FRACTURE-SEPARATION OF THE CAPITULUM HUMERI

This lesion occurs in patients between 5 and 15 years of age. If the fragment remains attached to the periosteum and the tendinous origin of the epicondylar muscles, it can become displaced and rotate 90 degrees. In this case there is no chance of spontaneous repair; healing can only be achieved with fibrous tissue, and cubitus valgus develops over time.

In adults this lesion is often accompanied by late paralysis of the ulnar nerve. A delayed operation focuses on the neurologic lesion rather than the skeletal deformity, as in the case of cubitus varus. Superficial anteposition is performed using three guidelines: protection of the medial cutaneous nerve of the forearm, the inadvertent section of which could trigger severe pain, excision of the medial septum, and the cutting of an epineural flap that, sutured at the epimysium, holds the nerve at the site of anteposition. During the operation, it is important to verify the freedom of movement of the nerve during elbow motion. We resort to deep muscle anteposition when pain is the main symptom or after incorrectly performed superficial anteposition.

FRACTURES OF THE PROXIMAL RADIUS AND THE RADIAL HEAD

Spinner (33) reports two instances of posterior interosseous nerve paralysis in cases of radial head fracture, confirming the anatomical vulnerability of the deep branch.

Spinner also agrees with other authors (36) as to the possibility of neural lesion during radial head resection. We have treated only one case of posterior interosseous nerve

paralysis caused by a complex fracture of the radial head; the patient showed no signs of recovery after 6 months.

MONTEGGIA LESION

Spinner (32) reports 4 cases of reversible paralysis of the posterior interosseous nerve resulting from a Monteggia fracture-dislocation. Morris (20) reported a particularly interesting case in which the irreducibility of the Monteggia lesion was due to the interposition of the radial nerve. The present study includes 3 such cases. In the first two, surgery revealed the hooking of the nerve at the radius, with almost full recovery after reduction of the dislocation. In the third case, the inveterate dislocation of the radial head caused irreversible paralysis of the nerve; this was recorded as a late complication of initial incorrect treatment of a Monteggia lesion (Fig. 4).

Paralysis of the posterior interosseous nerve has never been reported in congenital dislocation of the radial head (24).

OLECRANON FRACTURE

In olecranon fractures, the most frequent neurologic complication involves the ulnar nerve. In our experience this can happen in three situations: 1) in the tension-band technique, if the figure-8 wiring is placed too close to the olecranal groove, the nerve may suffer a foreign body reaction; 2) in pseudoarthrosis of the olecranon formerly fixed with a screw, cubitus valgus and neurologic deficit are often present; 3) in post-traumatic degenerative arthritis of the elbow, the involvement of the osteophytes inside the epitrochlear-olecranal groove provokes the symptoms and justifies anteposition.

ULNAR NERVE COMPLICATIONS CAUSED BY SKELETAL TRACTION OF THE OLECRANON

Among the traumatic lesions with several mechanisms (point, thermal agent, traction), the iatrogenic lesions caused by application of

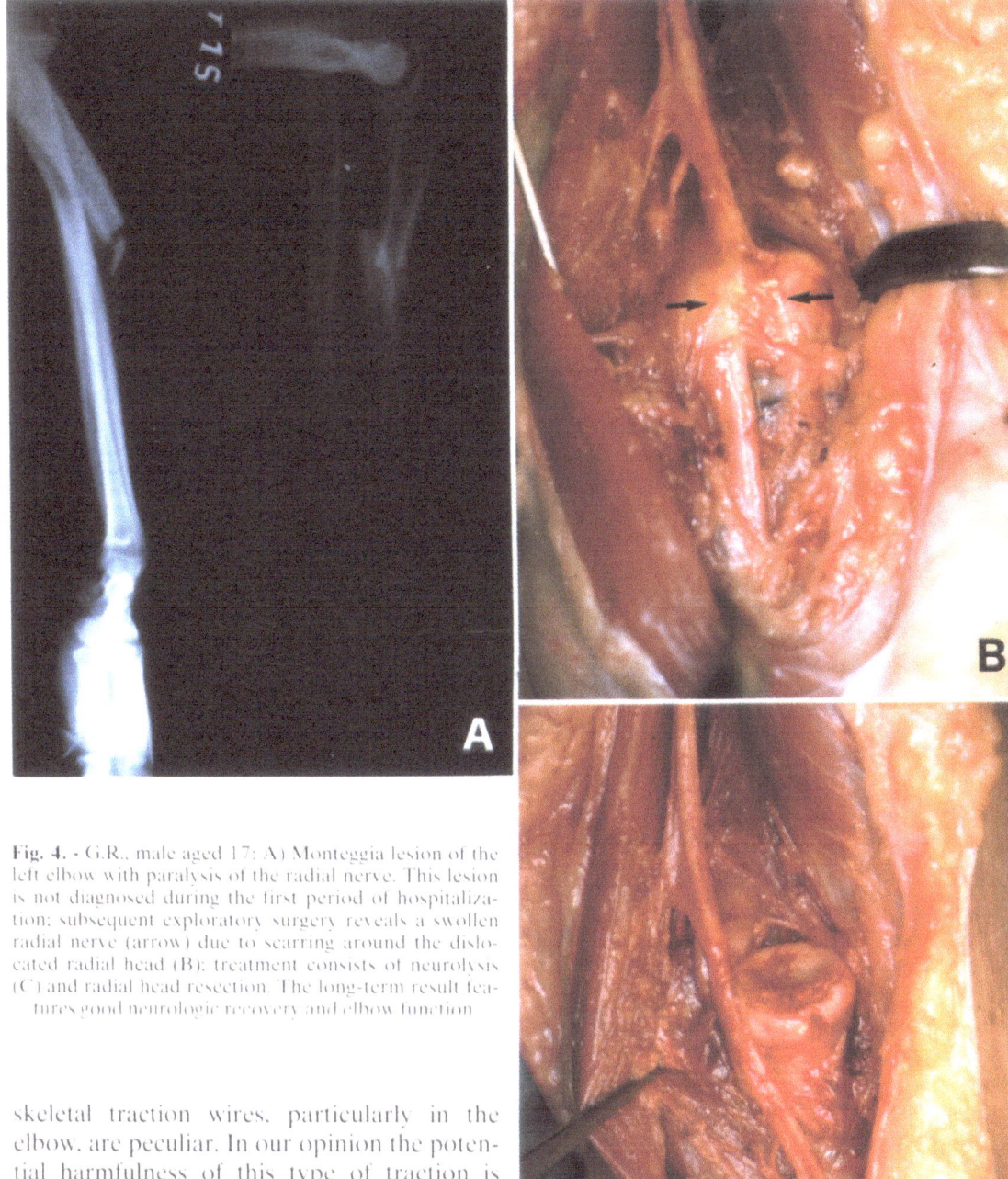

Fig. 4. - G.R., male aged 17: A) Monteggia lesion of the left elbow with paralysis of the radial nerve. This lesion is not diagnosed during the first period of hospitalization; subsequent exploratory surgery reveals a swollen radial nerve (arrow) due to scarring around the dislocated radial head (B); treatment consists of neurolysis (C) and radial head resection. The long-term result features good neurologic recovery and elbow function.

skeletal traction wires, particularly in the elbow, are peculiar. In our opinion the potential harmfulness of this type of traction is underestimated and it should be used with extreme caution in uncooperative patients. We treated six such cases, 2 of which surgically (13). The symptoms, such as acute pain and paralysis, can either appear early or late (2 cases), the latter probably because the traction wire is situated near the nerve but is not in direct contact with it. The three patients treated conservatively did not recover any sensory or motor function, while internal neurolysis yielded excellent results. In another case the lesion was linked to the pressure caused by a stirrup that was too tight. This lesion, despite the embarassment of its iatrogenic origin, should be adequately treated, and limited internal neurolysis corresponding to the crossing of the K-wire yields excellent functional results.

CONCLUSIONS

Neurovascular complications are a very important factor in the final functional outcome of traumas about the elbow. It is very important to realize that almost any lesion, except rare epiphyseal fracture-separation of the lateral epicondyle, may provoke a compartment syndrome that can lead to Volkmann's contracture.

Furthermore, as we chose to describe the most common neurologic complication for every type of fracture or dislocation, it became apparent that these should be diagnosed and treated early. Focusing attention exclusively on the fracture in a region like the elbow, through which the three nerves that govern hand function travel, may not be a wise choice if the overall function and not just perfect reduction and fixation of a fracture is the goal of treatment.

REFERENCES

1) ASHBELL T.S., KLEINERT H.E., KUTZ J.E.: Vascular injuries about the elbow. *Clin. Orthop.* 1967; **50**: 107-127.
2) AYALA H., DE PABLOS J., GONZALEZ J., MARTINEZ A.: Entrapment of the median nerve after posterior dislocation of the elbow. *Microsurgery* 1983; **4**: 215-220.
3) BONVALLET J.M.: Paralysie du nerf médian après incarceration dans une luxation du coude. *Ann. Chir.* 1977; **31** (4): 345-349.
4) EATON R.G., GREEN W.T.: Volkmann's Ischemia. A volar compartment syndrome of the forearm. *Clin. Orthop.* 1975; **113**: 58-64.
5) FLOYD III W.E., GEBHARDT M.C., EMANS J.B.: Intra-articular entrapment of the median nerve after elbow dislocation in children. *J. Hand Surg.* 1987; **12-A** (5): 704-707.
6) FOURRIER P., LEVAL J.P., COLLIN J.: Incarcération du nerf médian au cours d'une luxation du coude. *Rev. Chir. Orthop.* 1977; **63**: 13-16.
7) GURDJIAN E.S., SMATHERS H.M.: Peripheral nerve injury in fractures and dislocation of long bones. *J. Neurosurgery* 1945; **2**: 202.
8) GREEN N.E.: Entrapment of the median nerve following elbow dislocation. *J. Ped. Orthop.* 1983; **3**: 384-386.
9) HALLET J.: Entrapment of the median nerve after dislocation of the elbow. *J. Bone Jt Surg.* 1981; **63-B**: 403-412.
10) HEPPENSTALL R.B., SAPEGA A.A., SCOTT R., SHENTON D., PARK S.Y., MARIS J., CHANCE B.: The compartment syndrome. An experimental and clinical study of muscular energy metabolism using phosphorus nuclear magnetic resonance spectroscopy. *Clin. Orthop.* 1988; **226**: 138-155.
11) HOLDEN C.E.A.: Compartmental syndromes following trauma. *Clin. Orthop.* 1975; **113**: 95-102.
12) JONES E.T., LOUIS D.S.: Median nerve injuries associated with supracondylar fractures of the humerus in children. *Clin. Orthop.* 1980; **150**: 181-186.
13) LANDI A., DE LUCA S., LUCHETTI R., DE SANTIS G., SORAGNI O., SACCHETTI G.L.: Particular aspects of lesions in continuity of peripheral nerves. *J. of W.P.O.A.*, in press.
14) LANDI A., DE SANTIS G., SACCHETTI G.L., CIUCARELLI C., LUCHETTI R., BEDESCHI P.: Utilità della TAC nella valutazione della sindrome di Volkmann degli arti. *G.I.O.T.* 1989; **15**: 553-566.
15) LIPSCOMB P.R., BURLESON J.R.: Vascular and neural complications in supracondylar fractures of the humerus in children. *J. Bone Jt Surg.* 1955; **37-A** (3): 487-492.
16) MANNERFELT L.: Median nerve entrapment after dislocation of the elbow. Report of a case. *J. Bone Jt Surg.* 1968; **50-B**: 152-155.
17) MARTIN D.F., TOLO V.T., SELLERS D.S., WEILAND D.J.: Radial nerve laceration and retraction associated with a supracondylar fracture of the humerus. *J. Hand Surg.* 1989; **14-A** (3): 542-546.
18) MATEV I.: A radiological sign of entrapment of the median nerve in the elbow joint after posterior dislocation. A report of two cases. *J. Bone Jt Surg.* 1976; **58-B**: 353-355.
19) MERLE D'AUBIGNÈ R., VALENTIN P.: Résultat des réparations tronculaires du médian et du cubital. *Acta Chir.* 1965; 743-754.
20) MORRIS A.H.: Irreducible Monteggia lesion with radial nerve entrapment. A case report. *J. Bone Jt Surg.* 1974; **56-A** (8): 1744-1746.
21) MUBARAK S., HARGENS A.R., OWEN C.A., GARETTO L.P., AKESON W.H.: The wick catheter technique for measurement of intramuscular pressure. *J. Bone Jt Surg.* 1976; **58-A**:

1016-1020.

22) MUBARAK S., OWEN C.A., HARGENS A.R., GARETTO L.P., AKESON W.H.: Acute compartment syndromes: diagnosis and management with the aid of the wick catheter. *J. Bone Jt Surg.* 1978; **60-A**: 1091-1095.

23) MUBARAK S., CARROL N.C.: Volkmann's contracture in children: aetiology and prevention. *J. Bone Jt Surg.* 1979; **61-B** (3): 285-293.

24) NIEMANN K.M.W., GOULD J.S., SIMMONS B., BORA F.W. JR.: *The pediatric upper extremity. Diagnosis and management.* W.B. Saunders Co. Philadelphia, 1986, pag. 219.

25) POSTACCHINI F., MORACE G.B.: Fratture dell'omero associate a paralisi del nervo radiale. *G.I.O.T.* 1988; **14**: 467-477.

26) PRITCHARD D.J., LINSCHEID R.L., SVIEN H.J.: Intra-articular median nerve entrapment with dislocation of the elbow. *Clin. Orthop.* 1973; **90**: 100-103.

27) PRITCHETT J.W.: Entrapment of the median nerve after dislocation of the elbow. *J. Pediat. Orthop.* 1984; **4**: 752-753.

28) RANA N.A., KENWRIGHT Y., TAYLOR R.G., RUSHWORTH G.: Complete lesion of the median nerve associated with dislocation of the elbow joint. *Acta Orthop. Scand.* 1974; **45**: 365-369.

29) SACCHETTI G.L., DE SANTIS G., CASERTA G., CAVANA R., LANDI A.: Intrappolamento del nervo mediano dopo lussazione di gomito. *Atti S.E.R.T.O.T.*, in press.

30) SAINT CLAIRE STRANGE F.C.: Entrapment of the median nerve after dislocation of the elbow. *J. Bone Jt Surg.* 1982; **64-B**: 224-225.

31) SPEAR H.C., JANES J.M.: Rupture of the brachial artery accompanying dislocation of the elbow or supracondylar fracture. *J. Bone Jt Surg.* 1951; **33-A** (4): 889-894.

32) SPINNER M., FREUNDLICH B.D., TEICHER J.: Posterior interosseous nerve palsy as a complication of Monteggia fracture in children. *Clin. Orthop.* 1968; **58**: 141-145.

33) SPINNER M.: *Injuries to the major branches of peripheral nerves of the forearm.* W.B. Saunders Co. Philadelphia, 1974 pag. 112-113.

34) SPINNER M., SCHREIBER S.N.: Anterior interosseous nerve paralysis as a complication of supracondylar fractures of the humerus in children. *J. Bone Jt Surg.* 1969; **51-A**: 1584-1586.

35) STEIGER R.N., LARRICK R.B., MEYER T.L.: Median nerve entrapment following elbow dislocation in children. *J. Bone Jt Surg.* 1969; **51-A**: 381-385.

36) STRACHAN J.C.H., ELLIS E.W.: Vulnerability of the posterior interosseous nerve during radial head resection. *J. Bone Jt Surg.* 1971; **53-B**: 320-323.

37) WATSON-JONES R.: Primary nerve lesions in injuries of the elbow and wrist. *J. Bone Jt Surg.* 1930; **12-B**: 121-140.

38) WATSON-JONES R.: *Fractures and joint injuries.* Churchill Livingstone, New York, 1976; 5ª ed., p. 604.

39) WHITESIDES T.E. JR., HANEY T.C., MORIMOTO K., HIROSHI H.: Tissue pressure measurements as a determinant for the need of fasciotomy. *Clin. Orthop.* 1975; **113**: 43-51.

40) ZIPERMAN H.H.: Acute arterial injuries in the Korean War. *Ann. Surg.* 1954; **139**: 1-8.

Isolated traumatic lesions
of the musculocutaneous nerve

L. Celli - C. Rovesta - A. Balli - M.C. Marongiu

INTRODUCTION

Traumatic lesions of the musculocutaneous nerve are uncommon.

In Sunderland's study (14) of war injuries of the peripheral nerves, the musculocutaneous nerve is affected in only 1-3% of the cases. The reason for this is that the nerve has a short, deep course and is protected by muscular and bony structures.

The musculocutaneous nerve is more frequently affected by the trauma that causes brachial plexus lesions.

Out of the 362 surgical revisions of the brachial plexus we performed from 1971 to 1988, 98 patients (27%) had lesions of the musculocutaneous nerve. These were either isolated or associated with lesions of the lateral secondary trunk or other nearby nerves (median, radial, axillary).

The purpose of this study is to discuss the *isolated* lesions of the musculocutaneous nerve that, in our experience, are caused by one of three mechanisms:

— repeated microtrauma (nerve tunnel syndrome)
— indirect trauma
— direct trauma.

ANATOMICAL REFERENCES

The musculocutaneous nerve is composed of fibers from the C5 and C6 nerve roots, and often a small contingent from the C7 nerve root. The nerve originates from the lateral secondary trunk, proceeds downward and laterally to the median nerve, and after supplying the ramus for the coracobrachialis muscle, it perforates it (perforating nerve of Casserio) (Fig. 1), arriving at the space between the biceps and the anterior brachialis, which it in-

nervates. Proceeding downward between these two muscles, it approaches the skin in order to cross the deep fascia in the anterolateral portion of the elbow. Distally it becomes subcutaneous and turns into the lateral cutaneous nerve of the forearm, innervating the dermatome of its two terminal anterior and posterior branches (15).

There can exist some anomalies in the origin and course of the nerve. For instance, in 3-6% of the population it originates di-

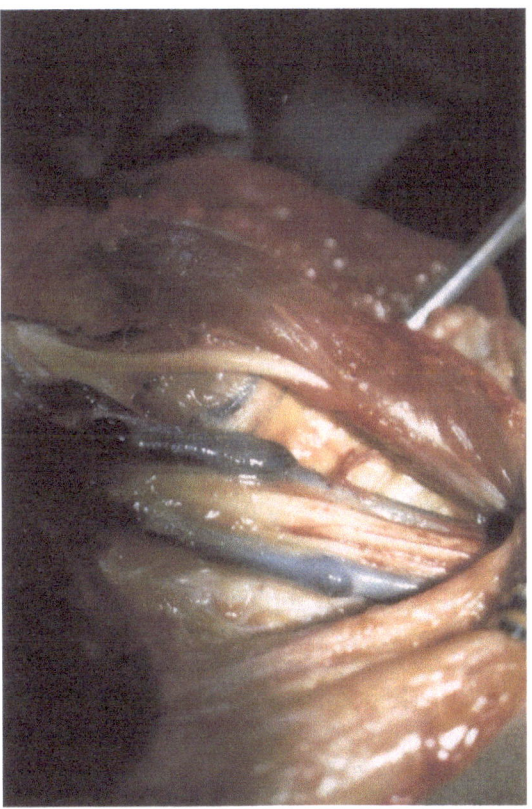

Fig. 1. - The musculocutaneous nerve, which originates from the lateral secondary trunk, perforates the coracobrachialis muscle.

rectly from the median nerve, while in 14% it circumvents the belly of the coracobrachialis without perforating it (10).

LESIONS CAUSED BY REPEATED MICRO-TRAUMA (NERVE TUNNEL SYNDROME)

The nerve is very vulnerable to compression at its point of entrance into the coracobrachialis muscle. When fully contracted, this muscle can act as a pair of pliers and compress the nerve. Hypertrophy and overwork of the biceps and anterior brachialis can contribute to the onset of compression syndrome. Braddon and Wolfe described this rare disease in an athlete (3). The risk of compression is even higher if shoulder abduction and retroposition, which tense up both the coracobrachialis muscle and the musculocutaneous nerve, are added.

Clinical picture

Subjective features

Pain in the subcoracoid region radiates to the volar surface of the arm and the anterolateral surface of the forearm. It intensifies when the elbow is flexed against resistance (i.e. lifting weights). The limb tires easily and may have paresthesia and tingling at night.

Objective features

There are no changes in muscle trophism. Pain can be evoked by palpation of the subcoracoid area (positive Tinel sign) and contraction of the coracobrachialis against resistance (anteposition and adduction of the arm). The biceps reflex may be impaired, and there is hypesthesia of the anterolateral surface of the forearm (Fig. 2).

The EMG, which is negative in the primary phase, may show a normal coracobrachialis muscle yet slight neural damage in the biceps and the anterior brachialis.

Motor and sensory conduction in the Erb-axilla pathway may be slower compared to the contralateral limb (16).

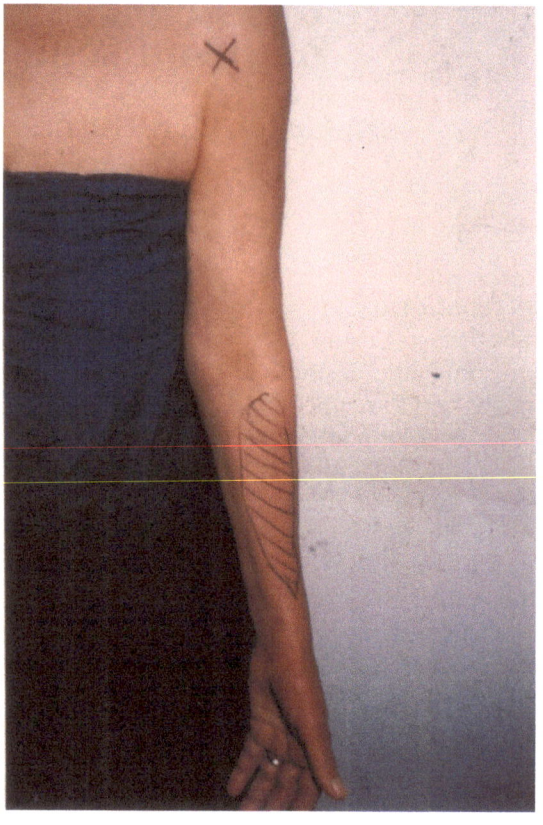

Fig. 2. - The elbow flexor muscles tire easily in cases of musculocutaneous nerve compression at the coracobrachialis muscle. Other symptoms are a positive Tinel sign in the subcoracoid area, and tingling and hypesthesia in the lateral region of the forearm.

Differential diagnosis

Musculocutaneous nerve tunnel syndrome must be compared to:

C5-C6 cervicobrachialgia. In this case the differential diagnosis is based on the following criteria:

— functional limitation of the spine, movement of which may evoke pain in the corresponding distribution;

— involvement of muscles other than the elbow flexors (deltoid, supraspinatus, brachioradialis)

Tendinopathy of the long head of the biceps. Criteria are as follows:

— pain in the biceps sulcus that intensifies at elbow and shoulder movements which subject the long head of the biceps to passive and active traction. The pain subsides after an intraarticular infiltration;

— absence of motor and sensory deficits and normal EMG.

Materials and methods

From 1983 to 1988 we observed 3 cases of musculocutaneous nerve tunnel syndrome. In all three cases, pain was first felt after prolonged exertion of the upper limb involving repeated contraction of both coracobrachialis and elbow flexors.

In two of the patients, curtailment of manual labor, medical treatment, and electrotherapy on the biceps led to regression of pain and full recovery of elbow flexion in 6 months.

In the remaining case, persistence of pain and increased functional limitation led us to prescribe surgery. The isolation of the musculocutaneous nerve after its emergence from the lateral secondary trunk revealed an anomaly in the course of the axillary artery in that it followed the nerve through the coracobrachialis.

A combination of neurolysis and arteriolysis led to complete remission of pain and recovery of the force of contraction after 2 months (7).

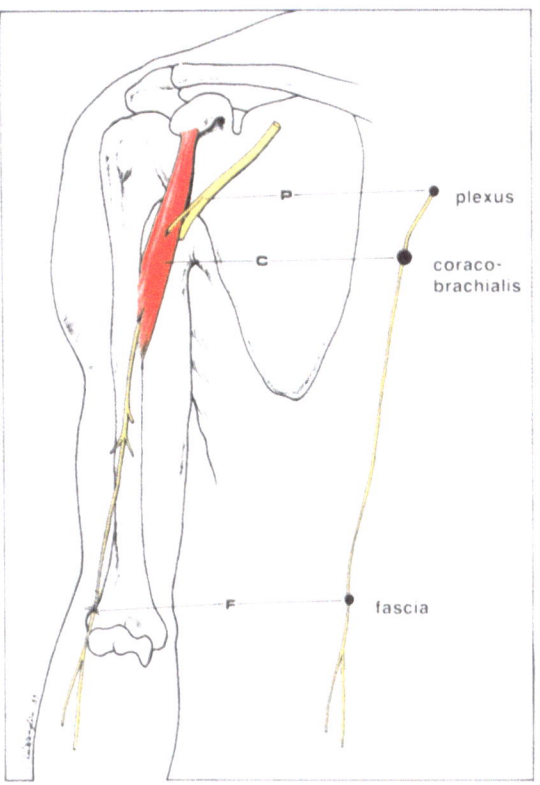

Fig. 3. - The musculocutaneous nerve has three points of attachment: the main one at its entrance into the coracobrachialis (C), the second at its point of origin from the lateral secondary trunk of the plexus (P), and the third at its passage through the brachial fascia (F).

LESIONS CAUSED BY INDIRECT TRAUMA

The musculocutaneous nerve has its main point of attachment at its entrance into the coracobrachialis muscle (C), plus two others at its extremes — its origin at the lateral secondary trunk of the plexus (P) and its entrance into the brachial fascia of the sensory branch (F) (Fig. 3).

Movements that pull these points away from each other cause *traction* of the nerve, and are listed as follows:

— *abduction and retroposition of the shoulder* tighten the axillary neurovascular bundle and may damage the nerve at its proximal attachment. This may be aggravated if the elbow is extended (13) (Fig. 4A).

— *retroposition and external rotation of the shoulder* completely loosen the fibers of the coracobrachialis muscle and cause traction of the musculocutaneous nerve. In this situation the muscular opening closes down on the already stretched nerve. Chances of nerve lesion are very high (Fig. 4B).

— *extension of the elbow* leads to traction of the musculocutaneous nerve at its entrance into the antebrachial fascia (16). The terminal sensory branch of the nerve may be injured (Fig. 4C).

The rapid execution of these movements, either alone or together, can cause traction injury to the nerve, which can then be aggravated by compression at the coracobrachialis and the plexus. Direct compression may occur in the arm (11) or on the terminal sensory branch in the elbow (5).

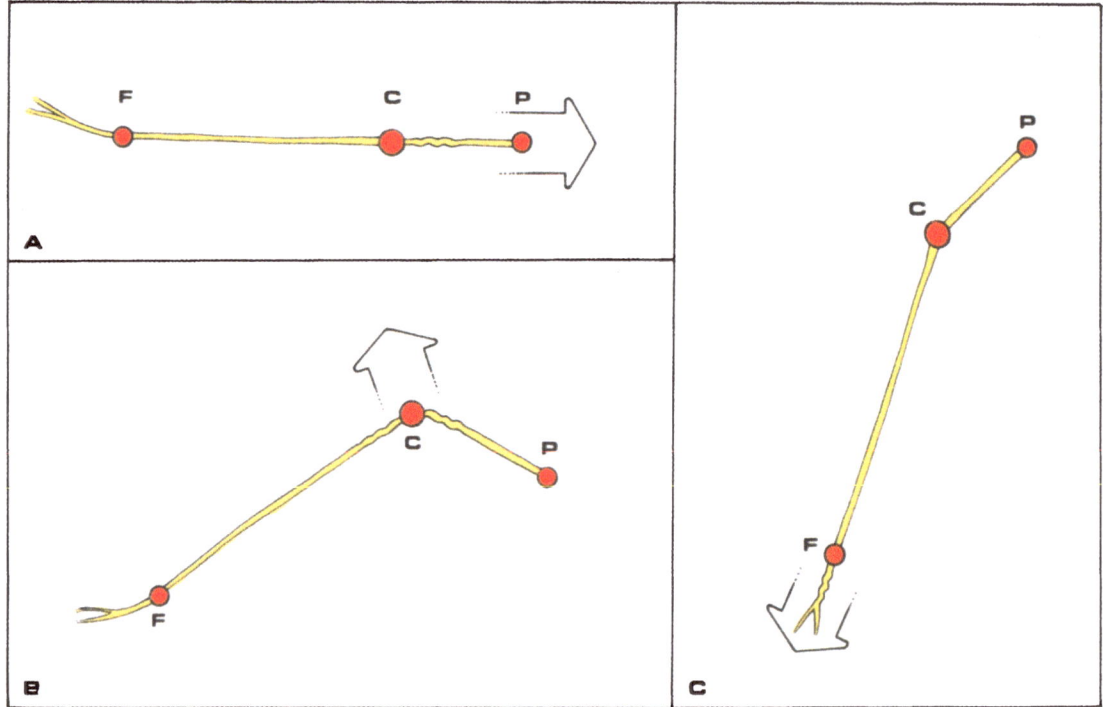

Fig. 4. - Indirect mechanisms of injury: A) *Abduction and retroposition of the shoulder* tighten the neurovascular bundle, causing traction of the musculocutaneous nerve from P to C. B) *Retroposition and external rotation of the shoulder* tighten the coracobrachialis muscle (C), causing traction of the musculocutaneous nerve. C) *Elbow extension* leads to traction of the nerve in its passage through the antebrachial fascia (F).

Clinical picture

Subjective

There is pain on the anterolateral surface of the arm and in the lateral portion of the forearm, where hypesthesia can occur. The main clinical feature is severe hyposthenia when the elbow is flexed.

Objective

Severe hypotrophy of the flexor muscles of the arm rarely compromises the active flexion capacity of the elbow, thanks to the compensation of the brachioradialis, epitrochlearis, and epicondylar muscles (Fig. 5A).

Hypesthesia of the lateral forearm is always present. The Tinel sign is positive in the subcoracoid region (Fig. 5B), and the EMG reveals neurologic damage in both the biceps and the anterior brachialis.

In case of compression and stretching of the terminal sensory branch, there is no motor deficit.

Differential diagnosis

It is necessary to differentiate between traumatic lesion of the musculocutaneous nerve and *traction lesion of the brachial plexus*. In a C5-C6 lesion, deficits occur in the infraspinatus, supraspinatus, deltoid, and brachioradialis muscles in addition to the elbow flexors.

In lesions of the lateral secondary trunk, deficits also affect the pronator teres and the flexor carpi radialis, with widespread hypesthesia even in the thumb and index fingers.

The differential diagnosis with *rupture of the long head of the biceps* is less difficult. A diagnosis of tendon rupture is confirmed when the anterior brachialis muscle is functioning normally, a muscular mass is detached

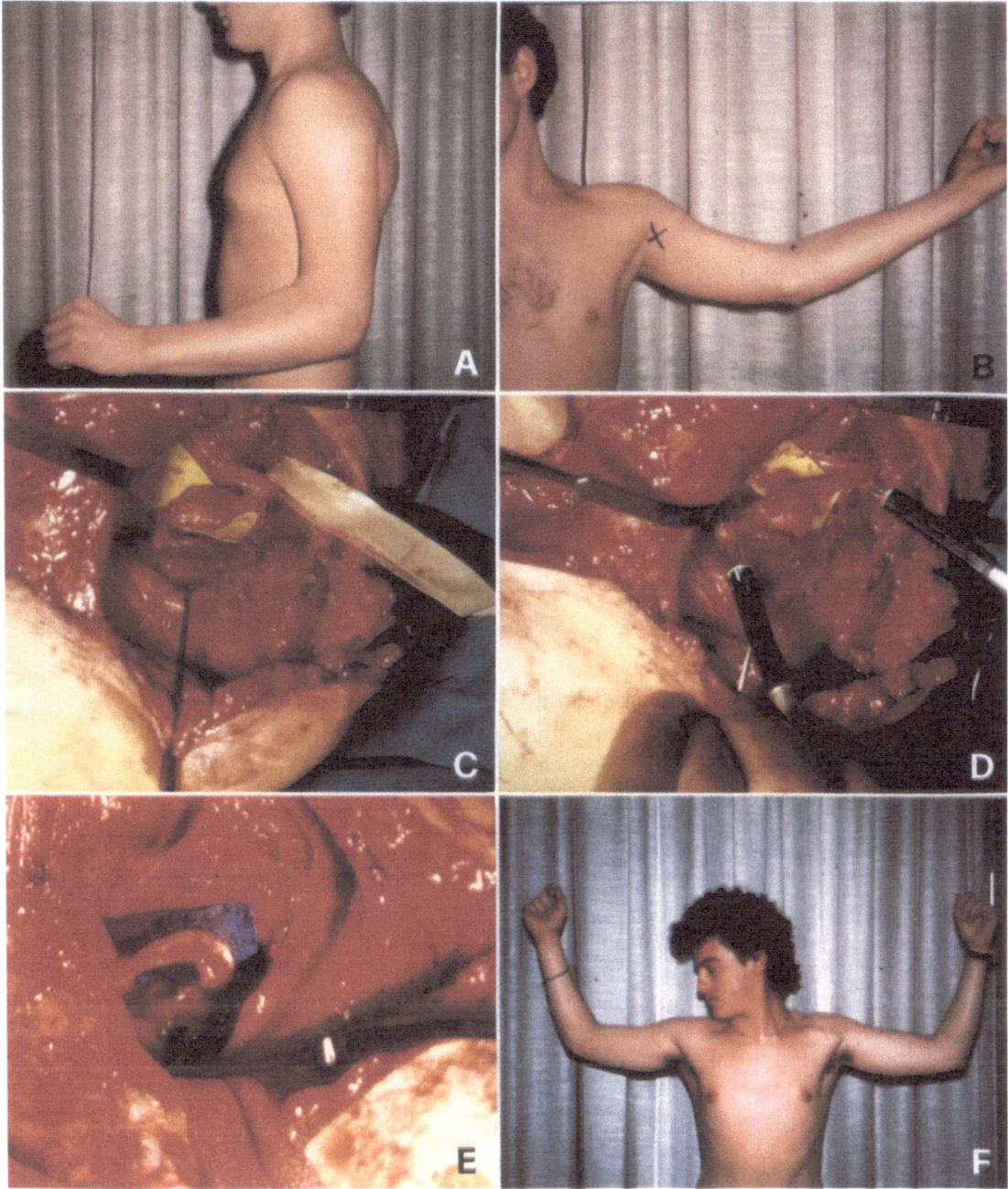

Fig. 5. - Lesion of the musculocutaneous nerve at its entrance into the coracobrachialis muscle. A) *Preoperative view*: severe hypotrophy of both the biceps and the anterior brachialis; elbow flexion is still possible because of the compensation of the brachioradialis and epicondylar muscles. B) Positive Tinel sign at the entrance of the nerve into the coracobrachialis. C) *Operative view*: large neuroma at the entrance of the coracobrachialis. D) EMG of the damaged nerve section during the operation. E) Replacement of the damaged section with two grafts. F) *Postoperative view*: clinical examination one year after surgery shows good recovery of strength and trophism of the biceps and anterior brachialis muscles.

distally, there is no sensory deficit, and the EMG shows no neurologic damage.

Materials and methods

This study consists of four cases of isolated traction injury of the musculocutaneous nerve treated from 1980 to 1988. The mechanism of injury was clear in two cases (retro-position and external rotation with shoulder abduction against resistance).

These four patients were treated with surgery 2-8 months after injury, after there had been either no (3 cases) or only slight (1 case) spontaneous recovery.

Surgical treatment was limited to lateral neurolysis in the last case because a continuous anatomical and electrophysiologic lesion was found operatively; in the other cases the nerve was completely severed, and therefore reconstructed with grafts (Table 1).

Table 1

Patient	Age	Preop.	Operation	Follow-up	Postop.
D.S.	18	M_0	2 grafts (8 cm)	12 months	M_5
R.L.	18	M_0	2 grafts (7 cm)	13 months	M_4
B.S.	36	M_1	neurolysis	10 months	M_5
B.M.	26	M_0	2 grafts (10 cm)	8 months	M_5

LESIONS CAUSED BY DIRECT TRAUMA

Gunshot wounds and fractures of the humerus (14) are common causes of direct lesion of the musculocutaneous nerve, but other iatrogenous causes have also been reported: internal fixation of the proximal humerus, and, more commonly, operations to stabilize habitual shoulder dislocation (1, 2, 6).

In the latter case, the trauma can occur in various ways: 1) inadvertent section of the nerve; 2) stretching of the nerve during exposure of the area to be operated on (Bristow and Laterjet techniques); 3) injury to the nerve during the transfer of the tip of the coracoid process and the corocoid muscles (especially the coracobrachialis) onto the glenoid.

The individual anatomical characteristics of the nerve can make it prone to injury. At its origin, when it branches off from the lateral secondary trunk and enters immediately into the coracobrachialis, it is vulnerable to traction if the coracoid process shifts (10).

Clinical picture

The extent of sensory and motor deficit depends on the severity of the neurologic damage and is the same as in the previously described lesions.

Diagnosis can be difficult because of concomitant lesions.

Material and method

This study comprises three iatrogenous lesions of the musculocutaneous nerve treated from 1980 to 1988. Two of these were partial, temporary lesions following anterior stabilization of the shoulder, while the remaining lesion was a complete rupture inflicted during internal fixation of a humeral fracture using the anterior transdeltoid-biceps approach.

This last lesion was treated surgically using nerve grafts, which yielded good muscular recovery after about a year.

CONCLUSIONS

Isolated traumatic lesions of the musculocutaneous nerve often occur at its point of entrance into the coracobrachialis muscle. Nerve tunnel syndrome is rare; isolated traumatic traction lesion is more common. When faced with pain and limitation of elbow flexion, which is too frequently attributed to spinal or musculotendinous disease of the shoulder and arm, isolated traumatic lesions of the musculo-cutaneous nerve should always be considered as a possible cause.

In shoulder surgery, and especially in anterior stabilization, direct trauma to the nerve can be avoided by isolating it. If the nerve enters into the muscle prematurely (5% of patients), it may be stretched during execution of the Bristow or Latarjet techniques. In these cases a different method of anterior stabilization should be used (i.e. plastic surgery of the soft tissues).

REFERENCES

1) BACH B.R., O'BRIEN S.J., WARREN R.F., LEIGHTON M.: An unusual neurological complication of the Bristow procedure. *J. Bone Jt Surg.* 1988; **70-A**: 458-460.

2) BATEMAN J.E.: Nerve injuries about the shoulder in sports. *J. Bone Jt Surg.* 1967; **49-A**: 785.

3) BRADDOM R.L., WOLFE C.: Musculocutaneous nerve injury after heavy exercise. *Arch. Phys. Med. Rehabil.* 1978 (1972?); **5**: 383.

4) DUNDORE D.E., DE LISA J.A.: Musculocutaneous nerve palsy: an isolated complication of surgery. *Arch. Phys. Med. Rehabil.* 1979; **60**: 130.

5) HALE: Handbag parestesia. *Lancet* 1976; 470.

6) JEROSCH J., CASTRO W.H.M., COLEMONT J.: A lesion of the musculocutaneous nerve. A rare complication of anterior shoulder dislocation. *Acta Orthop. Belg.* 1989; **55**: 230-232.

7) LUGLI M.G., ROVESTA C., CELLI L.: *Sindromi canalicolari del nervo muscolocutaneo. Atti XII Congresso Nazionale SIRC.* Monduzzi Editore, Bologna, 1986, **1**, 169-174.

8) MAGGI G., FUSARO I., PRIOLI L.: Distacco del capo breve del bicipite brachiale e paralisi del nervo muscolocutaneo in lussazione traumatica della scapolo-omerale (descrizione di un caso). *Chir. Org. Mov.* 1985; **70**: 389-392.

9) MIGLIORINI A., LICOPOLI R., DALMONEGO G.: Neuropatia isolata del nervo muscolocutaneo. *Eur. Med. Phys.* 1984; **20**: 33-36.

10) MORELLI A., PETRUCCI F.S., CECCHI M., MANUPASSA J., PAJARDI G., BEUT F.J.: Le paralisi isolate del nervo muscolo-cutaneo. *Riv. Chir. Mano* 1987; **24**: 369-378.

11) NEIDHARDT J.P., MORIN A., AUTISSIER J.M., LATARJET M.: L'entrée du nerf musculo-cutane dans le coraco-brachial. Applications chirurgicales. Societé de Chirurgie de Lyon 1968; 268-276.

12) PERRICONE G., PRIOLI L., FUSARO I.: Paralisi isolata post-traumatica del nervo muscolocutaneo in sportivi. *Med. Sport.* 1983; **36**: 171-174.

13) PITKOW R.B.: Partial neuroapraxia of the biceps brachil motor nerve simulating tendon rupture. *J. Bone Jt Surg.* **60A**: 1148.

14) SOK MIN KIM, GOODRICH J.A.: Isolated proximal musculocutaneous nerve palsy: case report. *Arch. Phys. Med. Rehabil.* 1984; **65**: 735-736.

15) SUNDERLAND S.: *Nerves and nerve injuries.* Churchill Livingstone, Edinburgh, 1978.

16) TESTUT L.: *Anatomia Umana.* UTET, 1923, vol. 6.

17) TROJABORG W.: Motor and sensory conduction in the musculocutaneous nerve. *J. Neurol. Neurosurg. Psychiatr.* 1976; **39**: 890-899.

18) WEIDMANN E., HUGGLER A.H.: Die Läsion des Nervus musculo-cutaneus bei der operativen Behandlung der habituellen Schulterluxation. *Orthopäde* 1978; **7**: 192-193.

Nonunion of elbow fractures

E. Sartori - G. Sallemi - G. Iacomelli

Nonunion is very uncommon in elbow fractures (distal humerus, olecranon, and radial head), the most frequent outcomes of which are stiffness and malunion.

We found only one reported case of nonunion of the radial head (16) because resection of this structure is widely practiced.

Slightly less rare is nonunion of the distal humerus, with an incidence of about 2% (1, 5, 8, 11, 12, 13).

Nonunion of the olecranon has also become quite rare since therapy in extension, which actually yielded excellent results on the average, and internal fixation with inadequate devices were abandoned (2, 10).

NONUNION OF THE DISTAL HUMERUS

The classification of nonunions of the distal humerus is almost identical to that of acute fractures (9, 11, 16). Their treatment varies according to the fracture site and the condition of the articular surfaces.

We therefore distinguish between articular and extraarticular nonunions.

Supracondylar nonunions are usually treated with plate and screws and autogenous bone grafts. The technique must follow the basic principles of operative treatment for acute fractures (14, 16).

In cases of articular nonunion the articular surfaces must be reconstructed as well as possible, then the articular fragment is fixed to the metadiaphyseal portion of the bone using condylar screws and lateral and medial compression plates or Y plates. The nonunion gaps are then filled with cancellous autogenous bone grafts.

Postoperative management depends on the stability of the fixation. In both supracondylar and isolated condylar fractures, internal fixation using interfragmentary screws or a D.C.P. allows mobilization within the first 10 days.

In both T fractures and cases of unstable fixation because of osteoporosis or repeated surgical intervention, mobilization is postponed for at least three weeks to allow both wound and edema to heal (13).

NONUNION OF THE ULNA

The classification of nonunions of the olecranon is also based on that of the corresponding fractures, too (3, 4, 15). Type I includes transverse nonunions that involve less than 50% of the articular surfaces. Type II are extraarticular, generally minor nonunions caused by avulsion fractures. Type III are transverse nonunions which involve more than 50% of the articular surfaces. Type IV are stable oblique nonunions, while type V are the result of comminuted fractures.

Since type I and II nonunions usually involve one small fragment, the best results are achieved by simply removing it, then carefully reinserting the triceps tendon onto the olecranon using transosseous sutures on the opposite cortex (4).

Transverse and oblique nonunions can be treated using various methods. Good results are obtained with cancellous screws. The proximal fragments must be perforated in order to get a grip on the screw, which must be long enough to provide an adequate hold on the medullary canal of the ulnar metaphysis. The screw should be at least twice or three times as long as the nonunited fragment. Sometimes a washer may be used to keep the head of the screw from penetrating into the tip of the olecranon. The threads must reach

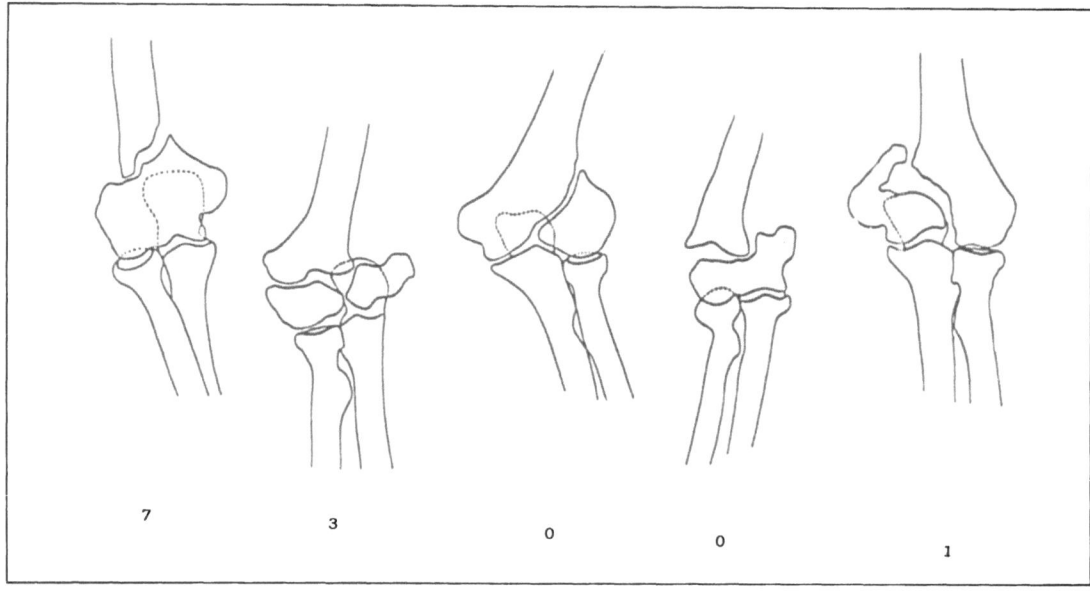

Fig. 1. - Distribution of the nonunions of the distal humerus (11 cases) according to Mitsunaga's classification.

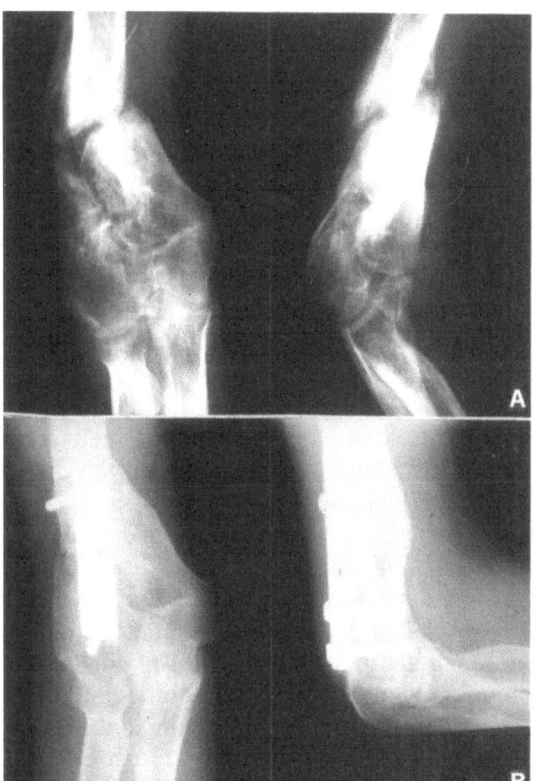

Fig. 2. - AP and lateral x-rays of the right elbow of a 36-year-old male. Residual supracondylar nonunion of a T fracture treated conservatively (A). Treatment with plate and cancellous bone graft (B).

past the nonunion line or the fragment may become displaced. Good results can be achieved with tension band wiring, bicortical screws, or plate and screws in more oblique fractures (14, 16).

Postoperative management requires immobilization at 90 degrees of flexion followed by (after 5-6 days) active mobilization between 0 and 90 degrees. If the fixation is not stable enough, the period of immobilization is lengthened. In type V nonunions, if reconstruction of the articular surfaces of the olecranon is possible, the fragments must be fixed using plate and screws. In elderly patients, if articular surface reconstruction is impossible or if the cartilage is severely damaged, the best results can be achieved by excising the fragments and fixing the proximal and distal segments with a shorter articular surface (4).

MATERIALS AND METHODS

We studied 11 cases of nonunion of the distal humerus, above all supracondylar, treated over a 25-year period (Fig. 1).

The initial treatment had been conservative in 8 cases and surgical in 3 (Fig. 2). Inter-

Table 1
NONUNIONS OF THE DISTAL HUMERUS

Period studied: 1962-1987		
Cases 11	Initial treatment	8 conservative 3 surgical
Average age 42 (range 21-75)		
Males 7	Females	4
Right 6	Left	5
Open 2		
Closed 9		
	Treatment for nonunions	1 interfragmentary screw and bone graft 10 plate and bone graft
Healing in 10 cases (3 of which after reoperation) Residual infectious nonunion in 1 case		

Table 2
NONUNIONS OF THE OLECRANON

Period studied: 1962-1987		
Cases 20	Initial treatment	4 conservative 10 inadequate fixation 5 poorly executed fixation 1 iatrogenous (posterior approach)
Average age 32 (range 17-78)		
Males 12	Females	8
Right 12	Left	8
Open 4		
Closed 16		
	Treatment for nonunions	3 excision of olecranal fragment 14 replacement of screws with tension band wiring 3 screws and bone graft
Healed 20		

nal fixation and cancellous bone grafts were used in all cases. The nonunion healed in 10 instances, but reoperation was necessary in 3 of these. Septic nonunion persisted in 1 patient (Table 1).

In the same period, we treated 20 olecranon nonunions (Fig. 3).

Their initial treatment had been conservative in 4 cases, and nonunion was the result of inadequate fixation in 10 cases and poorly executed fixation in 5 cases (Fig. 4).

The remaining patient had suffered iatrogenous nonunion (Table 2).

CONCLUSIONS

Nonunion of the radial head is very rare. Nonunion of the distal humerus can cause severe disability due to the pain and functional limitation associated with it. Because of the rarity of this lesion (2%), there is no do-

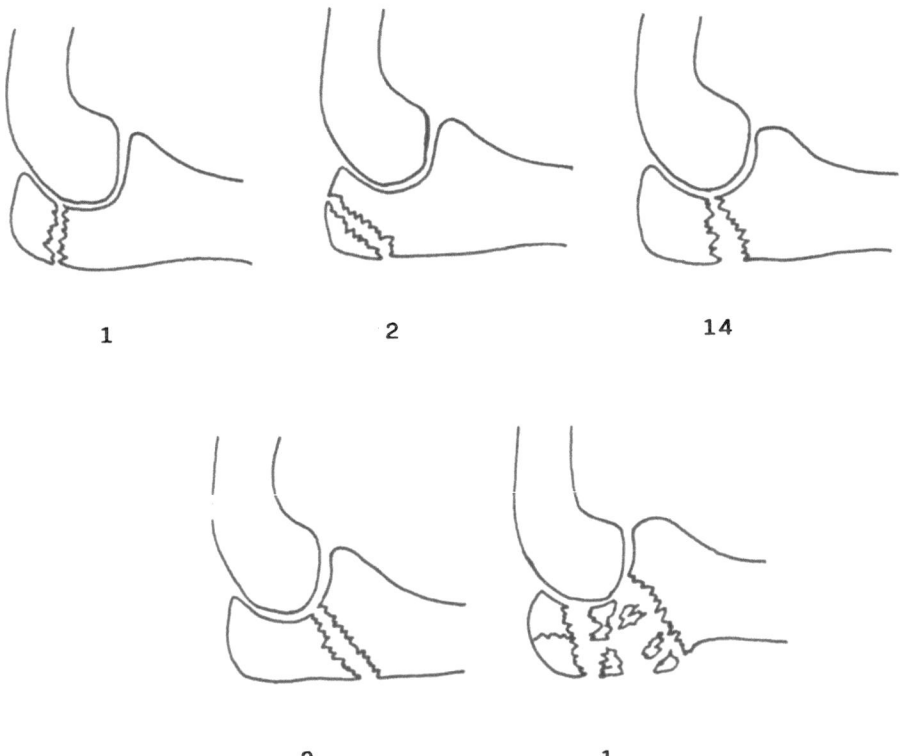

Fig. 3. - Distribution of olecranon nonunions (20 cases) according to a modified version of the Colton classification.

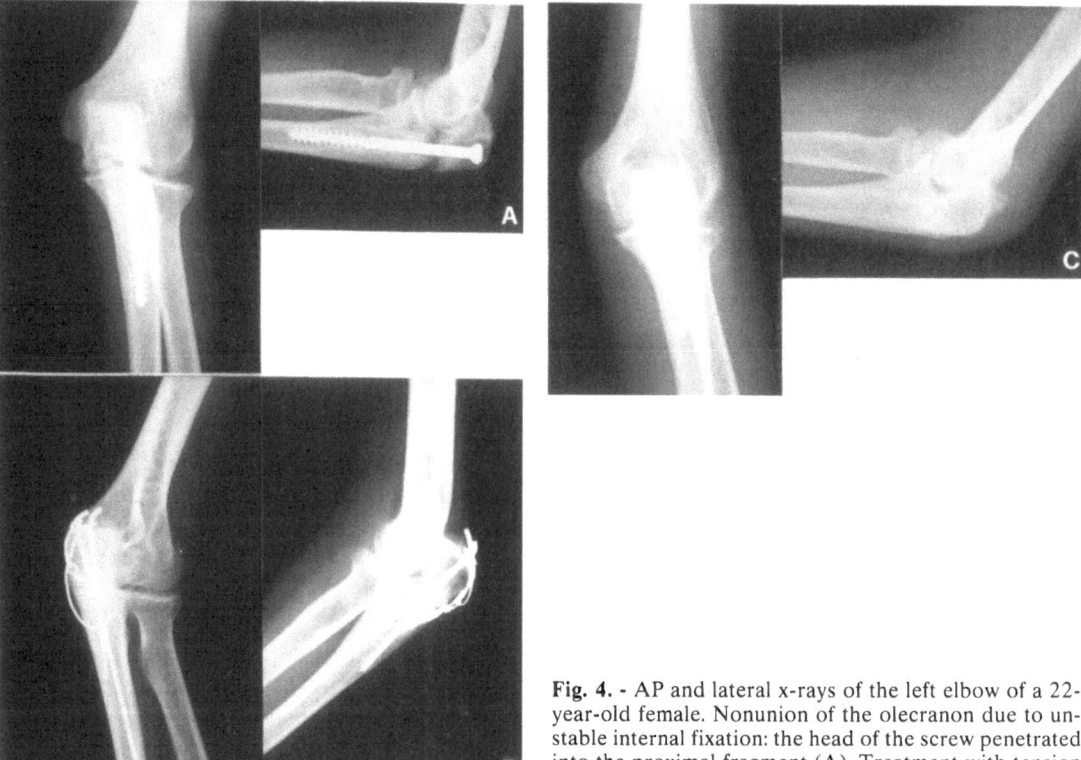

Fig. 4. - AP and lateral x-rays of the left elbow of a 22-year-old female. Nonunion of the olecranon due to unstable internal fixation: the head of the screw penetrated into the proximal fragment (A). Treatment with tension band wiring (B). Final result (C).

cumentation of the relationship between initial treatment and nonunion.

However, extraarticular nonunion seems to be more often the result of conservative treatment, while articular nonunion occurs more frequently as a result of open reduction.

Both should be treated with stable fixation and bone grafts. Healing brings relief of pain; the final range of motion depends on the preoperative conditions.

Nonunion of the olecranon, which is less rare (5%), can derive from any type of treatment.

In recent years we have noticed the appearance of iatrogenous nonunions as a consequence of olecranon osteotomy following a posterior approach to the distal humerus (7, 17).

In nonunion types I and II, removal of the fragment yields excellent results. In the other types, treatment consists of stable internal fixation (cancellous screws, tension band wiring, interfragmentary screws or plate) and possibly cancellous bone grafts. As in nonunion of the distal humerus, the results depend mostly on the preoperative conditions.

REFERENCES

1) ACKERMAN G., JUPITER G.B.: Non union of the distal end of the humerus. *J. Bone Jt Surg.* 1988; **70-A**: 75-83.
2) CALANDRIELLO B.: Le pseudoartrosi della rotula, dell'olecrano e dei malleoli. *G.I.O.T.* 1981; Suppl., **7**: 147.
3) COLTON C.L.: Fractures of the olecranon in adults. Classification and management. *Injury* 1973; **5**: 121.
4) COONRAD R.W.: Non union of the olecranon and proximal ulna. In: *The elbow and its disorders* (B.F. Morrey ed.). W.B. Saunders, Philadelphia, 1985, pp. 400-413.
5) GIACCAI L.: Su di un caso di pseudoartrosi sovracondiloidea di omero trattato con particolare tecnica chirurgica. *Boll. e Mem. Soc. Tosco-Umbra Chir.* 1965; **26**: 747-756.
6) HORNE G., SIM P.: Non union of the radial head. *J. Trauma* 1985; **25** (5): 452.
7) JUPITER J.B. E COLL.: Intercondylar fractures of the humerus, an operative approach. *J. Bone Jt Surg.* 1985; **67**: 226-239.
8) KALENAK A.: Ununited fractures of the lateral condyle of the humerus. *Clin. Orthop.* 1977; **124**: 181.
9) LECESTRE P.: Les fractures de l'extremité inférieure de l'humerus chez l'adulte. *Rev. Chir. Orthop.* 1980; Suppl., **1**: 66.
10) MAES J.M., VAN VELTHOVEN V.: Clinical and statistical research on the occurence of pseudoarthrosis of ulna and radius in forearm fractures. *Acta Orthop. Belg.* 1977; **43**: 767.
11) MITSUNAGA M.M. E COLL.: Condylar non unions of the elbow. *J. Trauma* 1982; **9**: 787-791.
12) RISEBOROUGH E.J., RADIN E.L.: Intercondylar T fractures of the humerus in the adult. *J. Bone Jt Surg.* 1969; **51-A**: 130-141.
13) SIM F.H.: Non union and delayed union of the distal humeral fractures. In: *The elbow and its disorders* (B.F. Morrey ed.). W.B. Saunders, Philadelphia, 1985, pp. 340-354.
14) SOLHEIM K., VAAGE S.: Delayed union and non union of fractures: clinical experience with the asif method. *J. Trauma* 1973; **13**: 121-128.
15) WADSWORTH T.G.: Screw fixation of the olecranon after fracture of osteotomy. *Clin. Orthop.* 1976; **119**: 197-201.
16) WEBER B.G., CECH D.: *Pseudoarthrosis.* II. Huber Publishers, Bern, 1976.
17) ZINGHI G.F. E COLL.: Le fratture dell'estremità inferiore dell'omero nell'adulto. *G.I.O.T.* 1988; **14**: 215-223.

Radial head fractures: long-term results of resection

F. Postacchini - G.B. Morace

Resection of the radial head is a common treatment for comminuted or displaced fractures. Despite its wide use it is still very controversial (5, 6); however, only a few authors (2, 3, 7) have analyzed the long-term results. The main controversy regards the proximal shifting of the radius, which is responsible for such severe biomechanical deformation of the proximal and distal radioulnar joints that arthroplasty might be indicated instead of simple resection (1, 4, 8).

This study analyzes the long-term clinical and radiographic results of resection of the radial head in order to obtain useful information as to its effectiveness.

MATERIAL AND METHODS

From 1961 to 1983, 46 patients with radial head fracture were either treated at the Clinica Ortopedica dell'Università "La Sapienza" in Rome or brought under observation after surgical treatment elsewhere.

Of these patients, 22 were reviewed after an average of 14.8 years (range 8-28). The average age of 19 patients, 10 females and 9 males, was 35 (range 22-57) at the moment of fracture, while the remaining 3 patients were between 9 and 11 years old.

Twelve patients had comminuted radial head fractures; 8 had displaced radial neck fractures, and two had a marginal fracture of the radial head with a displaced fragment. In these last two cases only the displaced fragment was removed. In addition to the radial head fracture, four patients had elbow dislocation, two had a fracture of the olecranon, and one a proximal ulnar fracture.

Surgery was performed an average of 6 days after the trauma. The average period of postoperative immobilization was 20 days.

Radiographs of the elbow and wrist were done on all patients reviewed. The clinical criteria were as follows: pain, valgus deformity, range of joint motion, strength of elbow pronation-supination and flexion-extension and wrist flexion-extension. On the basis of the overall evaluation of these criteria, the results were rated excellent, good, fair, or poor. Furthermore, the patients were asked to express their opinion of the result on a scale of 0-100. A score of 0-60 was considered poor, 61-75 fair, 76-90 good, and 91-100 excellent.

We divided the patients into three groups on the basis of age and the presence of associated lesions. Group I consisted of 12 patients with isolated radial head fractures (Fig. 1). Group II included 7 patients with other lesions as well, and group III consisted of 3 patients who had undergone radial head resection at the age of 9 or 10 (Fig. 2).

RESULTS

Of the 12 patients in group I, only 4 reported pain in the elbow after prolonged physical exertion. Two of these had marginal fracture of the radial head treated with removal of the displaced fragment. Two patients reported occasional paraesthesiae in the ulnar nerve distribution. Seven patients regained full active and passive range of motion, three had a moderate reduction, and the remaining two regained an overall range of up to 150 degrees (Table 1). The two patients treated with partial excision of the radial head showed the following reductions in range of motion: flexion-extension - 40 and 70 degrees, respectively; pronation-supination - 55 and 120 degrees, respectively. A moderate decrease in the strength of pronation-supination of the

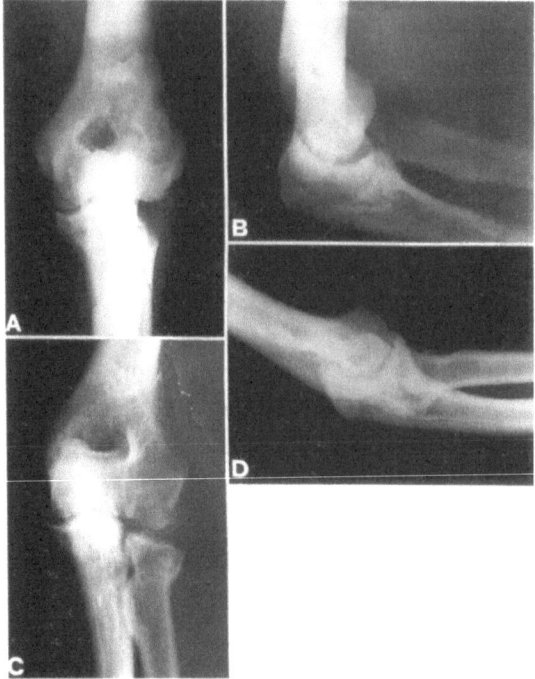

Fig. 1. - Radiographs of an isolated fracture of the radial head in a 34-year-old patient shortly after injury. A,B) After resection of the radial head. C,D) 12 years later, a kind of reformation of the radial head can be seen. Elbow mobility is normal.

the three patients.

The radiographs of four patients (2 from group I and 2 from group II) who had limited range of elbow motion revealed evident signs of degenerative arthritis throughout the joint, accompanied by rapid bone growth out of the radial fragment in 2 cases. Clear arthritic changes were seen in 2 of the 3 patients in the third group.

The radiographs also revealed a distal radioulnar subluxation in 18 of the 22 patients, which had not been found during the clinical examination. The extent of the subluxation was between 1 and 6 mm in all cases. Only one patient, who had undergone radial head resection at the age of 9, complained of pain and reduced wrist mobility; in addition to a radioulnar subluxation of about 6 mm,

forearm and flexion-extension of the elbow was found in 4 cases.

In the second group only one patient complained of pain in the elbow, especially in full supination. The range of motion of the elbow (Table 1) was considerably reduced in 2 cases, while in another 2 it was only slightly reduced. Two patients also showed a slight decrease in muscle strength.

Of the 19 patients in groups I and II, 16 showed a 5-17 degree (average 11°) increase in the valgus angulation of the elbow.

In group III, 2 patients reported frequent pain even at rest that was occasionally accompanied by paraesthesiae in the ring and little fingers, and all three suffered severe limitation of flexion-extension and pronation-supination (Table 1). A decrease in the strength of flexion-extension of the elbow and pronation-supination of the forearm was found in 2 cases. Because of the severe limitation of flexion-extension, it was not possible to determine the degree of valgus angulation in any of

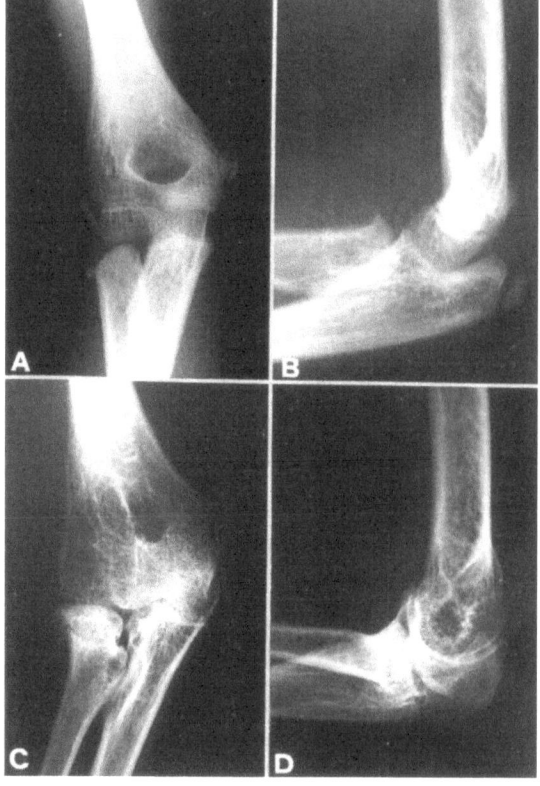

Fig. 2. - Radiographs of an isolated fracture of the radial head in a 9-year-old patient shortly after injury. A,B) After surgery. C,D) 18 years after radial head resection, both degenerative changes and severe valgus angulation can be seen in the elbow. Considerable reduction of the range of flexion-extension and pronation-supination.

Table 1
RANGE OF JOINT MOTION IN THE THREE GROUPS OF
PATIENTS

	Flexion-extension		
	I	II	III
Normal	4	–	–
Reduced			
5-20	4	3	–
25-40	1	3	–
45-60	1	–	1
More than 70	2	1	2

	Prono-supination		
	I	II	III
Normal	3	2	–
Reduced			
5-20	3	–	–
25-45	1	2	1
50-80	3	1	1
90-170	2	2	1

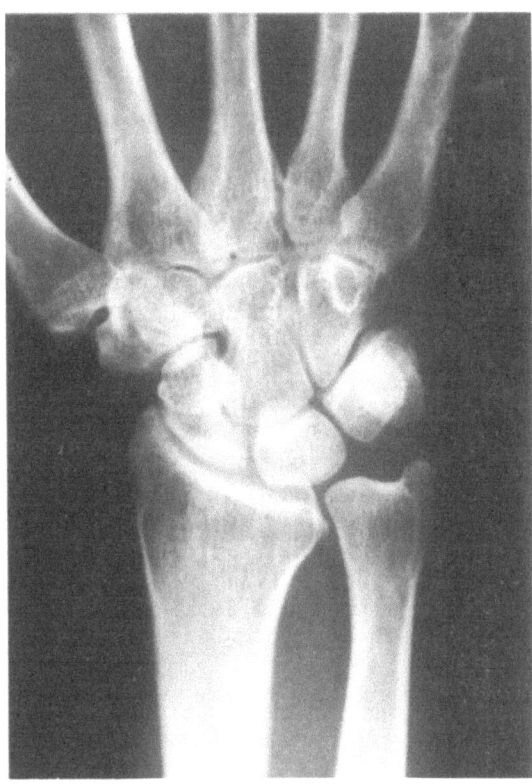

Fig. 3. - Distal radioulnar subluxation of 3 mm in a 58-year-old patient who underwent radial head resection at the age of 40.

Table 2
OVERALL RESULTS IN THE THREE GROUPS OF
PATIENTS WITH RADIAL HEAD FRACTURE

	I	II	III
Excellent	4	2	–
Good	3	1	–
Fair	3	2	–
Poor	2	2	3

the x-rays showed clear signs of radiocarpal degenerative arthritis and ankylosis of the carpal bones. No relationship between extent of subluxation and clinical picture was found in the other patients, and no other patient reported a reduction of wrist mobility. Distal radioulnar crossunion was found in two patients, accompanied by severe limitation of pronation-supination.

The average score given by the patients was 85 in group I, 80 in group II, and 52 in group III. None of the patients of the first two groups had changed his or her everyday activity or occupation for physical reasons.

The overall results, based on both the subjective and objective evaluations, were satisfactory in about half of the patients from groups I and II (Table 2). In group I (isolated radial head fractures), if we do not consider the two patients with marginal fracture of the radial head treated with removal of the displaced fragment, more than two-thirds of the group had satisfactory results. The two patients referred to had one fair and one poor result.

All three patients in group III had a poor result.

CONCLUSIONS

On the basis of the above results, the following conclusions can be drawn:

Resection of the radial head is a valid treatment for displaced or comminuted radial head fractures.

The result depends upon the effort of the patient in the delicate rehabilitation phase as well as the presence of associated lesions.

The distal radioulnar subluxation does not affect the result. As a matter of fact, in this study no relationship was found between the subluxation (present in 82% of cases) and either the extent of the proximal shifting of the radius or pain and reduced wrist mobility.

The results appear to be stable over time, as indicated by the high percentage of satisfactory results in the adult patients, who were reviewed after an average of 15 years.

For the marginal displaced fractures of the radial head, complete resection seems to be the most suitable treatment. The two patients with this type of fracture who were treated with simple removal of the displaced fragment had one fair and one poor result.

Resection of the radial head is not indicated for growing patients, except when there is no other feasible option. In all three of the children who underwent this treatment, the results were unsatisfactory as far as elbow function; moreover, one of them showed marked degenerative changes in the wrist.

REFERENCES

1) CARN R.M., MEDIGE J., CURTAIN D., KOENIG A.: Silicone rubber replacement of the severily fractured radial head. *Clin. Orthop.* 1986; **209**: 259-269.

2) COLEMAN D.A., BLAIR W.F., SHURR D.: Resection of the radial head for fracture of the radial head. Long-term follow-up seventeen cases. *J. Bone Jt. Surg.* 1987; **69-A**: 385-392.

3) GOLDBERG I., PEYLAN J., YOSIPOVITCH Z.: Late results of excision of the radial head for an isolated closed fracture. *J. Bone Jt Surg.* 1986; **68-A**: 675-679.

4) MARTINELLI B., D'INCECCO L.: La protesi di Silastic nelle fratture del capitello radiale: Controlli a distanza. *G.I.O.T.* 1980; **6**: 387-391.

5) MIKIC Z.D., VUKADINOVIC S.M.: Late results in fractures of the radial head treated by excision. *Clin. Orthop.* 1983; **181**: 220-228.

6) MILLER G.K., DRENNAN D.B., MAYLAHN D.J.: Treatment of displaced segmental radial head fractures. Long-term follow-up. *J. Bone Jt Surg.* 1981; **63-A**: 712-717.

7) STEPHEN I.B.M.: Excision of the radial head for closed fracture. *Acta Orthop. Scand.* 1981; **52**: 409-412.

8) SWANSON A.B., JEAGER S.H., LA ROCHELLE D.: Comminuted fractures of the radial head. The role of silicone-implant replacement arthroplasty. *J. Bone Jt Surg.* 1981; **63-A**: 1039-1049.

Prosthetic replacement for radial head fractures

B. Martinelli

INTRODUCTION

As an alternative to resection in cases of radial head fracture that is too severe for internal fixation (Fig. 1), we have used replacement with internal prostheses made of Silastic for over 15 years.

We prefer prosthetic replacement to simple resection because it restores the normal length of the radius, ensures elbow stability, and does not cause pain in the distal radioulnar joint.

HISTORICAL REFERENCES

The first attempt at replacement of the radial head with an internal prosthesis was made by Speed-Kellog in 1940 using a component made of Vitallium.

In the years that followed, both materials and shapes changed (Marino-Zuco metal prosthesis, Cherry acrylic prosthesis, and reinforced acrylic prosthesis). More recently, the Swanson prosthesis made of Silastic (a silicone compound) has become the most widely used component in the world.

PROSTHESIS

The Swanson prosthesis made of Silastic (Fig. 2) is a flexible, one-piece component in the shape of the radial head: concave on the inside to cover the end of the resected radius and equipped with an extension for intramedullary insertion. The prosthesis is available in three sizes to allow for increased bone loss in proportion to the type of fracture.

Implantation technique

1) The Kocher lateral approach (the most anatomical) is used.

2) The resection must be as conservative as possible.

3) The Denucé quadrate ligament, the key element of the proximal radioulnar joint, must not be damaged; the orbicular ligament, which many argue must be left intact, is in reality closely attached to the joint capsule, which must be opened longitudinally up to (and including) the radial neck.

4) The size of the prosthesis must be the same as that of the original radial head, the reconstruction of which may be useful.

5) The preparation of the medullary canal, which will house the stem of the prosthesis, must be done very carefully using a hand perforator (curved if possible) while holding the elbow in varus angulation and slowly pulling the radial fragment laterally.

6) The prosthesis is pressed in with the thumb, however, the flexible stem cannot enter a medullary canal that has not been sufficiently reamed.

7) The neck of the prosthesis can cover the proximal end of the radius only if the radial neck has been left completely intact by the resection, which is not always possible.

8) When resection of a portion of the radial neck is necessary and a prosthesis with a longer head is not available, the prosthesis should be only partially inserted so that it will occupy the entire space and thus prevent the radius from shifting proximally.

9) At the conclusion of the operation, the elbow can be wrapped in a simple bandage.

Postoperative management

Passive mobilization may begin the day after surgery.

Active mobilization may begin after 8

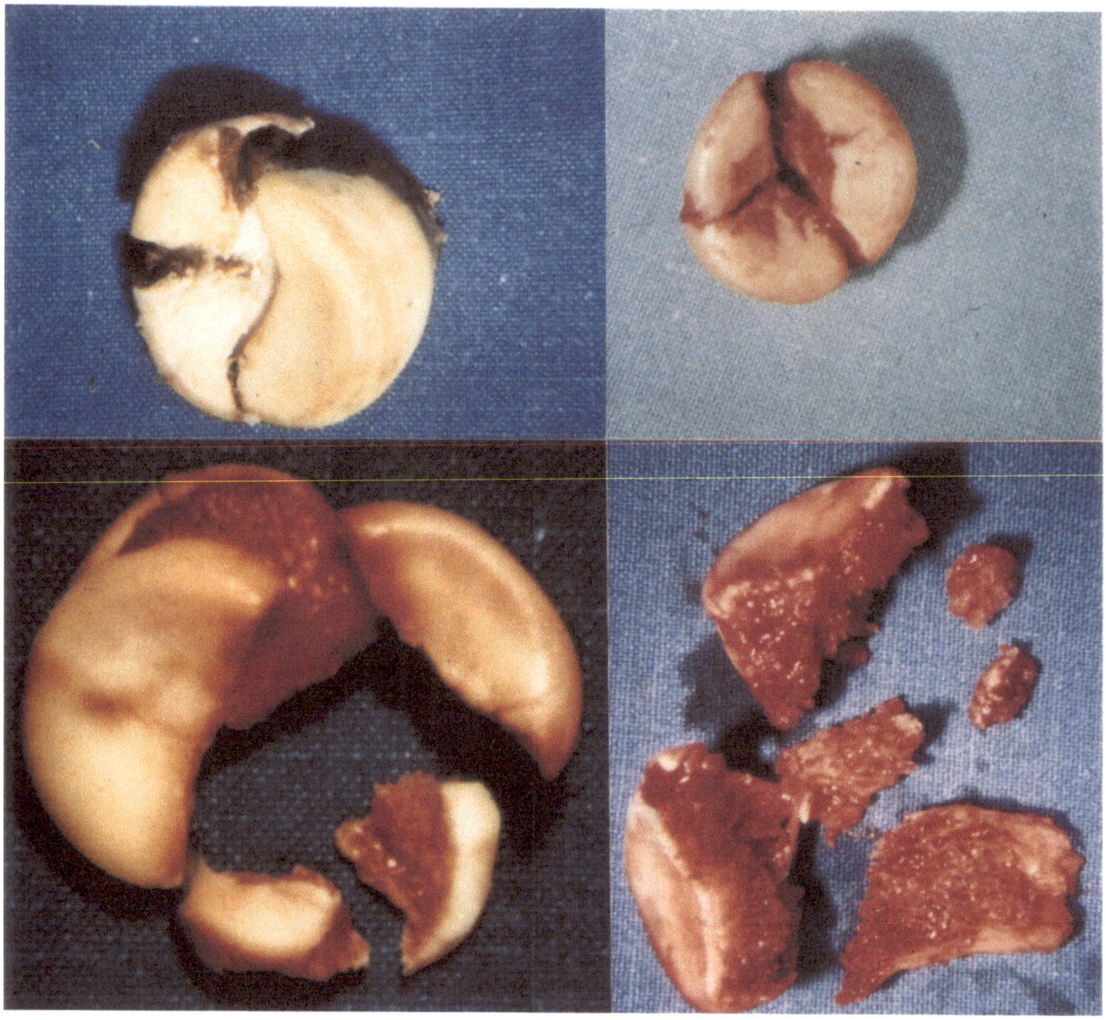

Fig. 1. - Examples of radial head fractures that are too severe to be treated with internal fixation.

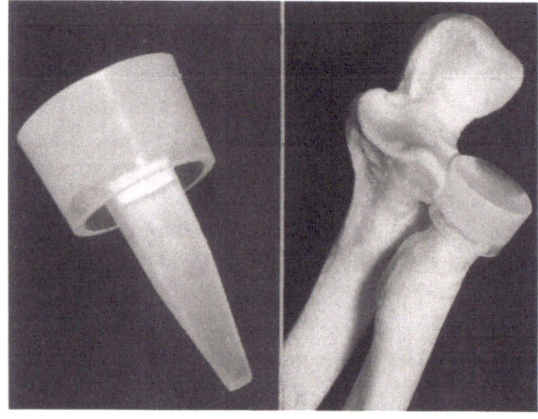

Fig. 2. - Internal prosthesis made of Silastic: available in
3 sizes — small, medium, and large.

days and should include flexion-extension and especially pronation-supination.

Full elbow mobility should be regained within three weeks.

MATERIALS AND METHODS

We treated 55 patients for radial head fractures that were too severe for internal fixation. There were 20 males and 35 females; the age distribution is as follows:

Males	Females
age 20-30= 2	age 20-30= 4
31-40= 2	31-40= 4
41-50= 6	41-50= 1

51-60= 4   51-60= 8
61-70= 4   61-70= 6
71-80= 2   71-80= 12

Table 1

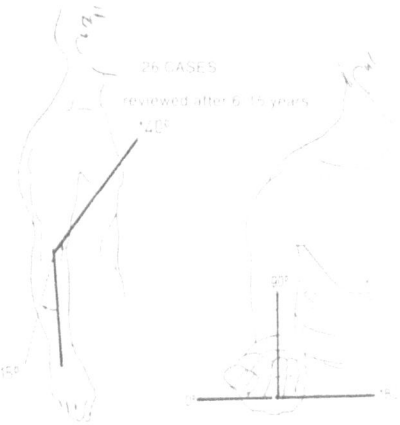

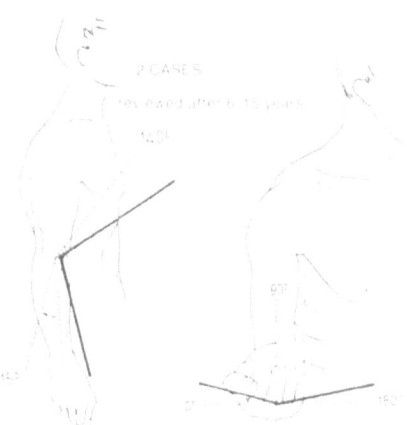

Forty of the fractures treated were isolated; of the rest, 8 were accompanied by elbow dislocation, 5 by wrist fracture, and 2 by fracture of both olecranon and coronoid as well as dislocation.

We were able to review 28 cases of isolated fracture, 2 cases with elbow dislocation, 1 case with wrist fracture, and 1 case with olecranon and coronoid fracture plus dislocation.

We will now discuss the cases of isolated fracture of the radial head because they make up the bulk of the study, because we believe the internal prosthesis is highly indicated for this lesion, and because these patients can begin mobilization immediately after surgery, an important factor in the outcome.

The follow-up period ranges from 3 to 15 years after surgery.

Three criteria were used in the clinical evaluation: pain, range of flexion-extension and pronation-supination, and strength, which was determined by the patient's postoperative ability to lift weights with the elbow both flexed and extended compared to previous ability in everyday activity.

Pain: no internal prosthesis was reported as painful.

Range of motion: 26 patients regained full range of flexion-extension and pronation-supination; 2 patients regained a range of only two-thirds (Table 1).

Strength: all patients had full recovery of strength, even those who engaged in manual labor before injury.

Two of the 26 patients with full recovery of range of motion reported occasional joint block more than 8 years after surgery; surgical revision was required.

A series of **radiographs** taken over several years were comparable to those taken immediately after surgery, showing the durability of Silastic. Nevertheless, after 4 years the *prosthesis* (Fig. 3) may begin to deteriorate, showing height decrease, crepitus, detachment of the stem, and fragmentation. *The proximal end of the resected radius* reacts to the deterioration of the prosthesis by forming ossifications, sometimes loose and sometimes crowning the site of the implant.

The capitulum humeri reacts in various ways, with widespread atrophy of the subchondral cancellous bone sometimes accompanied by ulceration of the cartilaginous surfaces; there is a double image of the joint on the x-ray, and secondary arthritic degeneration appears (Fig. 4).

One of the **complications** that necessitated prosthetic revision was the occasional joint block (2 cases): the prosthesis had fragmented, causing the occasional interposition of pieces of Silastic into the joint space. The surgery (Fig. 5) required to remove the fragments of the prosthesis revealed the presence of a fibrous tissue that had filled both the medullary canal and the space left by the fragmented prosthesis, despite the lack of macroscopic signs of phlogistic reaction.

The **histologic report** confirmed the macroscopic evidence: the Silastic, broken into minute fragments, had infiltrated into the capsular and periprosthetic tissue as well as the synovial membrane. Macrophagic cells due to the foreign body were present, but there were no significant phlogistic occurrences (Fig. 6).

Confirming the above observations, the patients recovered normal elbow function just a few days after removal of the remains of the prosthesis.

DISCUSSION

From a clinical standpoint, replacement of the fractured radial head with an internal prosthesis made of Silastic has a high prob-

ability of success and is quite durable, thus fulfilling the requirements of both patient and surgeon. From a radiologic standpoint, however, the Silastic prosthesis is shown to have a limited life, with signs of degeneration appearing about 4 years after implantation. Nevertheless, we would like to emphasize the clinical tolerance of the articular structures of the elbow for this device, even in cases of fragmentation of the prosthesis and follow-up periods of more than 15 years.

At this point we would like to address the reasons why the prosthesis is so vulnerable to deterioration. We believe that there are three possible causes:

1) **Variations in the composition of Silastic.**

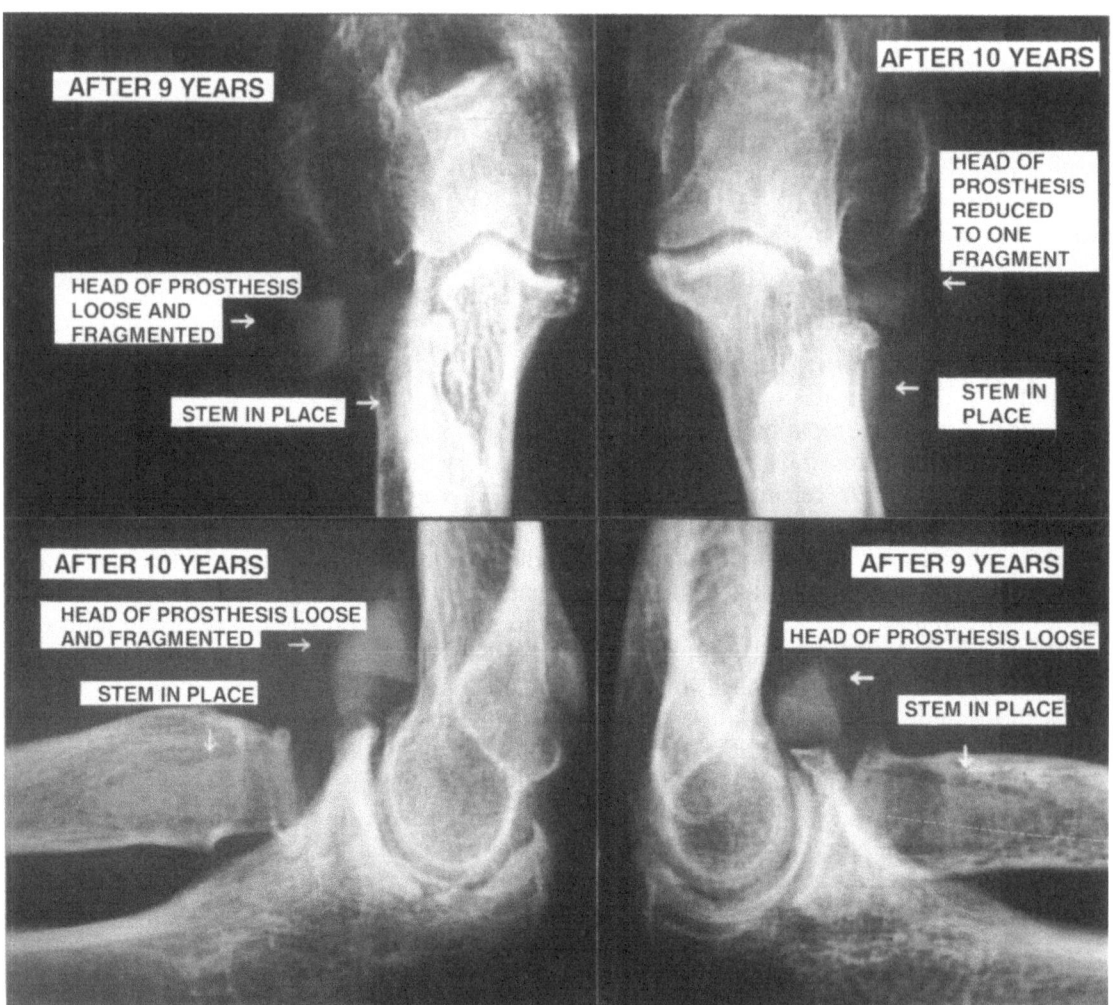

Fig. 3. - Examples of follow-up x-rays showing deterioration of the prosthesis.

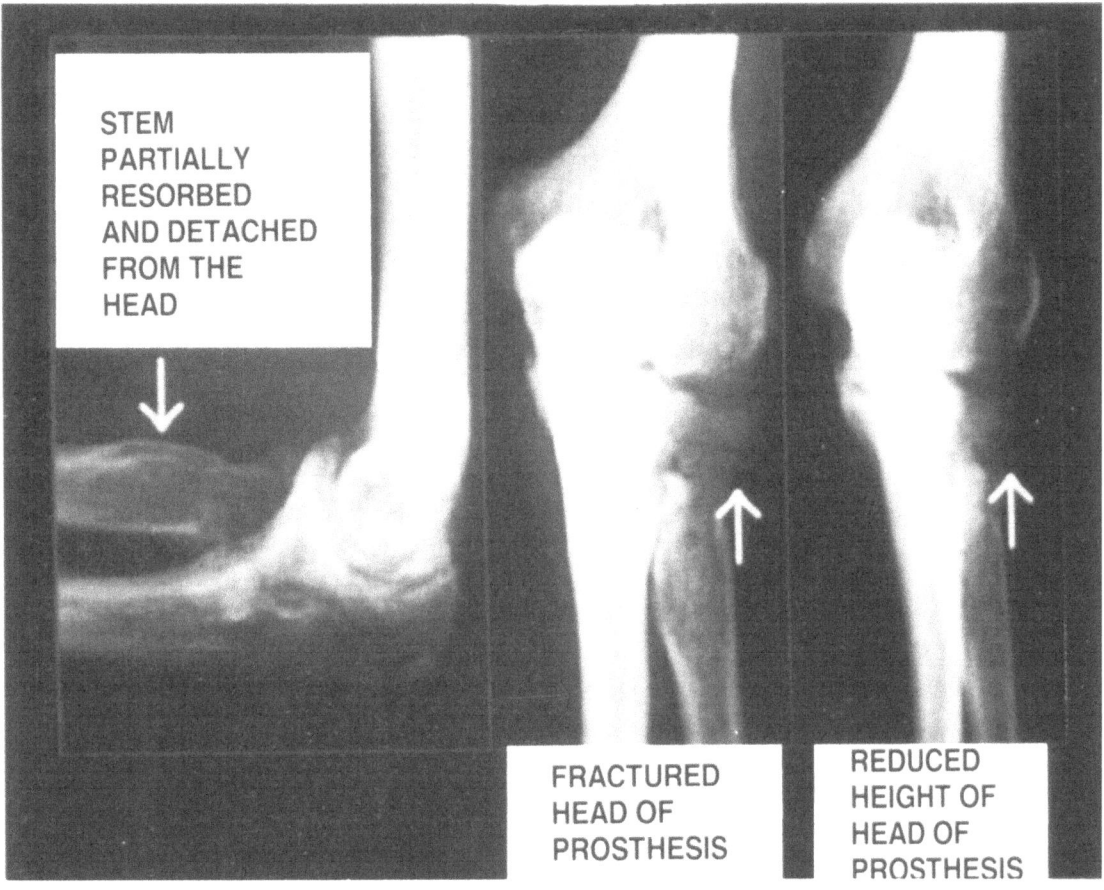

Fig. 4. - Follow-up x-rays after 15 years: despite the deterioration of the prosthesis and the other articular components, elbow function is normal.

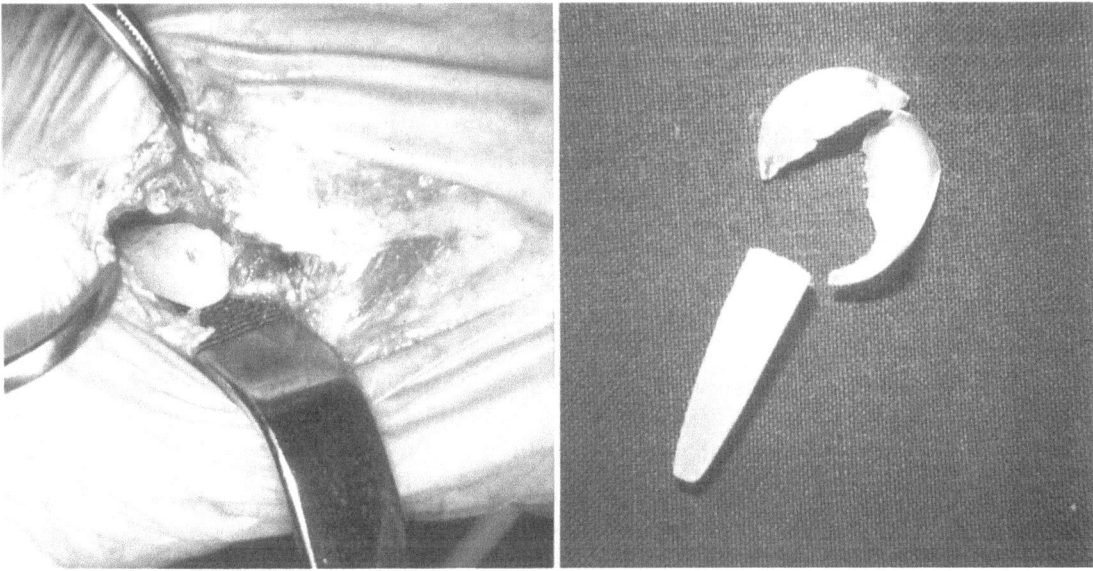

Fig. 5 - Operative view (*left*) of the removal of prosthetic fragments (*right*).

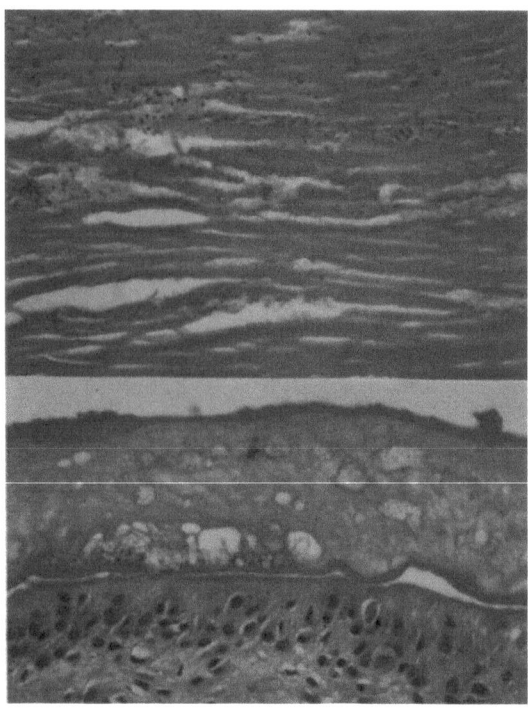

Fig. 6 - Histologic specimens reveal the "crushed" Silastic in the capsule, the synovial membrane, and the fibrous tissue occupying the space left by the disintegrated prosthesis. Granulomatous formations due to presence of a foreign body are clearly visible; there are no significant signs of phlogosis.

Some fluids present in the blood provoke oxidation, hydrolysis, imbibition, and dilution of this material; the silicone hardens, causing decreases in its weight-bearing and stress capacity, as well as disgregation and fragmentation.

2) **Mobility of the prosthesis.**

The greater the mobility of the prosthesis, the greater the wear on it, causing a reaction to the foreign body consisting of the formation of interface tissue that further increases mobility, which in turn increases wear, and so on, creating a vicious circle.

3) **The biomechanics of the humeroradial joint.**

The extent and direction of the forces acting upon the radial head change with both the movement of the forearm (flexion-extension and pronation-supination) and, obviously, the effort of biceps traction, thus everyday activity can cause an array of stresses (compression, shear, and torsion) that contribute to the wear on the Silastic and prime it for rupture.

CONCLUSIONS

When the radial head is too severely fractured for internal fixation, its replacement with an internal prosthesis made of Silastic guarantees a good clinical result. It is indicated for recent fractures and should be performed soon after the trauma.

Very early mobilization is essential for a good outcome. If the radial head fracture is complicated by other lesions (wrist fracture, olecranon and coronoid fracture, elbow dislocation), the result could be compromised by immobilization.

Nevertheless, it should be pointed out that in radial head fractures with elbow dislocation, simple resection does not guarantee stability; in this instance prosthetic replacement is highly indicated.

We agree with those who believe that resection of the radial head should be avoided because an articular component cannot be "simply" eliminated without provoking imbalances in the joint, but when resection is the only feasible option, we believe that prosthetic replacement has all the same advantages. The clinical results confirm this as well as the tolerability of Silastic, in spite of its degeneration over time.

The surgeon may never be satisfied with the radiographic result, but in our experience both surgeon and patient have always been happy with the clinical result.

In proposing prosthetic replacement, we feel it is our duty to inform the patient that the Silastic prosthesis will promote rapid functional recovery, prevent proximal shifting of the radius, and will not be rejected by the body, but has a limited life and might require further surgery in order to remove the fragmented component; all this will not, however, compromise joint function.

Adoption of this treatment should nonetheless be limited to isolated acute comminuted lesions, for which the only other option is resection, and to acute lesions accompanied by dislocation which are still unstable even after reduction and resection.

In any case, mobilization should always begin a few hours after surgery if complete functional recovery is to be achieved.

REFERENCES

1) ASSENNATO G., PERUGIA L.: Sul trattamento delle fratture del capitello radiale secondo la metodica di Marino-Zuco. *Atti S.O.T.I.M.I.* 1960; **5** (1).

2) CHERRY J.C.: Fracture of the head of the radius treated by excision and substitution of an acrylic head. *J. Bone Jt Surg.* 1953; **35-B**: 486.

3) MARTINELLI B.: Chirurgia sostitutiva dell'estremo prossimale del radio con endoprotesi. *Chir. Org. Mov.* 1975; **62**: 181.

4) MORREY B.F., AN K.N., STORMONT T.J.: Force transmission through the radial head. *J.Bone Jt Surg.* 1988; **70-A**: 250.

5) SPEED-KELLOG: Ferrule caps. (vitallium) for head of radius. *Surg. Gynec. Obstet.* 1941; **73**: 845.

6) SWANSON A.B., JAEGER S.H., LA ROCHELLE D.: Comminute fractures of the radial head. *J. Bone Jt Surg.* 1981; **63-A**: 1039.

Arthroscopic arthrolysis

P. Montemagni - G. Carnazza

INTRODUCTION

Arthroscopy of the elbow was performed for the first time by Burman on a cadaver in 1932 (1), and used for the first time as a diagnostic examination by Watanabe in 1971 (2) on a patient suffering from arthrosynovitis. Subsequently, McGinty (3) in 1982, Hempfling (4) in 1983, and Eriksson (6) in 1984 dedicated themselves to setting some standards for arthroscopic technique as well as indications for its use on the elbow.

Recently, at the Congresso Internazionale di Artroscopia in Rome in May of 1989, Lindenfeld (7), Berner (8), and Saito (9) presented their new contribution to the field of arthroscopy in diseases of the elbow regarding the treatment of rheumatoid arthritis.

CLINICAL EXAMINATION AND IMAGING STUDY

The clinical examination can reveal sites of damage and functional limitation. **Palpation** of the areas corresponding to the lateral and medial epicondyles may reawaken the pain reported by the patient.

Listening closely during passive or active elbow movements can provide further clues as to possible articular problems. The degree of active movement (flexion-extension and pronation-supination) should always be measured and then compared with the contralateral elbow.

Standard **radiographs** (AP and lateral) should be taken, possibly rounded out by two functional lateral views in full flexion and extension in order to check articular congruity. The lateral projection provides a tangential view of the olecranon and can reveal small le-

sions that would otherwise go unnoticed. Sometimes xerography can be useful for showing possible calcifications on the tendinous insertions.

Arthrography is not very helpful, while a **CAT scan** provides a close look at the articular cartilage, showing even the smallest lesions in detail.

APPROACHES

The elbow joint in encased in two distinct joint capsules: an anterior one, which is wider and easily accomodates the standard 4.5 mm arthroscope, and a posterior one, which is narrower and therefore must be penetrated with a 2.4 mm needlescope.

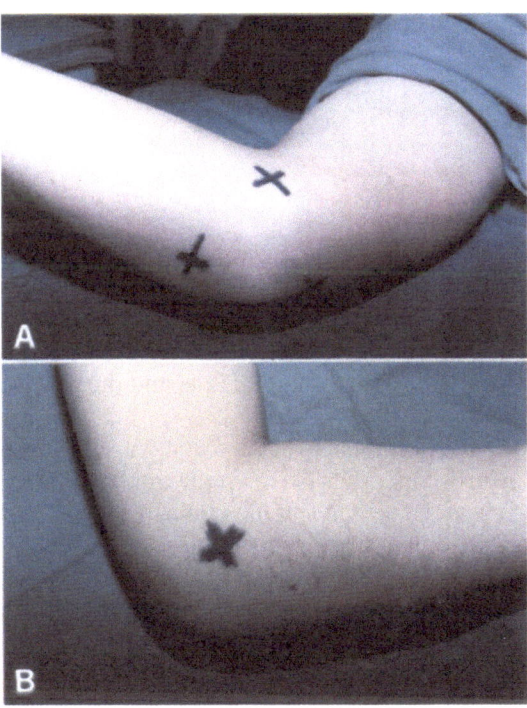

Fig. 1. - A) Medial approach. B) Lateral approach.

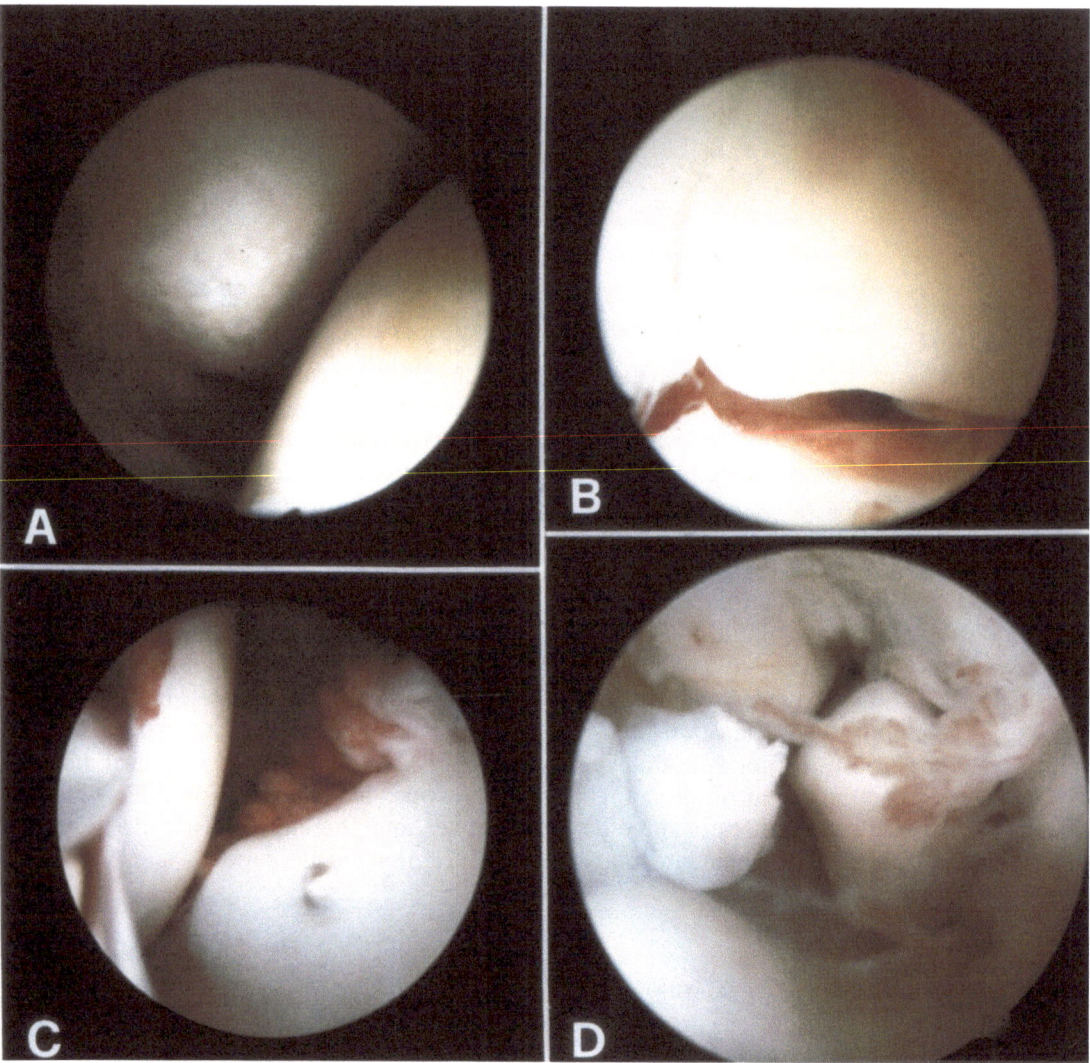

Fig. 2. - Arthroscopic diagnosis of the anterior compartment. A) Humeroradial joint. B) Humeroulnar joint. C) Degenerative synovitis. D) Loose bodies.

The most commonly used approaches are the medial one, the lateral one, and the posterior one.

The medial approach, usually used for the arthroscope, runs between the medial epicondyle and the center of the joint (Fig. 1A).

The lateral approach, used for the instrumentation, begins right above and in front of the radial head (Fig. 1B).

The seldom used posterior approach goes right through the triceps tendon.

Arthroscopically, the elbow is divided into the anterior, posterior, and lateral compartments.

The anterior and lateral compartments can be viewed through the medial and lateral windows. Care should be taken to avoid the median and ulnar nerves and the radial artery. We can in this way study the humeroradial, radioulnar, and humeroulnar joints and make diagnoses regarding the anterior compartment (Fig. 2 A-D). The posterior compartment can be viewed through the posterolateral window, penetrating directly above the olecranon process, or through a posterior window piercing the triceps tendon.

In this area it is also possible to examine the region that corresponds to the olecranon

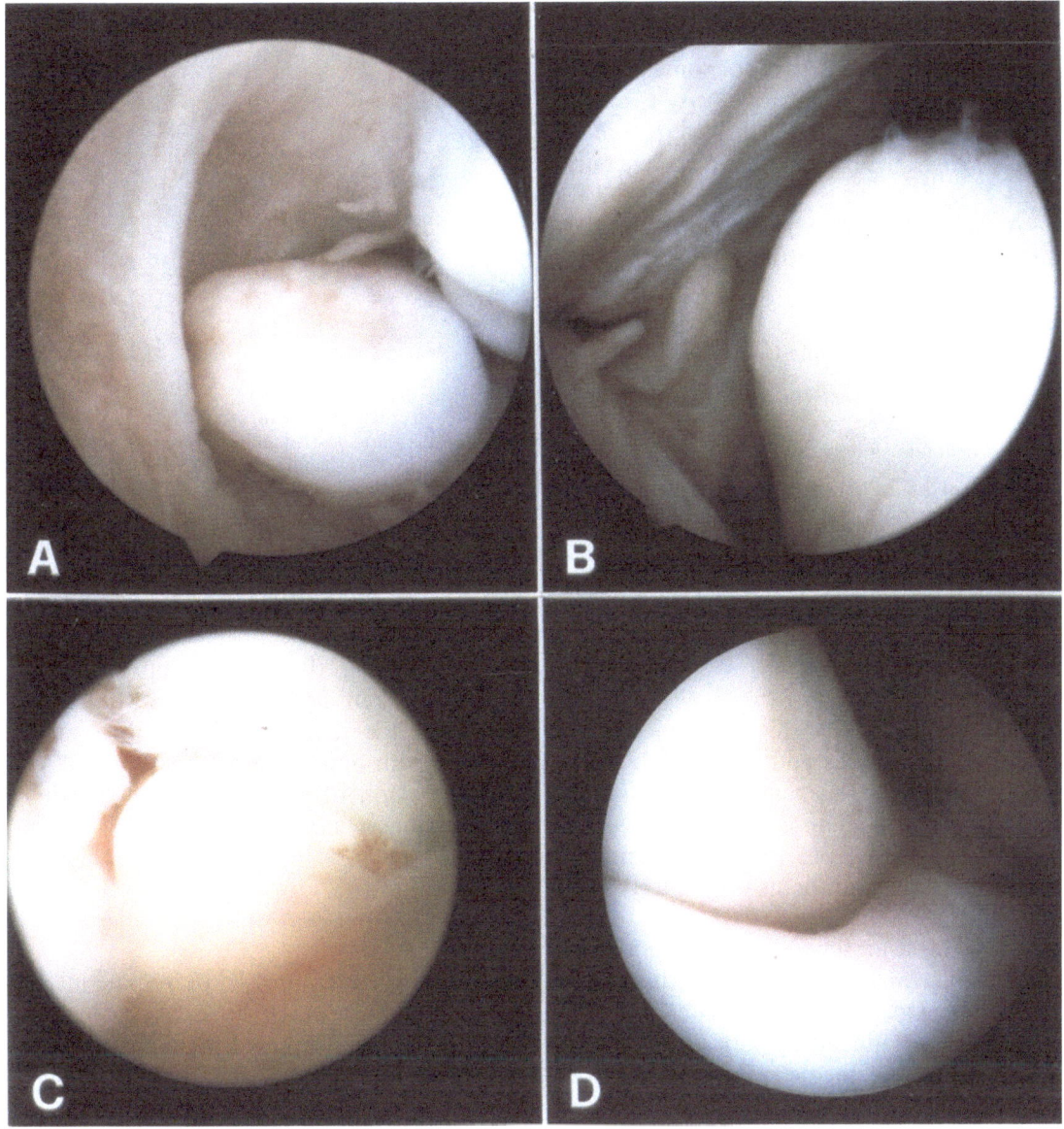

Fig. 3. - Arthroscopic diagnosis of the posterior compartment. A) Loose bodies in the posterior compartment. B) Olecranon process. C) Oblique view of the humerus and ulna. D) Olecranon fossa.

fossa and the retro-olecranon bursa as well as make diagnoses regarding the posterior compartment (Fig. 3 A-D).

INDICATIONS

Elbow arthroscopy is indicated if either loose bodies or primary degenerative arthritis is suspected.

The loose bodies can be the manifestation of **osteochondrosis dissecans**, **synovial chondromatosis**, or **osteochondral detachment**.

Removal of the non-radiopaque loose bodies and *debridement* of the accompanying reactive synovitis can relieve the symptoms.

Arthroscopy is also indicated in cases of post-traumatic stiffness normally appearing after radial head fracture, when conservative treatment (physical therapy and mobilization under anesthesia) does not lead to satisfactory recovery of elbow mobility.

Finally, arthroscopy (especially arthroscopic surgery) can be used for some resistant forms of lateral epicondylitis.

The results achieved using *lateral epicondylar release* have so far been very encouraging.

According to our experience, elbow arthroscopy is indicated for the syndromes listed in Table 1.

Table 1

Indications
— Osteochondrosis dissecans
— Synovial osteochondromatosis
— Post-traumatic stiffness
— Lateral epicondylitis

OPERATIVE TECHNIQUE

The patient lies on his back with elbow flexed to 90 degrees and upper limb in the type of balanced suspension used for the shoulder. The patient is usually put under general anesthesia, but local, peripheral, or block anesthesia can be used in purely diagnostic arthroscopy.

The joint is loosened by inserting a spinal needle anterior and proximal to the medial epicondyle. Once the joint is dilated, the arthroscope is introduced by way of the medial approach and the needle in flow is inserted by way of the posterolateral approach (Fig. 4). In this way the anterior and lateral compartments can be examined and the following syndromes can be diagnosed:

— *erosion* of the radial head
— degenerative *synovitis*
— *osteochondrosis* dissecans of the capitulum humeri
— *loose bodies.*

Then, by switching the positions of the arthroscope and the needle in flow, it is possible to examine the posterior compartment and diagnose:

— *synovial reaction*
— non-radiopaque *loose bodies.*

The posterior and lateral approaches are used for the instrumentation.

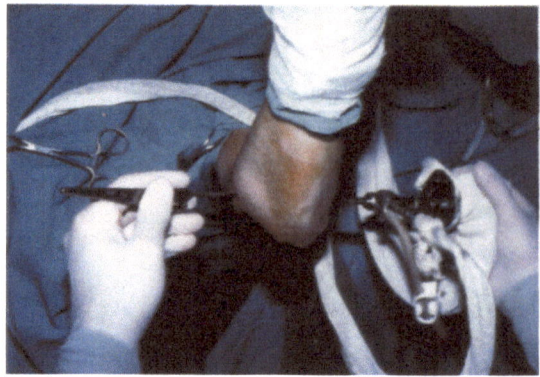

Fig. 4. - Introduction of arthroscope by way of the medial approach and instrumentation by way of the posterolateral approach.

Use of the posteromedial approach should be avoided because of the proximity of the ulnar nerve, which runs posteriorly near the medial epicondyle.

When using the lateral approach care must be taken not to damage the motor branch of the radial nerve, but this can be avoided with appropriate dilatation and 90-degree flexion of the elbow, both of which move the nerve medially.

PATIENTS AND TREATMENT

This study is comprised of 39 patients, 23 males and 16 females, whose average age was 48 and who were treated for a degenerative syndrome of the elbow using **arthroscopic release.**

The patients' occupational and sports activity is listed in Table 2.

Table 2

Patients	
Males 23 - Females 16	
Average age: 48 (20-67)	
Sports activity	7
Manual labor	19
Sedentary job	13

The diagnoses were as follows: 6 cases of osteochondrosis dissecans, 15 of synovial chondromatosis, 8 of post-traumatic stiffness, and 10 of lateral epicondylitis.

Arthroscopic release consists of the following elements:

resection of the fibrous adhesions,

synovectomy,

chondroplasty,

excision of the osteophytes,

removal of the loose bodies.

Osteochondrosis dissecans can be clearly shown by a **CAT** scan of the joint.

The CAT scan reveals a small osteochondritic area on the lateral condyle and a loose body.

The indicated surgical treatment is **arthroscopic debridement.**

After the unbridling of the articular defect, the necrotic tissue is excised with the arthroscopic cutter. Finally, suction and decompression are done by means of lavage and the use of a motorized instrument (Table 3).

The small, scattered loose bodies in cases of *synovial chondromatosis* can be removed with arthroscopic suction.

Sometimes there is only one large (2-3 cm) loose body. In this case, it can be removed with an arthroscopic grasper (Fig. 5).

Peripheral reactive synovitis is treated by removing the hypertrophic tissue with a motorized instrument (Fig. 6).

Table 3

Debridement
— Correction of articular defect
— Unbridling of the articular defect
— Resection of the enucleated fragment and articular suction and decompression

Post-traumatic stiffness can characterize several different pathologic conditions. It occurs above all in cases of malunion of the radial head, bringing with it pain and limitation of pronation-supination. Stiffness can also arise following prolonged cast immobilization and surgical treatment of forearm fractures. In these instances stiffness is triggered by anterior capsular retraction that causes limitation of elbow flexion-extension.

In these cases, the functional x-rays of the fully flexed and extended elbow reveal a reduction in functional capacity; the arthrography shows narrowing of the anterior capsule.

Furthermore, arthroscopy can expose changes in the articular cartilage and chronic inflammation of the synovial tissue.

Arthroscopic treatment involves the **release** of the adhesions that limit joint move-

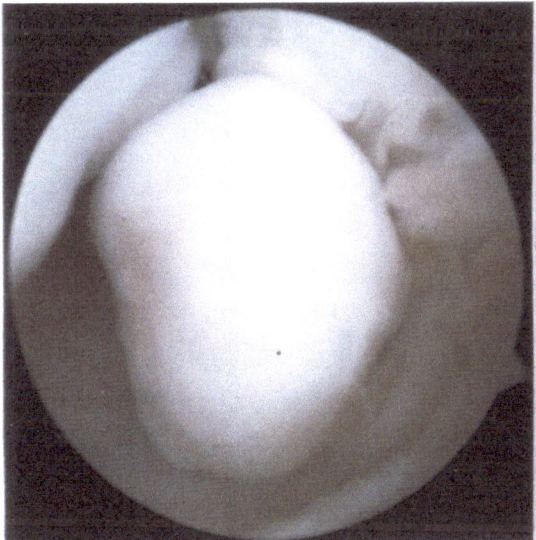

Fig. 5. - Loose body in the anterior compartment.

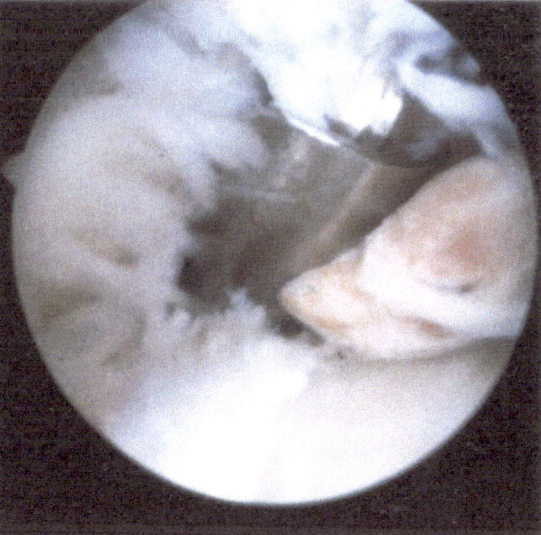

Fig. 6. - Arthroscopic treatment of reactive synovitis.

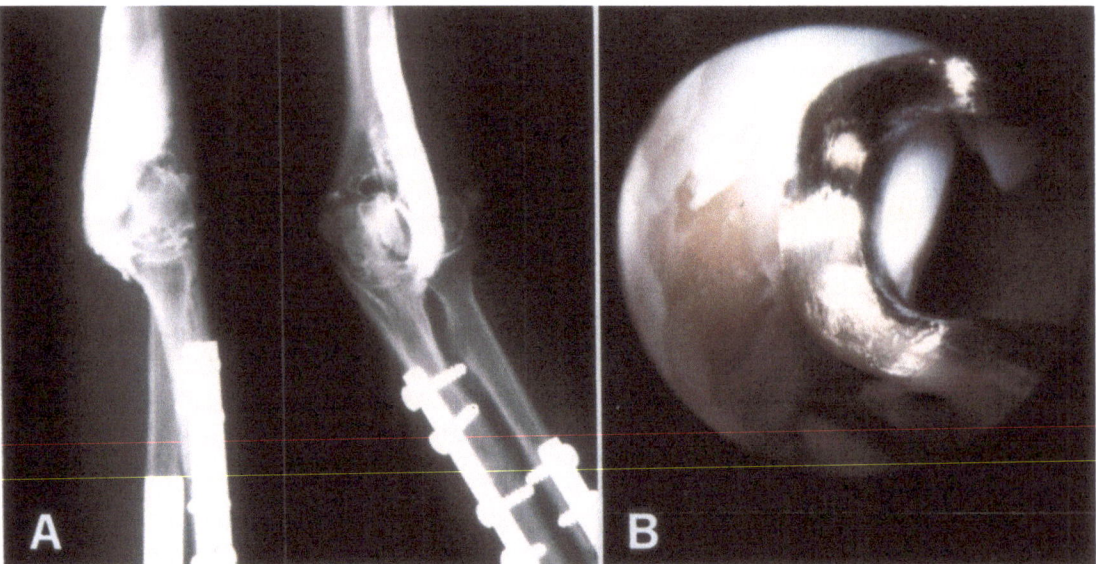

Fig. 7. - Post-traumatic elbow stiffness. A) Arthrography. B) Arthroscopic treatment.

ment, the resection of possible osteophytes, and the synovectomy of the anterior compartment (Fig. 7).

Finally, we would like to discuss the arthroscopic treatment, called **lateral epicondylar release**, for lateral epicondylitis that does not respond to conservative treatment.

The arthroscope is introduced by way of the medial approach and the surgical in-strumentation from the radial side. Synovectomy of the anterior compartment is done first, followed by release of the extensor tendons and resection of their insertional aponeuroses (Fig. 8).

This treatment allows an almost immediate recovery of the normal range of elbow motion and provides relief of lateral epicondylar pain (Fig. 9).

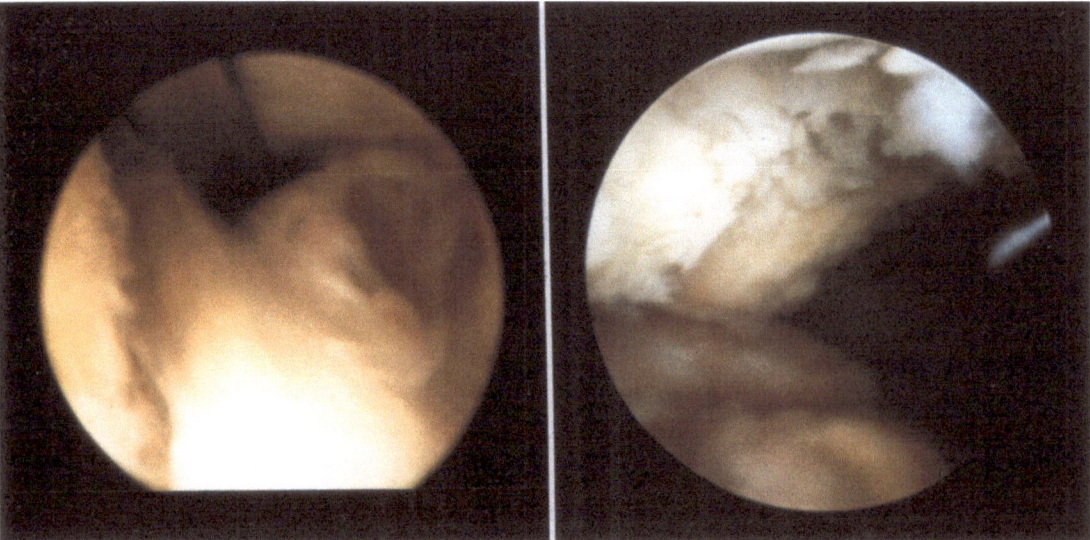

Fig. 8. - Lateral epicondylar release.

Fig. 9. - Arthroscopy after resection of the aponeurosis of the tendinous insertion.

RESULTS

The results were classified on a 50-point scale which assigned 20 points to pain and 30 to function (Table 4).

Eight excellent results were achieved, 18 good, 10 fair, and 3 poor (Table 5).

Table 4

50-point scale	
Pain	20 points
Function	30 points

Table 5

Results	
Excellent	8
Good	18
Fair	10
Poor	3

The positive results (excellent and good) made up 66% of the total, and were attained in those cases of synovial chondromatosis and lateral epicondylitis that were treated with *debridement* and *release*.

The negative results (fair and poor) made up 34% of the total and occurred mostly in cases of osteochondrosis dissecans and post-traumatic stiffness, which are no longer treated arthroscopically save in exceptional circumstances.

CONCLUSIONS

Arthroscopic release can provide both functional benefit and relief of pain in some degenerative syndromes of the elbow.

Elbow arthroscopy is easy to perform and involves minimal trauma.

In our experience with this technique we have never had any vascular or neurologic complications. Arthroscopy yielded the best results in cases of pain and functional limitation due to loose bodies and lateral epicondylitis, resulting in improved functional capacity and relief of pain. The least satisfactory results of arthroscopy occurred in the treatment of osteochondrosis dissecans and post-traumatic stiffness, in which pain relief was not accompanied by increased joint mobility.

All patients with a positive result were able to resume both work and sports after a very short time and were very satisfied with the outcome.

Even though this was a fairly small case study, the results do confirm the promise of **arthroscopic release** in the treatment of degenerative syndromes of the elbow, provided that this treatment is limited to carefully selected cases and performed by an expert team.

REFERENCES

1) BURMAN M.: Arthroscopy of the elbow joint: a cadaver study. *J. Bone Jt Surg.* 1932; **14**: 349.
2) WATANABE J.: Arthroscopy of small joints. *J. Jap. Orthop. Ass.* 1971; **45**: 908.
3) McGINTY J.: Arthroscopic removal of loose bodies. *Orthop. Clin. North Am.* 1982; **13**: 313.
4) HEMPFLING H.: Endoscopic examination of the elbow joint from the dorsoradial approach. *Clin. Orthop.* 1983; **121**: 331.
5) ERIKSSON E., PITMAN M.: Arthroscopy and arthroscopic surgery of joint other than the knee. In: *Textbook of arthroscopic surgery* (O. Connor's ed.). Lippincott Co., Philadelphia 1984, p. 311.
6) ERIKSSON E., DENTI M.: Diagnostic and operative arthroscopy of the shoulder and elbow joint. *It. J. Sports Traumat.* 1985; **7**(3).
7) LINDENFELD T.N.: *The medial approach for elbow arthroscopy.* Communication Congress I.A.A., Rome, May 1989.
8) BERNER W., SÜDKAMP N., LOBENHOFFER P.: *Disorders of the elbow treated by arthroscopy.* Communication Congress I.A.A. Rome, May 1989.
9) SAITO T., KOSHINO T., OKAMOTO R.: *Results of arthroscopic synovectomy through lateral approaches for rheumatoid elbow.* Communication Congress I.A.A., Rome, May 1989.

Reconstruction of the post-traumatic elbow

T.G. Wadsworth

Surgical reconstruction of the acutely injured elbow is often necessary to give the best opportunity for subsequent function, in particular the following injuries:
— unstable lateral humeral condylar fractures in the child;
— displaced segmental fractures of the adult capitulum;
— displaced intraarticular lower humeral fractures and displaced fractures of the olecranon in the adult;
— adult radial head fractures and Monteggia injuries with displacement of the radial head.

Supracondylar fracture of the humerus in the child may require stable fixation, either by percutaneous pin fixation or open reduction prior to fixation, especially in the presence of vascular trauma. In cases of severe cubitus varus at skeletal maturity, following on supracondylar fracture, corrective lower humeral osteotomy may be indicated.

Certain intraarticular fractures, particularly of the lower humerus, can lead to considerable stiffening of the elbow, sometimes of the forearm as well. Stiffness is quite often due to mechanical obstruction as a result of bony deformity as well as soft tissue changes, in particular to the anterior capsule; adhesion formation anteriorly, posteriorly, and within the joint can also be a problem. However, even isolated injury to the radial head in the adult can give a similarly disappointing functional result, usually caused by unnecessary and unwise prolonged immobilisation. Whenever possible, displaced intraarticular fractures involving the elbow joint should be properly reduced and internally fixed; subsequent very early active motion is usually the best regime to avoid important stiffness of the elbow and proximal radioulnar joints.

Surgical release, properly timed, can often give a pleasing result: in some, appropriate soft tissue release is enough, in others resection of bone is necessary, particularly anteriorly at the lower humerus. When bone has to be resected, bleeding from the bone can be minimised by the application of "bone wax". Where there is important restriction of extension and flexion, it is usually best to use a lateral approach so that the anterior and posterior aspects of the elbow joint can be dealt with; sometimes it is necessary to additionally use a medial approach. In those individuals with important lack of extension only of the elbow due to soft tissue changes of thickening and contracture of the anterior capsule, anterior capsulotomy can be a useful surgical procedure.

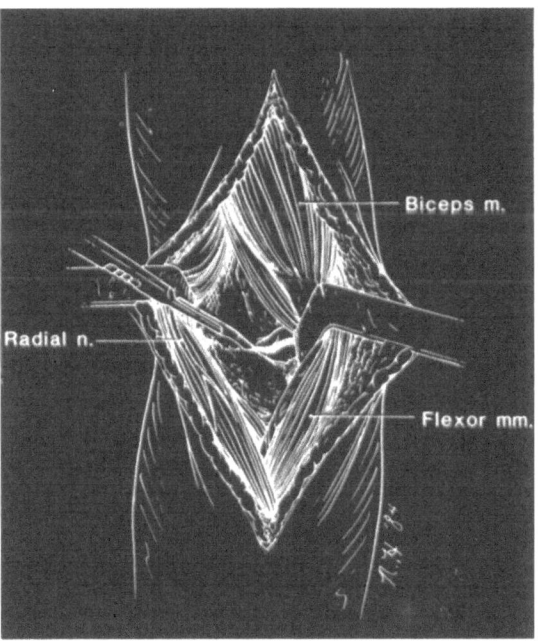

Fig. 1. - Anterior capsulotomy for post-traumatic flexion contracture of the elbow. This can give pleasing results in the well-chosen case (courtesy of Dr. James R. Urbaniak).

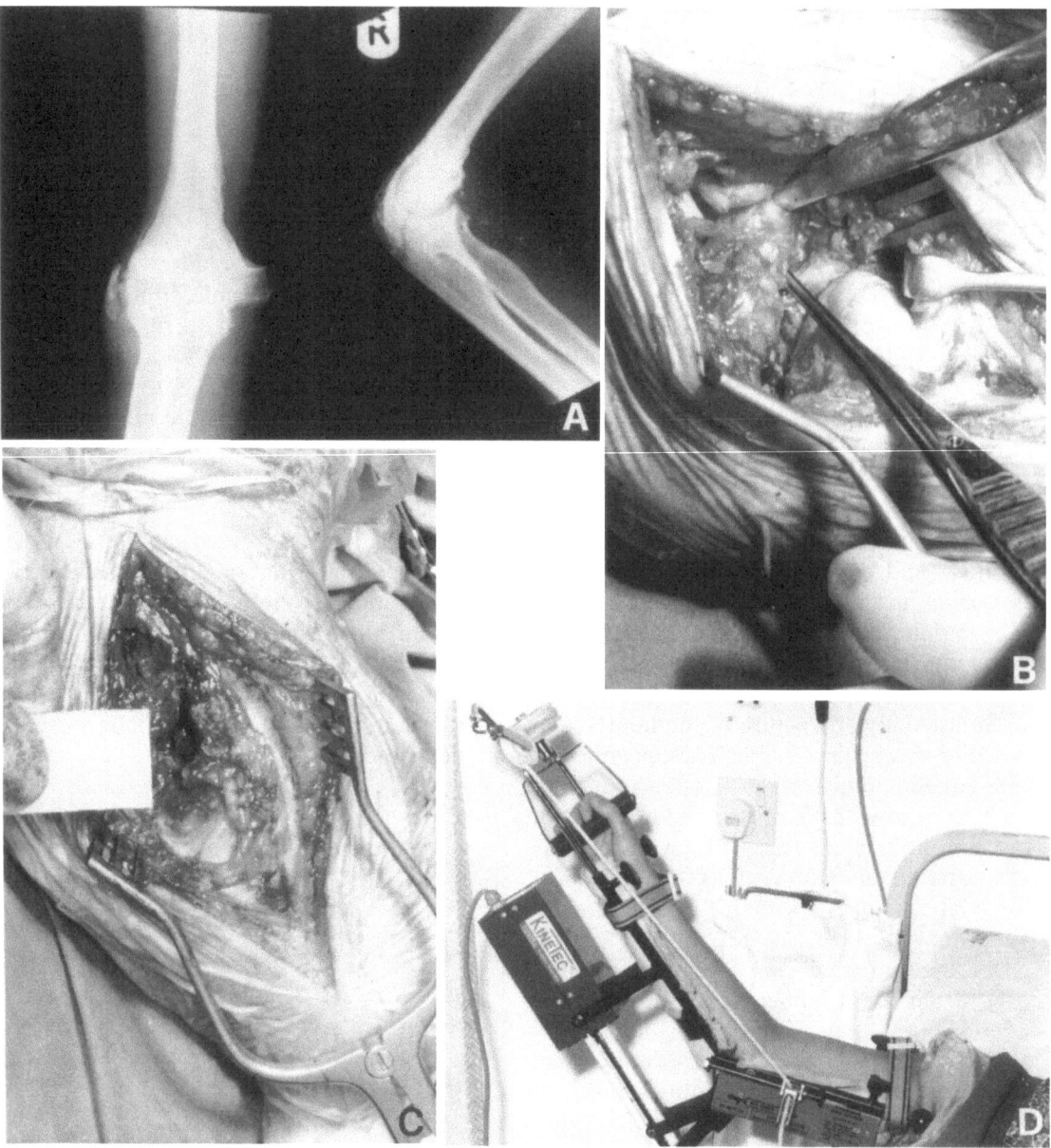

Fig. 2. - More extensive surgical release is required when there is bony deformity and severe anterior and posterior adhesions in addition to thickening and contracture of the anterior capsule. Here, bone has been resected anteriorly from the humerus, then being covered with bone wax; anterior and posterior adhesions have been released. This lady was managed postoperatively on a passive motion machine, movement being increased by 35 degrees.

In all patients after surgical arthrolysis, a very intensive active exercise programme is mandatory: nowadays, a passive motion machine can be a useful adjunct in the management of these awkward cases. Progressive osteoarthritis of the elbow and proximal radioulnar joints can be an important long-term result of intraarticular fractures of the elbow; in fact, most patients with arthritis of the elbow are suffering from rheumatoid disease.

In those suffering from osteoarthritis, lower humeral fenestration arthroplasty can be considered, described by Outerbridge and

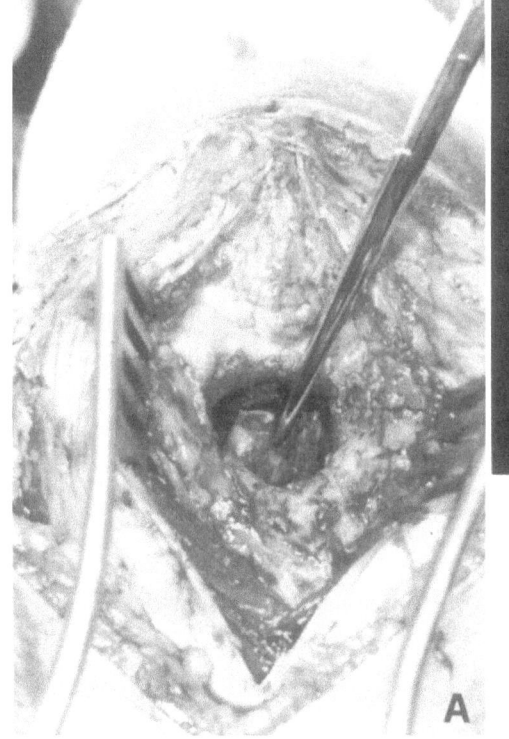
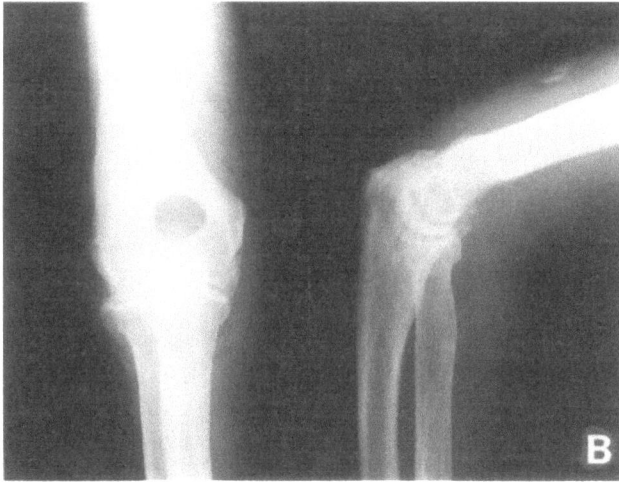

Fig. 3. - Painful and disabling post-traumatic osteoarthritis of the elbow may be relieved by lower humeral fenestration arthroplasty, the Outerbridge-Kashiwagi
operation. Surgery is simple, a posterior triceps splitting
approach being used: posterior osteophytes in the olecranon fossa are resected, a disc of bone removed from
the fossa and any anterior loose bodies can be removed
through this window.

Kashiwagi. A posterior triceps splitting incision is used: osteophytic formation in the olecranon fossa is resected and a 1.5 cm
diameter window is opened to communicate
with the anterior joint cavity. Interestingly,
loose bodies lying anteriorly can easily be
removed through the lower humeral window.
In terms of pain relief, modest improvement
in motion and increased function, this can be
a worthwhile and simple procedure.

In more severe cases of osteoarthritis of
the elbow, consideration may have to be given
to prosthetic replacement of the joint. Available elbow prostheses are fully constrained,
semi-constrained, or non-constrained.

An example of the non-constrained variety is the Wadsworth II elbow prosthesis.
The articulating surface is concavo-convex;
the prosthesis has humeral and ulnar stems
and is made of Titanium: the proximal articulating surface is metal and the distal surface is
high-density polyethylene, trapped in the re-
mainder of the metal ulnar component.

The author has described a posterolateral
approach to the elbow joint which gives excellent exposure: a curved posterior skin incision is made with a lateral convexity, a tongue
of triceps tendon, distally based, being reflected. The ulnar nerve is identified and protected, and if necessary, the cubital tunnel can
be surgically released. Usually, the radial
head is resected and the lower humerus and
the olecranon and proximal ulnar nerve shaft
are appropriately prepared; then, the humeral
and ulnar components are cemented in position. Postoperatively, the elbow is immo-
bilised in a well-padded posterior p.o.p. splint
with the elbow at 90 degrees and the forearm
in zero position; this is used intermittently
after the first five days and at that time an active exercise programme is begun, the splint
being discarded at four weeks post-surgery. It
is unwise to insert an elbow prosthesis in
those patients who have to go back to a heavy
manual job.

All available elbow prostheses at this time
are really on clinical trial; failure for any reason may result in the necessity for resection
arthroplasty or even arthrodesis of the elbow
joint; however, many patients do have a pleasing result from elbow prosthesis surgery, particularly if this is non-constrained.

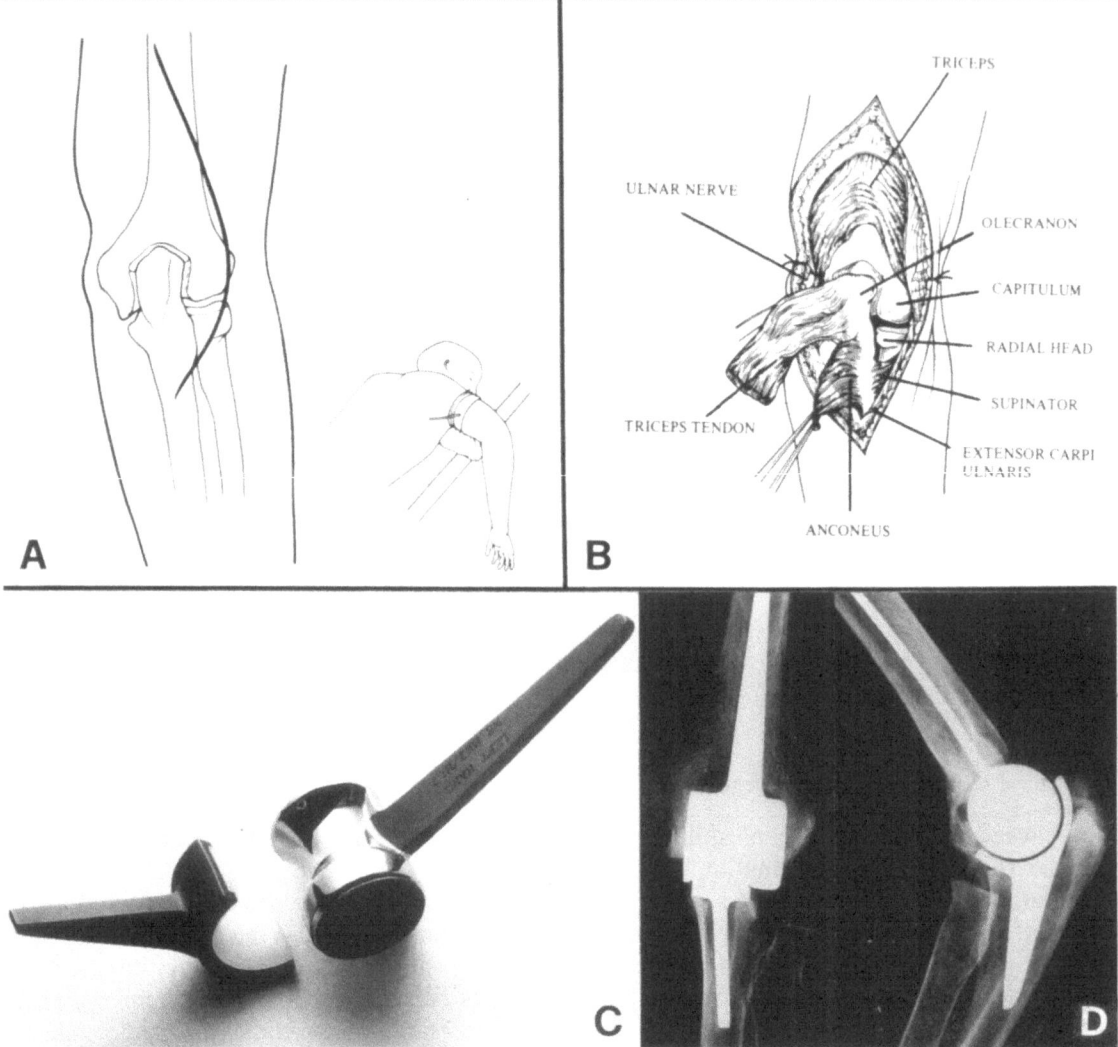

Fig. 4. - In more severe cases of post-traumatic osteoarthritis, prosthetic replacement of the elbow joint may be required. Here, a Wadsworth II non-constrained has been inserted, using the posterolateral approach.

REFERENCES

1) GLYN J.J., NIEBAUER, J.J.: Flexion and extension contracture of the elbow. Surgical management. *Clin. Orthop. Rel. Res.* 1976; **117**: 289.
2) KASHIWAGI D.: Osteoarthritis of the elbow. In: *Elbow Joint.* D. Kashiwagi (ed.). The Netherlands: Elsevier Science Publishers B.V. (Biomedical Division), Excerpta Medica (International Congress Series 678), 1985.
3) MORREY B.F.: *The elbow and its disorders.* W.B. Saunders Company, Philadelphia, 1985.

4) URBANIAK J.R., HANSEN P.E., BEISSINGER S.F., AITKEN M.S.: Correction of post-traumatic flexion contracture of the elbow. *J. Bone Jt. Surg.* 1985; **67**-A: 1160.
5) WADSWORTH T.G.: A modified postero-lateral approach to the elbow and proximal radio-ulnar joints. *Clin. Orthop. Rel. Res.* 1979; **144**: 151.
6) WADSWORTH T.G.: *The elbow.* Churchill Livingstone, London and New York, Edinburgh, 1990, 2nd ed.

The use of arthroplasty in elbow trauma

W.A. Souter

HISTORICAL BACKGROUND - EARLY DISASTERS

Radiographic appearances of the type illustrated in Fig. 1 not unnaturally gave the elbow arthroplasties of the early 1970's an unenviable reputation for inherent disaster.

Although the immediate postoperative results were beguilingly brilliant with regard to pain relief and recovery of movement, within 5 years, 75% were showing evidence of radiological loosening while over 40% exhibited major clinical instability (1).

Most of these early elbow replacements were performed on rheumatoid patients, but in the few cases undertaken for post-traumatic problems, the results were certainly no better, which was hardly surprising in view of the much greater stresses to which these patients were likely to subject the prosthesis and its fixation.

Loosening of the surrounding distal humeral shaft, which was then liable to fracture in the event of a fall, fracture of the prosthetic stem itself, the repeated necessity for revisions, and the totally flail nature of the pseudarthrosis if the prosthesis had finally to be removed, were all likely to render the supervision of the patient's subsequent clinical course something of a nightmare. Clearly fully constrained metallic hinge arthroplasty did not hold the answer, either for the severely eroded rheumatoid joint or for the post-traumatic elbow.

THE PROBLEM AND A POSSIBLE SOLUTION

It is generally accepted that the main cause of loosening of the original hinges was the high torsional force which had to be transmitted across the elbow in such activities as lifting a fairly heavy object between the palms of the hands where an internal rotational force must be generated on the humerus by the pectoral muscles and their synergists. This force is normally passed across the wide bone surface of the elbow into the forearm, any tendency for the elbow to buckle outwards being resisted by the tiebeam of the medial collateral ligament.

After the early hinge arthroplasties in which the collateral ligaments were completely excised, the only mechanism for passing this internal rotation force from arm to forearm was the cement-bone interface in the humerus, the latter acting as a box-spanner around the stem of the humeral component.

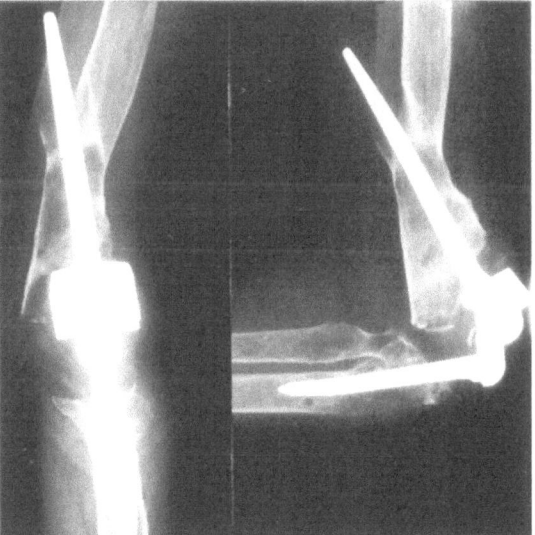

Fig. 1. - Radiograph of left elbow showing the extreme ballooning and thinning of the distal cortex which could be so disastrous after the original hinge arthroplasties. Here gross penetration of the antero-medial humeral cortex by the stem of the implant has occurred and it seems likely that this humerus has been the site of a previous pathological fracture.

A further factor in loosening may have been the posterior pull of such muscles as the brachioradialis when the elbow is flexed to 90 degrees. This is likely to displace the hilt of any hinge mechanism posteriorly relative to the long axis of the humerus.

Accordingly, if the slightest loosening had once been set up by torsional forces, there would be a tendency for this force to draw the hilt of the hinge posteriorly while tilting the tip of the humeral stem anteriorly against the anterior humeral cortex. Experience in fact showed that this was indeed what happened, as ballooning or frank perforation of the anterior humeral cortex opposite the tip of the humeral stem was frequently visible on radiographs.

Morrey (2) stresses that during movement of the elbow there is a cyclical reversal of the thrust on the humeral fixation from an anterior vector when the elbow is in extension to an increasingly posterior vector as full flexion is approached. This again could be a potent cause of loosening.

In order to address these problems, a joint research project was set up between Professor Paul's Bioengineering Unit of the University of Strathclyde, Glasgow, and by own clinical unit in Edinburgh, the engineer principally involved in the research being Dr. A.C. Nicol.

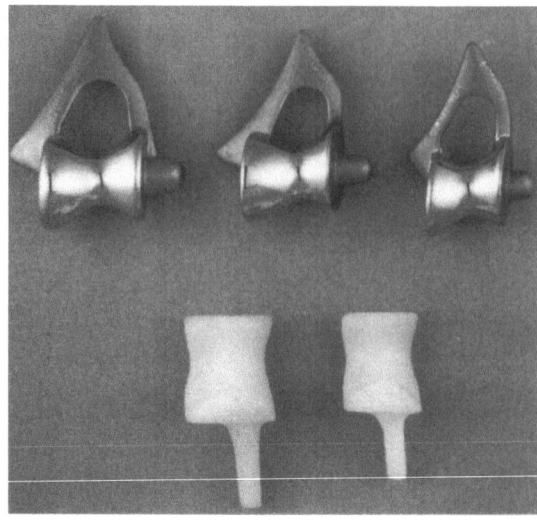

Fig. 3. - The humeral component is available in three sizes and the ulnar component in two. Each of the humeral components is compatible with either of the ulnar components and indeed the use of the medium humeral component along with the small ulnar component is fairly frequently required. The large humeral component is virtually always required in male patients.

By 1977 we were ready to start clinical trials with a prototype which, apart from a small early alteration to the coronoid process and the angle of the ulnar stem, still remains our standard prosthesis for the vast majority of the elbow replacements we undertake (Fig. 2).

Three sizes of this standard model are now available (Fig. 3).

In patients with extremely severe condylar erosion, bone coverage of the flanges of the standard implant may be incomplete or totally impossible. For such cases a longer-stemmed model is available (Fig. 4).

The rationale behind our own design of humeral component has been to carry fixation as far out to the extremity of the epicondyles as possible (Fig. 5) and to utilise in addition the whole arch of the supracondylar ridges so as to give maximal resistance to torsional stresses and changing anteroposterior vectors. The ulnar component is securely anchored in the excavated olecranon by a dovetailed keel which is continued distally into a short stem in the proximal ulnar shaft.

Since the prosthesis has been modelled as closely as possible on the contours and align-

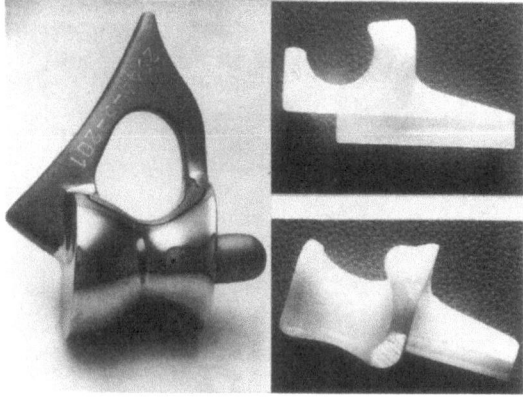

Fig. 2. - Standard model of Souter-Strathclyde elbow prosthesis. The articular surfaces of the humeral and ulnar components are modelled as closely as possible on those of the normal elbow joint. As the prosthesis is asymmetrical in shape, right and left models are required.

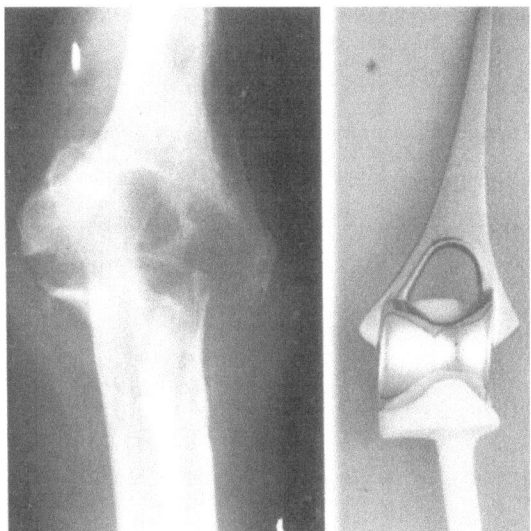

Fig. 4. - Radiograph of left elbow showing severe grade 5 rheumatoid erosion. Here the residual bone of the humeral condyles would be insufficient to cover the fixation flanges of the standard prosthesis. The long-stemmed model of the humeral component which is suitable for such cases is shown on the right. Note that the side fixation flanges are much smaller and more proximally sited.

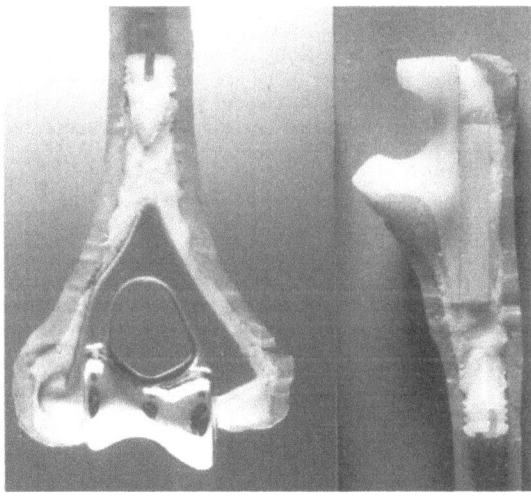

A   **B**

Fig. 5. - A) This hemi-section of distal humerus shows the excellent fixation which is achieved by the penetration of flanges and cement well out to the epicondyles of the humerus. This is supplemented by the extensive fixation offered by the countersinking of the whole metal stirrup of the prosthesis into the excavated supracondylar ridges. B) The hemi-section of the ulna shows the fixation of the ulnar component in the olecranon by a dovetailed keel which is prolonged into the proximal ulna by a short 2.5 cm stem. Note the Exeter cement restricters used in both bones to limit penetration and enhance the impaction of the cement.

ment of the normal elbow, we believe that the assembled joint very accurately mimics the biomechanics of the normal anatomical elbow.

IMPROVED RESULTS OF ARTHROPLASTY IN THE FIELD OF RHEUMATOID SURGERY

To date, our clinical experience has been very encouraging. Pain relief has been excellent and has been well-maintained at 5 years (Table 1).

Moreover these results have been reproduced successfully by a variety of units taking part in our field trial (Table 2).

Table 1
ELBOW ARTHROPLASTY IN ADULT RHEUMATOID DISEASE

Pain status	Before surgery	1 year after surgery	5 years after surgery
None	3	72	69
Occ. twinges	–	6	8
Mild	–	6	4
Significant	10	1	4
Severe	72	–	–
Total	85	85	85

Table 2
FIELD TRIAL OF ELBOW ARTHROPLASTY

Pain status	Before surgery	At latest follow-up (Mean 1.7 years)
None	–	63
Occasional	–	40
Mild	7	15
Significant	69	11
Severe	57	4
Total	133	133

Similarly favourable and reproducible results have been achieved with regard to movement (Table 3). Postoperative flexion, pronation, and supination have been very acceptable and only the recovery of extension has proved disappointing.

Such improvements were of course equally well-obtained through the use of the original hinge replacements, and the real question is whether the durability of the

Table 3
ELBOW ARTHROPLASTY IN ADULT RHEUMATOID DISEASE

	Home unit (n= 85)			Field trial units (n= 133)	
	Before surgery	1 yr after surgery	5 yrs after surgery	Before surgery	At latest follow-up (Mean 1.7 yrs)
Flexion	127	143	145	116	136
Pronation	49	64	67	54	73
Supination	47	65	68	50	65
Extension (Flex. deformity)	47	49	57	42	41

procedure has now been improved. We would submit that this is indeed the case. In our first 100 cases we encountered no primary loosenings and only 4 secondary loosenings resulting from a fracture of the medial epicondyle, a fracture of the olecranon, persistent dislocation, and a possible chronic infection or metal sensitivity. Our radiological loosening rate has also shown great improvement (Fig. 6), and we have witnessed none of the thinning and ballooning of the humeral shaft which was such a dangerous complication of the original hinge procedures. If we take a radiolucent line greater than 1 mm that shows some indication of activity as evidence of x-ray loosening, it would seem that we have

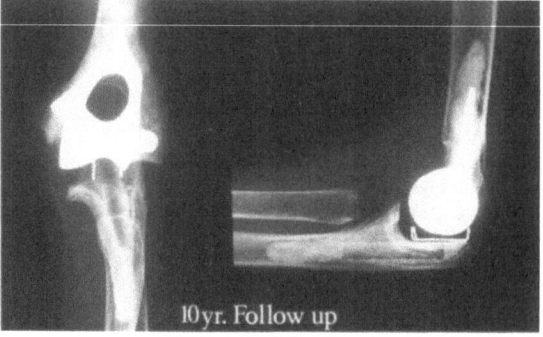

Fig. 6. - Radiograph of prosthesis *in situ* 10 years after the original operation. Note the absence of any cement line around the humeral flanges and stirrup. On the ulnar side, although thin cement lines are visible between the cement and the cut edges of olecranon and proximal face of the coronoid, none are seen in the depths of the olecranon nor around the cement plug in the proximal ulnar shaft.

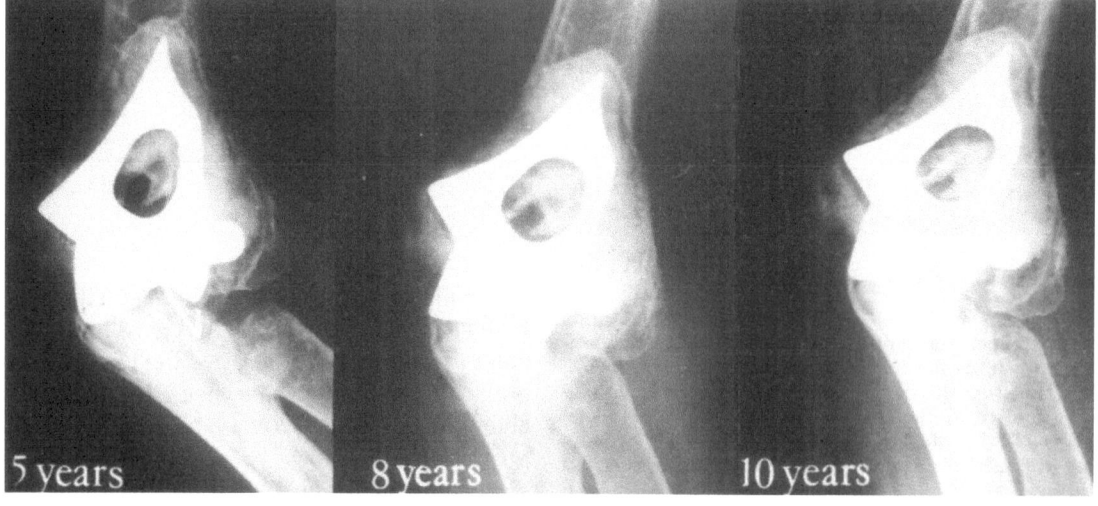

Fig. 7. - Radiographic follow-up on a female patient with definite radiological loosening of the humeral component at 5 years shows only very slow deterioration at 8 and 10 years. Moreover, at 10 years this patient still remains entirely symptom-free.

been able to contain our loosening rate within a figure of 11-12%.

Moreover, through advocating the use of our long-stemmed prosthesis should any fracture of the supracondylar ridges occur at surgery, and through the introduction of the large sized humeral component for use in male patients, we would hope that in the future our incidence of radiological loosening will be halved. I should stress that the elbows in which we have observed radiological loosening still remain largely symptom-free and exhibited very little evidence of further radiological deterioration during the 5-10 year follow-up period (Fig. 7).

THE NEED FOR A GRADUATED SYSTEM OF PROSTHESES TO MATCH THE FULL SPECTRUM OF ELBOW PATHOLOGY

In very severe grade 5 erosion (Fig. 4) it might be thought that the joint would be too unstable and the ligamentous destruction too great for an unlinked surface replacement to be successful. Apart from the need to resort to the use of the long-stemmed model of our humeral component, however, no great difficulty has been encountered in achieving satisfactory results in this type of case. Perhaps even more surprising was the relative ease with which we were able to obtain very satisfactory fixation and stability in a highly unstable and painful excision arthroplasty. In addition, successful results have also been achieved in the reconstruction of elbows destroyed by JCA even where preoperative bony ankylosis has existed for years (Fig. 8).

It is however important to realise that there are limitations to unlinked surface or condylar replacements of the elbow. Where complete disruption of the supracondylar ridges has occurred, or where there is actual loss of bone extending into the humeral shaft, or total loss of the ligaments, an unlinked prosthesis will not yield satisfactory results and the aid of custom built, linked modifications of our implant may be necessary (Fig. 9). In these, the HDP insert is slightly greater than a semicircle, so that it provides a snapfit over the waist of the metal trochlea. As the transmission of torsional forces is likely to be

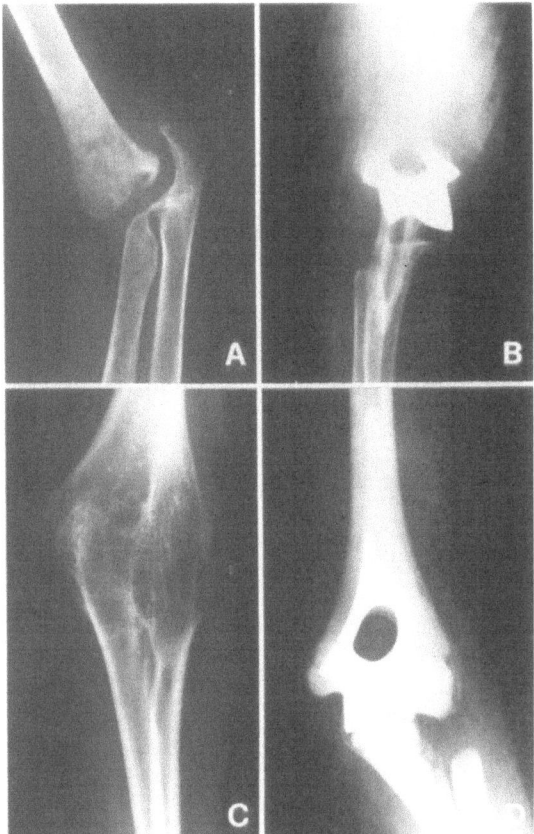

Fig. 8. - A,B) Radiographs of an elbow in which excision arthroplasty two years previously had resulted in a painful flail joint. This was successfully reconstructed using a long-stemmed prosthesis. C,D) Radiographs of elbow showing bony ankylosis resulting from juvenile chronic arthritis. Despite the fact that the elbow had been ankylosed for several years, stable reconstruction with our standard prosthesis was still possible as the ligaments were found to be essentially intact.

much greater with this type of prosthesis, the ulnar components are strengthened by metal backing and secured with 5-9 cm intramedullary stems. The stems we have used on the humeral side are 15 cm in length. It is important to match the prosthesis to the bone stock available (Figs. 10-11). Where the supracondylar ridges have been symmetrically preserved, flanges should be retained on both sides of the prosthesis for fixation. Where only the medial or more usually the lateral ridge remains, the prosthesis can be appropriately modelled. Where both ridges have been lost, the unsupported metallic shoulders of the implant are strengthened to avoid fatigue

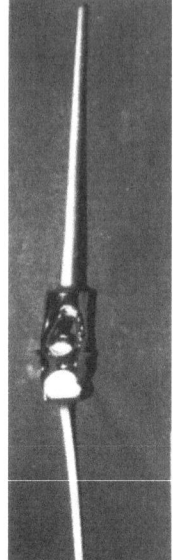
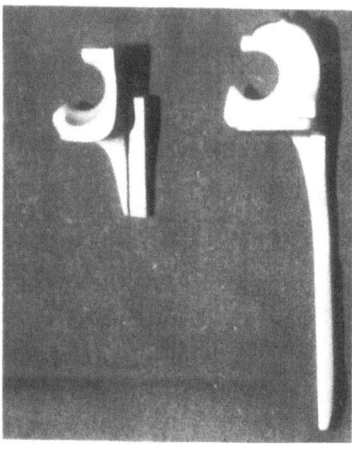

Fig. 9. - Snapfit model of prosthesis suitable for cases in which the ligaments or their attachments have been destroyed. The dimensions of the trochlear joint are modelled on the small standard implant. The humeral component has a 15 cm stem, while the ulnar component is metalbacked and equipped with a 5-9 cm stem according to the degree of bone destruction in the proximal ulna. The HDP insert in the ulnar component is slightly greater than a semicircle so that it provides a snapfit over the waist of the metal trochlea.

fracture. Finally where there has been loss of humeral shaft a cylinder of metal is incorporated in the prosthesis to maintain skeletal length.

Armed with this system of implants it should be possible to treat the whole spectrum of elbow pathology. For the vast majority of the rheumatoid patients (85%), the standard prosthesis (Figs. 2-3) should suffice. A further 14% may require the longer-stemmed humeral model (Fig. 4) and only about 1% will require the custom built snapfit joints shown in Fig. 11. The latter however are likely to play a much larger role in the management of post-traumatic cases.

POTENTIAL PROBLEMS WHICH MAY BE ENCOUNTERED IN APPLYING ARTHROPLASTY TECHNIQUES TO THE MANAGEMENT OF ELBOW TRAUMA

The greatly improved results of elbow arthroscopy in rheumatoid disease have natu-

rally led to a reexamination of the potential of total joint replacement in the management of the sequelae of trauma (3). Many questions remain to be answered. Will the scarring associated with trauma reduce postoperative movement? Will myositis ossificans be a problem? Will myositis recur? Will the incidence of loosening be much higher? Will the necessity to resort to linked implants have adverse effects on the durability of the re-

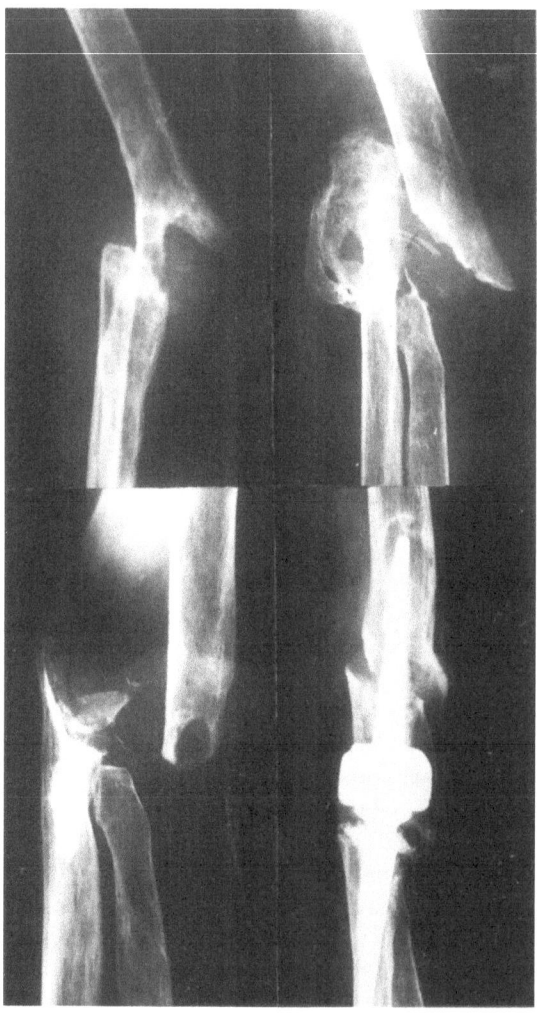

Fig. 10. - Radiograph illustrating the progressive bone destruction in the distal humerus which may occur spontaneously in severe rheumatoid arthritis, or as the result of severe elbow trauma, or again may be encountered in difficult revision surgery. Any of these humeral pathologies may be complicated by varying degrees of bone loss or perforation in the proximal ulna, including total loss of the olecranon.

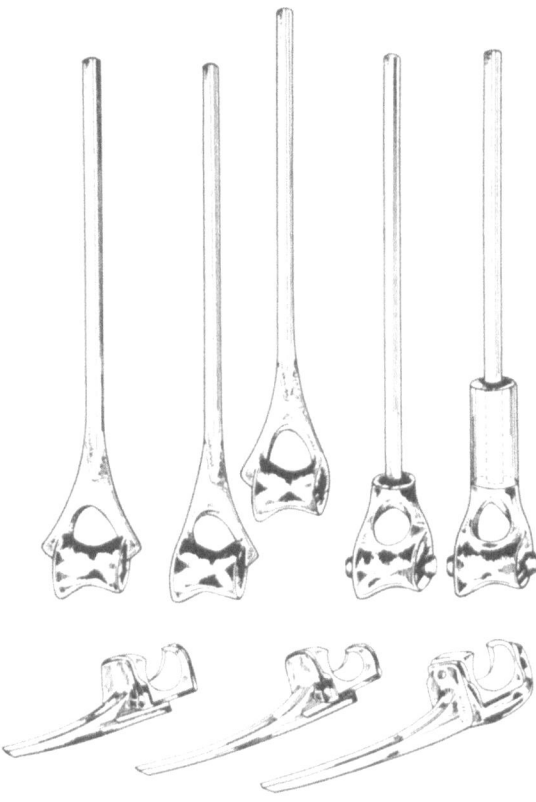

Fig. 11. - Graduated system of snapfit prostheses with which it should be possible to cope with the full spectrum of advanced elbow pathology. At present such prostheses are custom built, but it is hoped that they will shortly be available as "off the shelf" extensions to the standard range. It is important to match the appropriate prosthesis to the stages of bone destruction illustrated in Fig. 10 (see also in text). The ulnar component shown at the far right has no dovetailed keel but backing for use in patients with total loss of the olecranon.

◄

dylar fractures of the humerus.

5. Nonunion of high supracondylar comminuted distal shaft fractures of the humerus.

Any of the above may be complicated by distorsion, fragmentation, or complete absence of the olecranon.

As experience grows in this field it is conceivable that elbow arthroplasty might occasionally be applicable in the primary treatment of severe elbow injuries. To date however we have not undertaken any such procedures, our experience being entirely confined to secondary or tertiary reconstructive surgery.

sults? Will the incidence of infection rise unacceptably, expecially in initially compound injuries which have in any way been complicated by delayed wound healing or any frank element of infection? Only time and the careful observation of the growing clientele for this type of surgery will provide the answers. What we know already is that elbow arthroplasties in post-traumatic patients are technically much more difficult to do. Consequently, surgeons contemplating this form of treatment would be well-advised to serve their apprenticeship on rheumatoid patients.

POSSIBLE INDICATIONS FOR ELBOW ARTHROPLASTY AFTER TRAUMA

1. Malunion of intraarticular fractures with severe loss of movement.

2. Post-traumatic arthritis resulting in pain and severe loss of movement.

3. Myositis ossificans causing severe or total loss of movement.

4. Nonunion of trans, supra, or intercon-

Problems of malunion and post-traumatic arthritis

Where severe loss of elbow movement has occurred in the presence of a relatively mild degree of malunion, treatment should initially be by soft tissue release and appropriate recontouring of the bone. Where this fails, however, or where one is faced with irretrievable distortion of the articular surfaces, total joint replacement must be very seriously considered especially as the patient is likely to have a major degree of pain and disability. The major counterindication would be the patient's work if this involved significant impact stresses or the handling of vibrating tools, since in these circumstances early loosening of the prosthesis would be almost inevitable. In such cases, and where a change of occupation is impossible, it might be necessary to have recourse to the far from ideal solutions of excision arthroplasty or arthrodesis.

To date we have undertaken total elbow replacement for post-traumatic arthritis with major loss of movement in 7 patients. Our longest follow-up is in a young man who presented at the age of 26 painful post-traumatic arthritis resulting from a fracture one year previously (Fig. 12). Prior to surgery the patient had a range of movement of only 68-110 degrees. At his recent 8-year follow-up the joint remained pain-free and exhibited a range of movement from 40-147 degrees, or a gain of just over 70 degrees.

Even in our as yet very limited experience of arthroplasty for post-traumatic arthritis, it has become obvious that there are many technical difficulties and pitfalls over and above those likely to be encountered in the rheumatoid clientele.

A) Extensive scarring from the original injury and/or previous operative interven-

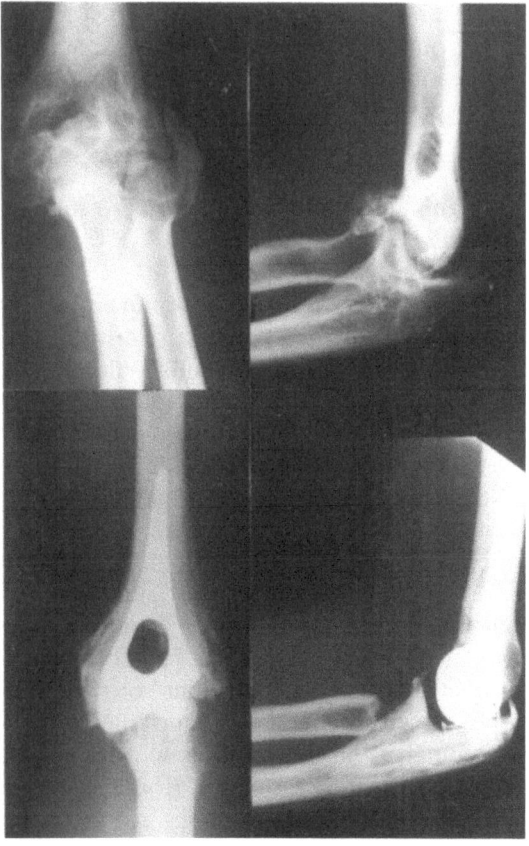

Fig. 12. - Radiograph of the left elbow of a 26 year-old man with well-established changes of post-traumatic arthritis one year after injury. The lower radiographs show the very satisfactory appearance of the elbow 8 years after total joint replacement.

tions may render further approaches to the elbow hazardous with regard to wound healing. Hence it may be necessary to alter the operative technique so as to limit as far as possible the need for extensive elevation of skin flaps. Where severe soft tissue injury has occurred, such scarring may be virtually circumferential. One of our patients was a 19-year-old man who was referred from Saudi Arabia 7 years after the original fracture. The elbow was covered with multiple extensive scars resulting from the original injury and from previous surgical intervention in Cairo. Moreover it exhibited only 80-100 degrees of rather painful movement. Although it was perfectly possible to carry out our standard arthroplasty procedure, I am afraid I was overzealous in attempting to remove all the fragments of bone from the front of the joint. Some of these were adherent to paper-thin scars on the cubital fossa. Postoperatively this scar tissue gave way with the formation of a joint sinus and the plastic surgeons had to be brought in to transpose a small flap from amid the preexisting scars to achieve adequate closure and thus avoid the almost certain complication of infection of the prosthesis had the sinus been allowed to persist for any length of time. In spite of all these problems, and of the necessity of keeping the elbow splinted for 3-4 weeks after surgery, a range of movement from 70-120 degrees was achieved.

B) Considerable distortion of the supracondylar ridges may have occurred at the time of surgery and this may render the fitting of our standard, or even our long-stemmed humeral component, extremely difficult. Nevertheless, with the aid of a high speed ball-headed burr it may be possible to carve out a satisfactory fixation channel from the distorted bone.

C) In one of our patients in whom the foregoing difficulty was successfully circumvented, and who initially appeared to achieve a very satisfactory postoperative range of movement, subsequent progressive loss of movement became a major problem. Unfortunately, this patient was from abroad and as a result we have no proper follow-up data. From correspondence, however, it would seem very possible that the virtually total loss of movement which eventually occurred had been due to myositis ossificans. If this was indeed so it was in very marked contrast to our experience with rheumatoid patients in whom myositis ossificans is virtually unknown.

D) Where major soft tissue contractures have followed the original injury there may be a need for formal lengthening of tendons or for muscle slide procedures. The presence of such soft tissue scarring may also explain why the remobilisation in the immediate postoperative convalescence has tended to be much more difficult than in the average rheumatoid patients. In one of our patients, a 33-year-old man, the original injury would seem to have been in the nature of a Monteggia fracture complicated by initially unrecognised damage to the condyles of the humerus. The joint had subsequently ankylosed in virtually full extension. This is an appalling disability for any patient, and total elbow replacement seemed amply justified. Postoperative mobilisation unfortunately proved much more difficult than had been anticipated, the posterior tissues being extremely tight so that V-Y lengthening of the triceps tendon was required. One year after surgery, a range of movement from 48-98 degrees is all that has been

achieved. Even this, however, still represents a major functional improvement.

E) The degree of malalignment of the fracture fragments of the humeral condyles may be such as to render the attachment of the collateral ligaments and their resulting tension so abnormal as to make it impossible to reestablish stability with an unlinked prosthesis. We in fact encountered this in a 23 year-old woman referred 6 years after her original injury, in which she had sustained a severe fracture-dislocation of the elbow with ulnar nerve involvement. Nonunion of the trochlear fragment complicated her convalescence and necessitated bone grafting. Transposition of the ulnar nerve was also required. At the time of her referral she still had a painful elbow which was clearly the site of severe post-traumatic arthritis resulting from considerable malalignment of the radial and ulnar compartments of the joint (Fig. 13). The range of movement was only 80-115 degrees. In view of the malalignment it was anticipated that it might be very difficult to get ligamentous stability with our standard prosthesis. Accordingly, a linked prosthesis was ordered for her. With the aid of this she has achieved a remarkable satisfactory range of movement

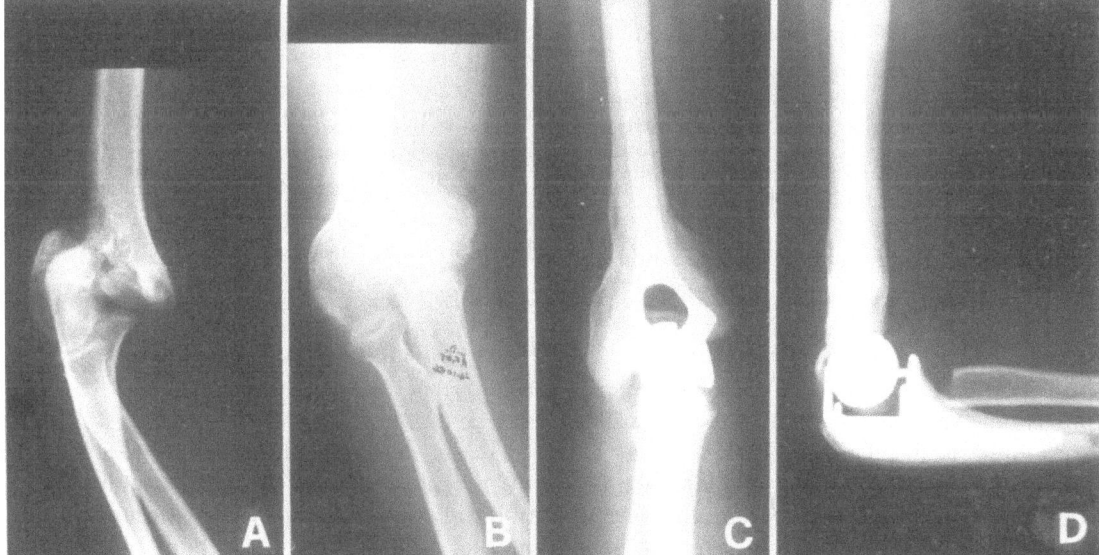

Fig. 13. - A) Radiograph of original comminuted fracture-dislocation of right elbow in a 23 year-old woman. B) Radiograph taken 6 years later showing malunion with marked malalignment of the medial and lateral humeral "condyles" with well-developed post-traumatic arthritis. C,D) Radiographs showing reconstruction of the elbow with a custom built snapfit prosthesis.

(58-138 degrees) and has complete relief of pain.

F) A past history of infection complicating the initial trauma greatly increases the hazards of secondary joint replacement. In the one case in our series in which this problem existed, a successful outcome was achieved under antibiotic cover and with the use of antibiotic impregnated cement, the reconstructive surgery being undertaken two years after the original injury.

G) Finally one of our cases represented the late result of a nonunion of a lateral condylar fracture sustained in childhood (Fig. 14). Somewhat contrary to our expectations, recontouring of the greatly distorted and ununited fragment to which the lateral ligament complex was securely attached, allowed it to be screwed back as an "epicondyle" with re-

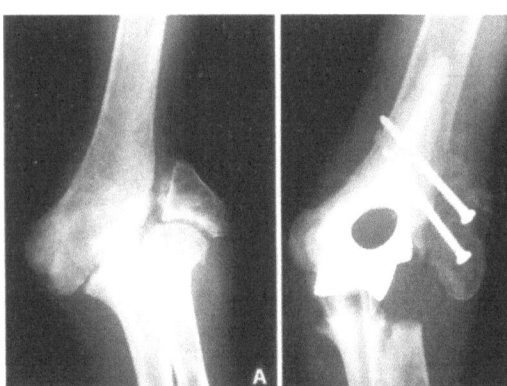

Fig. 14. - A) Radiograph of arthritic elbow in a 61 year-old man who had sustained a lateral condylar fracture in childhood. B) Successful and stable reconstruction using an unlinked long-stemmed model of prosthesis with recontoured fragment secured back as epicondylar attachment for lateral ligament.

sulting very adequate restoration of joint stability and a pain-free range of movement from 54-134 degrees.

The overall result with regard to pre and postoperative movement in the five patients on whom we have adequate follow-up data are summarised in Table 4. As these joints are all essentially pain-free, the functional gain to the patient has been enormous. In view of this, all the difficulties which have just been enumerated are to be regarded as a challenge and not a contraindication to employing total replacement arthroplasty in the secondary reconstruction of the traumatic elbow.

Table 4
ARTHROPLASTY IN POST-TRAUMATIC ARTHRITIS

Ankylosed cases: 2	
Pre.-op. position	Post-op. range
0	48-98°
82	30-120°
Cases with limited movement: 3	
Pre-op. range	Post-op. range
68-110°	40-148°
80-115°	50-138°
30-128°	54-134°

Problems related to myositis ossificans

After severe elbow trauma, myositis ossificans can be of massive extent. Moreover, the ligaments are likely to share in the ossification and hence will have to be excised, so that a linked implant becomes essential for the maintenance of stability. To date we have dealt with two such cases. Both proved technically difficult as it was necessary, especially in the second case, to carve out the normal bone contours from a great mass of newly formed bony buttresses (Fig. 15). Nevertheless, in both a very worthwhile arc of movement was reestablished, the first patient achieving 40-130 degrees, and the second 70-122 degrees. The situation with regard to the restoration of supination and pronation, however, has been much less satisfactory as further new bone formation in one patient has greatly limited pronation and supination, while in the second complete recurrence of the radioulnar synostosis has taken place.

Nonunion of trans, supra, or intercondylar fractures of the humerus

These can present appalling disabilities for patients who may have been subjected to multiple operations involving various types of internal fixation with or without bone grafting. Moreover, many years may have elapsed since the original injury before the patient is eventually seen by the arthroplasty surgeon. To date we have dealt with three such cases.

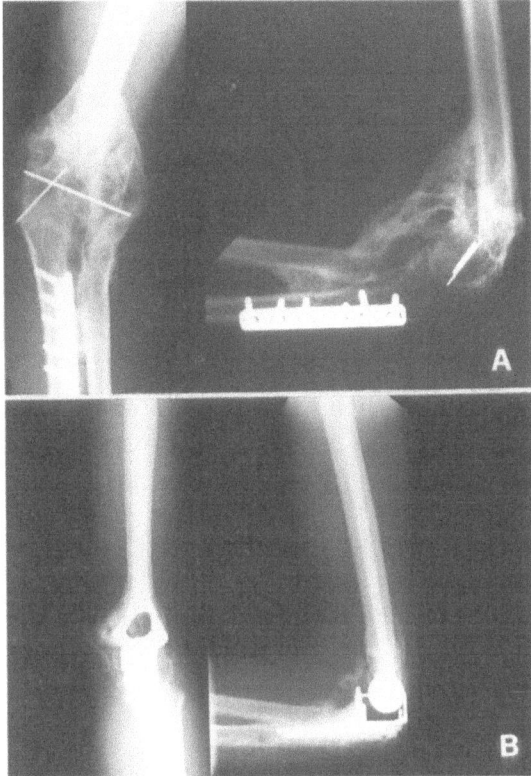

Fig. 15. - A) Radiographs of gross myositis ossificans following severely comminuted fracture-dislocation of right elbow in a 39 year-old man. B) Radiological appearance after radical excision of heterotopic bone and insertion of custom built snapfit joint. Although useful elbow movement was restored, the recurrence of radioulnar synostosis has resulted in complete loss of forearm rotation.

One of our patients, a 59 year-old woman, was seen 5 years after the original injury (Fig. 16). Active movement was from 15 degrees of hyperextension to 25 degrees of flexion. Passive movement on the other hand was from 25 degrees of hyperextension to 165 degrees of flexion. After satisfactory reconstruction with a custom built snapfit joint (Fig. 17), good, stable, pain-free movement from 15 to 130 degrees was reestablished. The rise in morale and quality of life accompanying such improved function can hardly be overestimated.

Another very similar situation was encountered in a 60 year-old man seen two years after the injury. Prior to arthroplasty he had active movement from 27 to 84 degrees and passive movement from 15 degrees of

hyperextension to 115 degrees of flexion. Postoperatively he has stable movement from 40 to 120 degrees.

Nonuniun of comminuted high supracondylar or distal humeral shaft fractures

If low supracondylar or intercondylar fractures can give rise to painful flail problems, nonunion of high supracondylar or low shaft fractures can result in completely devastating degrees of disability. Two such problems have been successfully dealt with.

The first of these was a 48 year-old nurse who had undergone multiple surgery over a 7-year period after injury. Her active movement was from 25 degrees of hyperextension to 122 degrees of flexion. After the fitting of a custom built implant and a four-year follow-up she has stable, pain-free movement from 8 to 140 degrees. She is absolutely delighted with the result and nurses full-time in a surgical ward.

Our second patient was a 23 year-old man who was referred 3 years after injury with active movement from 40 to 86 degrees and passive movement from 36 to 114 degrees. This disability resulted from a severe fracture-dislocation of the elbow in which some 10 cm of humerus were extruded from the arm onto the road. Although this segment of bone had been reapplied as a free graft, nonunion had occurred with gradual resorption of the dead bone (Fig. 18). Moreover, the situation had proved completely resistant to several further grafting procedures. Reconstruction with a custom built implant a few months ago has so far resulted in excellent healing with complete relief of pain and the restoration of a range of stable movement from 45 to 108 degrees.

SUMMARY AND CONCLUSIONS

1) From the foregoing survey of our current experience of the application of arthroplasty in traumatic lesions, it will be clear that the indications can in fact be quite wide-reaching, and the pathology to be treated highly variable. It therefore must be stressed

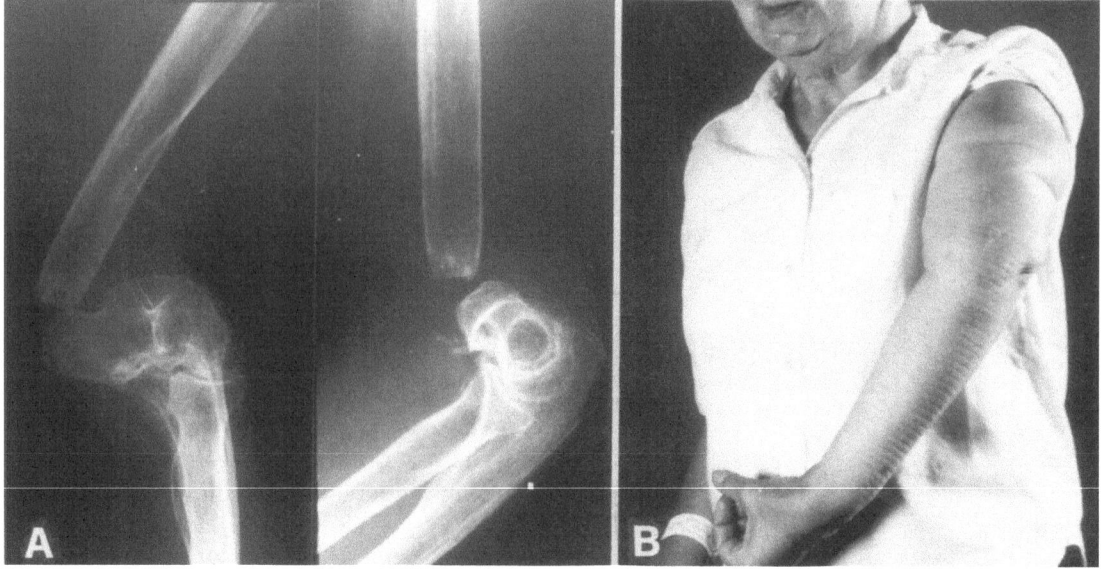

Fig. 16. - A) Radiographs of persistent nonunion of low supracondylar fracture of humerus in a 59 year-old female patient 5 years after injury. B) The marked clinical instability of the elbow is clearly apparent.

that before such cases are undertaken, the surgeon should establish a basis of very considerable experience in more routine elbow arthroplasty work and should be fully conversant with the various modifications of the implants which are avaliable on a custom built basis.

2) Careful preoperative planning is essential for a successful result.

3) It must be appreciated that these can be formidably difficult operations requiring 4 hours or more in theatre. Moreover, meticulous peroperative management of the soft tissues, especially with regard to the integrity and retensioning of the collateral ligaments, and unimpeachable postoperative supervision of the wound and skin flaps are vital to the success of the operation.

4) Provided all these points are kept in mind, total replacement arthroplasty can certainly salvage very useful function in elbows which have been the seat of intractable pain, disability and instability for many years.

▶

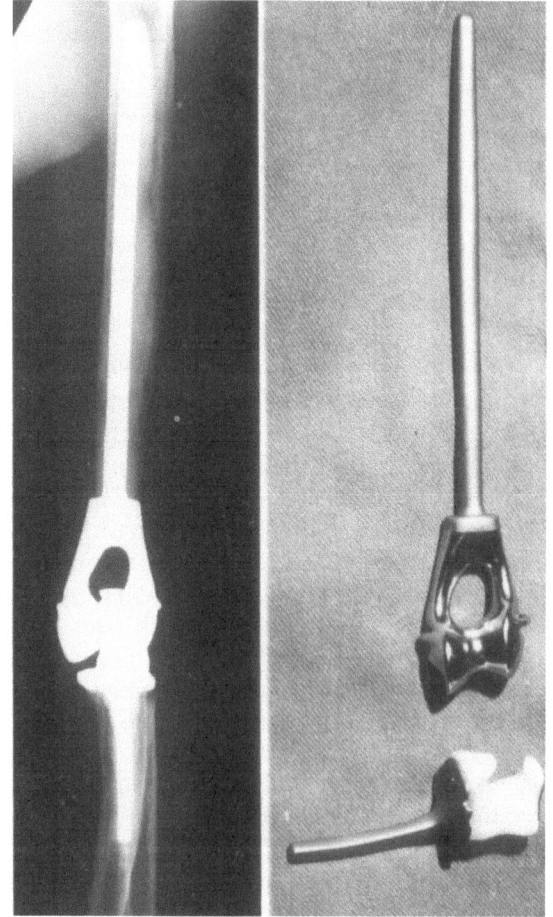

Fig. 17. - Radiograph of same elbow as in Fig. 16 after reconstruction with the snapfit prosthesis illustrated at right.

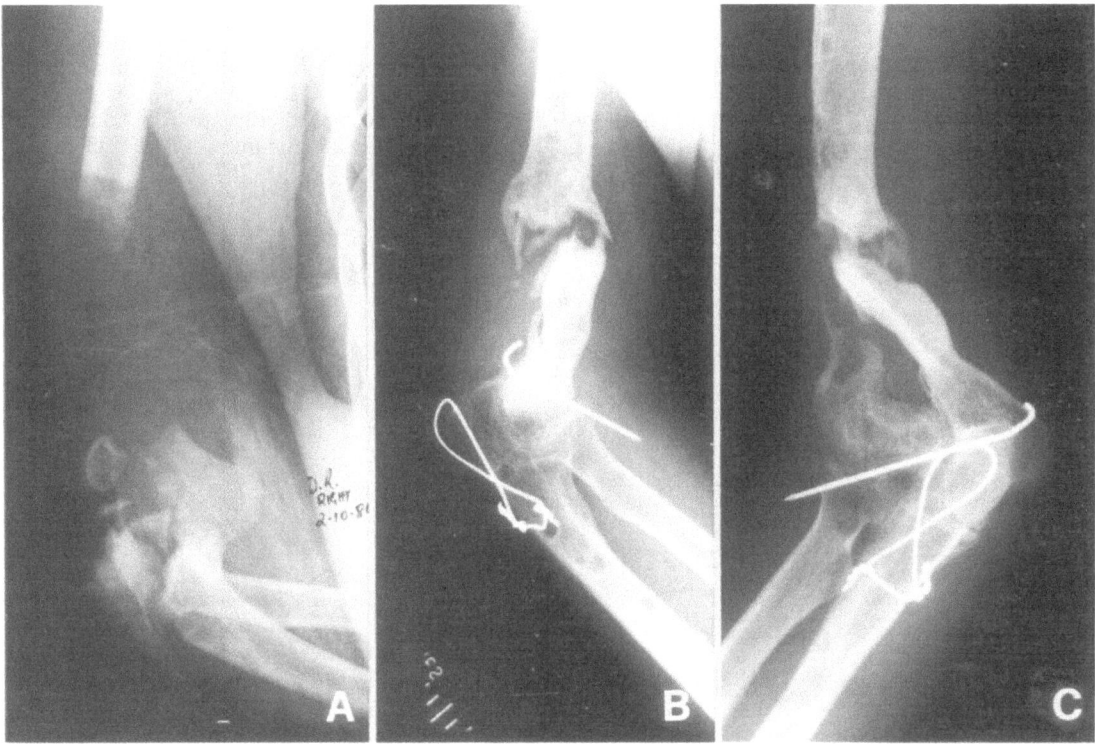

Fig. 18. - A) Radiograph of severely comminuted fracture of the elbow with loss of 10 cm segment of humerus. B,C) Radiographs taken three years after the initial injury showing persistent nonunion with necrosis and shortening of the initially extruded segment.

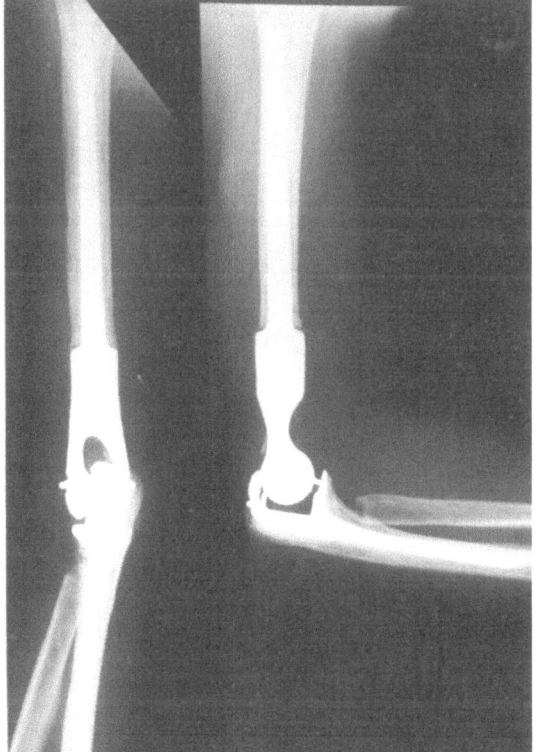

5) Whether the procedure will prove of acceptable durability in the post-traumatic elbow, only much more prolonged follow-up will determine. In view of this and of all the other at present unanswered questions already referred to, *the application of this technique should be pursued with caution.* Nevertheless, our results to date provide some grounds for optimism.

◄

Fig. 19. - Radiographs of elbow shown in Fig. 18 following reconstruction with custom built snapfit joint incorporating a cylindrical spacer in the shaft of the humeral component in order to maintain skeletal length.

REFERENCES

1) SOUTER W.A.: Total replacement arthroplasty of the elbow. In: *Joint replacement in the upper limb*. I. Mech: E. Conference Publications, 1977; **4**: 99-106.

2) MORREY B.F.: *The elbow and its disorders.*

W.B. Saunders Company, Philadelphia, 1985.

3) MITSUNAGA M.M., BRYAN R.S., LINSCHEID R.L.: Condylar nonunion of the elbow. *J. Trauma* 1982; **22** (9): 787-791.

Arthroplasty of the elbow joint

K. Tsuge

The stiff elbow with loss of function is quite common in our daily practice. This frequently occurs due to trauma but also due to rheumatoid arthritis, infectious arthritis, or osteoarthritis.

Until now, various methods have been attempted with the aim of restoring elbow function, but none of them have proved to be reliable. Over the last 20 years I have developed a new procedure of elbow arthroplasty, the results of which have been quite encouraging. In this chapter I would like to describe this procedure in detail.

SURGICAL PROCEDURE

The patient is placed in a supine position and a tourniquet is applied.

The incision begins several centimeters proximal to the elbow on the posterolateral side of the arm and proceeds distally to the lateral epicondyle. It then heads toward the base of the olecranon and continues distally along the posterior border of the ulna for 3-4 cm. The entire incision is about 12-13 cm long (Fig. 1).

Next, the subcutaneous tissue is separated on the medial side of the elbow to expose the ulnar nerve, which is protected from secondary injury by taping. Then, the periostal incision is made between the brachioradialis and the triceps muscles along the lateral supracondylar ridge, going to the base of the olecranon and then curving distally along the posterior border of the ulna.

The triceps muscle is then retracted medially to expose the attachment of the triceps tendon. The triceps attachment on the olecranon is detached subperiosteally with a scalpel, and the periosteum and its covering aponeurotic fibers are reflected ulnarward from

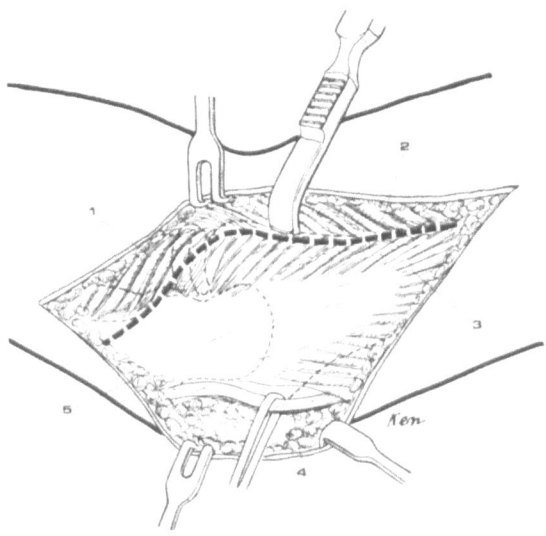

Fig. 1. - Skin incision and separation of the subcutaneous tissues. 1. Anconeus; 2. Brachioradialis; 3. Triceps; 4. Ulnar nerve; 5. Olecranon.

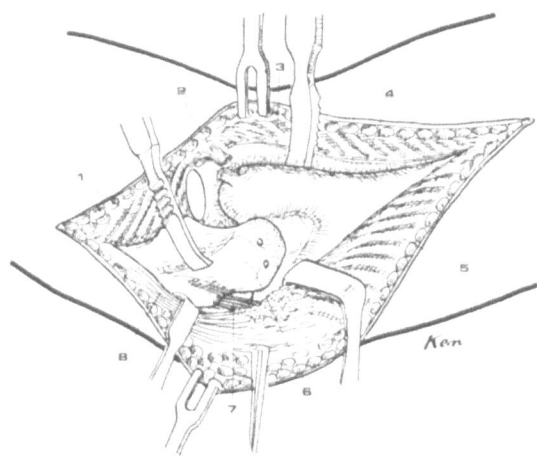

Fig. 2. - Exposure of the joint. 1. Anconeus; 2. Detached radial collateral ligament; 3. Extensor carpi radialis longus; 4. Brachioradialis; 5. Triceps; 6. Olecranon; 7. Ulnar collateral ligament; 8. Detachment of the periosteum from the ulna while maintaining the continuity of the former with the triceps tendon.

the olecranon, maintaining its continuity with the triceps tendon (Fig. 2).

Next, the brachioradialis and extensor carpi radialis longus muscles are stripped subperiosteally from the humerus anteriorly and distally, and the anconeus is stripped from the ulna and retracted laterally. At this point, the radial collateral ligament is exposed and incised in a z-shaped fashion. The elbow joint is opened with slight varus stress. Now the posterior and anterior aspects of the elbow are fully exposed.

Further stripping of the anterior joint capsule from the anterior aspect of the distal humerus and the coronoid process dislocates the elbow, facilitating observation of the en-

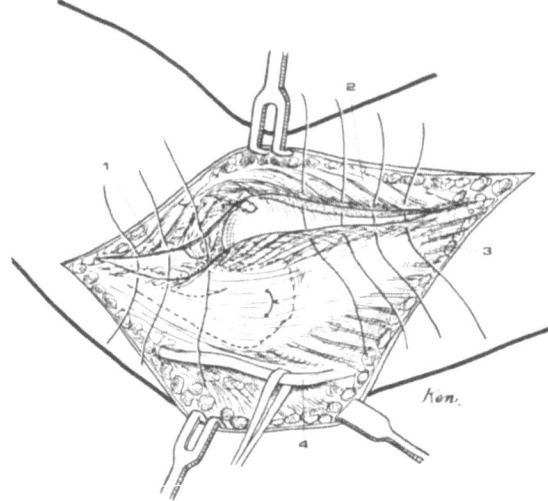

Fig. 4. - Closure of the wound. 1. Anconeus; 2. Brachioradialis; 3. Triceps; 4. Ulnar nerve.

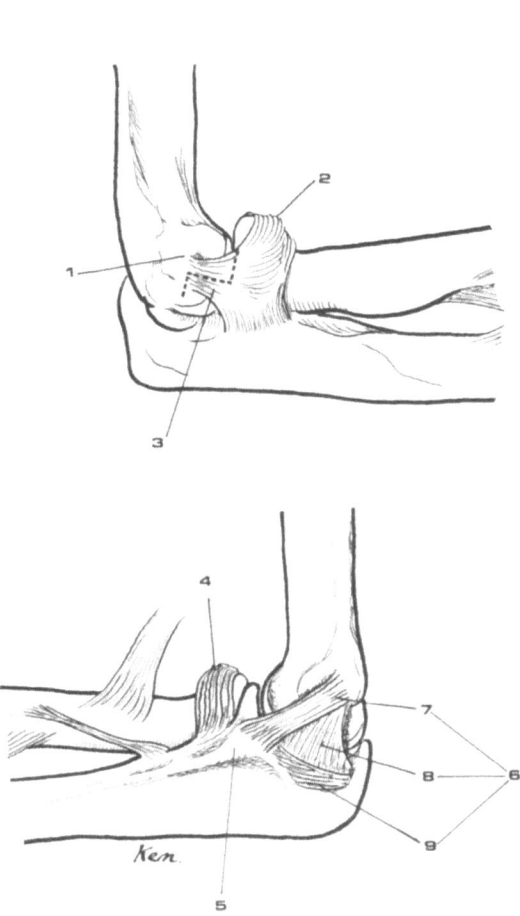

Fig. 3. - Anatomy of the ulnar and radial collateral ligaments of the elbow. 1. Lateral epicondyle; 2. Orbicular ligament; 3. Radial collateral ligament; 4. Orbicular ligament; 5. Tubercle of the coronoid process; 6. Ulnar collateral ligament; 7. Strong anterior cord-like part; 8. Weaker fan-like part; 9. Oblique part.

tire joint cavity and making it possible to remove all of the scar tissue and ossifications that impede elbow mobility. Necessary procedures can be performed under direct vision without any risk of injury to the arteries and nerves.

Figure 3 shows the anatomy of the radial and ulnar collateral ligaments. A z-shaped incision is made in the radial collateral ligament. The ulnar collateral ligament is made up of three parts: the strong anterior cord-like part, the weaker posterior fan-like part, and the oblique part. Of these, the latter two can be excised, but the anterior cord-like part should be preserved for the stability of the elbow.

After completing the necessary procedure, the tourniquet is released, haemostasis is achieved, and the wound is well-irrigated. Then, the radial collateral ligament is sutured, restoring the elbow to its normal position.

Two holes are then drilled into the tip of the olecranon, and the ulnarly retracted triceps muscle with its retaining periosteum of the olecranon is returned to its original position and sutured to the tip of the olecranon under slightly high tension (Fig 4). Finally, the periosteum and fascia of each muscle are sutured together and the wound is closed. If necessary, suction drainage should be performed.

At one time, the elbow was immobilized postoperatively in 90-degree flexion for 10

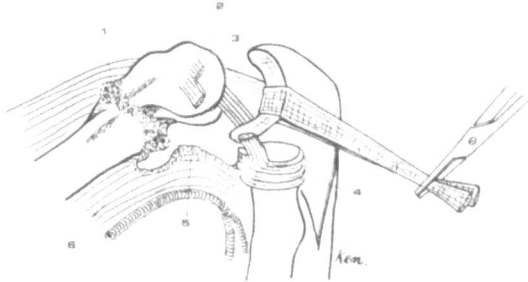

Fig. 5. - Exposure of the stiff post-traumatic elbow. 1. Bony prominence; 2. Detached radial collateral ligament; 3. Ulnar collateral ligament; 4. Orbicular ligament; 5. Scar tissue; 6. Brachialis.

days, after which active exercises were begun, but today a continuous passive motion unit is applied immediately after surgery. At the beginning, the elbow is usually moved from 45 degrees of extension to 75 degrees of flexion, then motion is increased by 10 degrees every 2-3 days, continuing for 7-10 days.

Figure 5 shows a schematic drawing of our procedure applied to the post-traumatic stiff elbow. Bony prominences on the posterior and anterior aspects of the supracondylar area are excised and the scar tissue of the anterior joint capsule is also removed until full range of elbow flexion and extension is achieved.

When performing arthroplasty using this procedure, the following points should be kept in mind:

1) Local tissue reactions such as heat, swelling, erythema, and tenderness must be minimized. X-ray pictures must be mature.

2) The biceps and triceps must be strong.

3) In intraarticular fractures, the procedure should be postponed until the bony union is satisfactory. In early cases, the stripping of soft tissues shoud be minimal.

4) Rheumatoid elbow and advanced osteoarthritic elbow are other good candidates for this procedure.

The merits of this approach are summarized as follows:

— Wide exposure can be obtained.

— No risk of jeopardizing vessels and/or nerves.

— Easy access to the joint under direct vision.

— Procedure is quite atraumatic.

— Rehabilitation can be commenced early.

— An artificial joint is not necessary. I believe that a true indication for artificial joint replacement in the elbow is very rare.

From my 20 years of experience, I can say that this procedure has many merits. I hope that it will be widely accepted and attempted so that a large number of patients may benefit from it.

REFERENCES

1) SUMIDA Y., MURAKAMI T., ADACHI N.: Elbow arthroplasty in our clinic. Selkeigeka to Saigaigeka. *Orthop. Traumatol.* 1982; **30**: 740-746.
2) TSUGE K., NAGAYAMA G.: Mobilization of the elbow joint: elbow arthroplasty. *Shujutsu* (in Japanese) 1965; **26**: 54-51.
3) TSUGE K., MURAKAMI T., YASUNAGA Y., KANAUJIA R.R.: Arthroplasty of the elbow. Twenty years' experience of a new approach. *J. Bone Jt Surg.* 1987; **69-A**: 116-120.

Post-traumatic elbow stiffness

M. Pizzetti - D. Fredella - A. Erriquez

The development of rigidity following elbow trauma is quite common and may result in severe disability.

Stiffness occurs most frequently in distal epiphyseal fractures of the humerus and in pure dislocations (Trillat and Dejour, Kerboul and Debruge, Fauvy *et al.*, etc.). It should be noted that there have been almost no reported cases of isolated stiffness during pronation-supination; thus the term "stiffness" refers exclusively to limitation of flexion-extension.

From a clinical standpoint, it is important to distinguish between stiffness caused by anatomical changes of the joint components and pure stiffness, in which the anatomical changes are minimal.

Physical therapy is quite effective in pure stiffness, yet simple conservative treatment can produce satisfactory results in cases of articular incongruity.

In some cases, the initial trauma is so violent and the reconstructive procedure so complex that elbow stiffness cannot be prevented.

The degree of stiffness is obviously an important factor in choosing the treatment and evaluating the final outcome.

This study uses the Vidal classification system (1979) (Table 1).

Table 1

Very severe stiffness	Range of motion from 180° to 150°
Severe stiffness	Range of motion from 150° to 120°
Moderate stiffness	Range of motion from 120° to 90°
Slight stiffness	Range of motion beyond 90°

Elbow stiffness should be viewed in absolute terms (stiffness in extension is very serious, while stiffness which does not allow flexion beyond 90 degrees is relatively insignificant) as well as in terms of its effect on the occupational and social life of the patient.

If the elbow is unable to extend because of stiffness, the hand loses almost all motor capability, whereas an elbow that has lost flexion capability beyond 90 degrees can still function normally in all everyday activities and most occupational activities.

In this study we have excluded the cases of severe articular incongruity in order to concentrate on cases of stiffness in which there are no significant anatomical changes in the joint components.

This study is based on 41 patients reviewed by us during the last five years, distributed as follows according to etiology (Table 2):

Table 2

Comminuted fractures	6	14.6%
Distal humeral epiphyseal fractures	12	29.2%
Olecranon fractures	5	12.2%
Pure dislocations	13	31.8%
Other trauma	5	12.2%

The patients were divided as follows according to the degree of stiffness (Table 3):

Table 3

Very severe stiffness	3	7.3%
Severe stiffness	22	53.2%
Moderate stiffness	11	27.3%
Slight stiffness	5	12.2%

The diagnosis of post-traumatic stiffness is usually made 4 months after the injury, when the three phases of rehabilitation — prophylaxis of unsatisfactory results, primary treatment, and final treatment — have been completed (Figs. 1-4).

In the elbow, prophylaxis mainly consists of making sure that immobilization is undergone with the elbow flexed to 90 degrees and the forearm in zero position.

Equally important in this stage is mobilization of the fingers, and wrist when possible. This measure helps prevent the algoneurodystrophy that sometimes complicates, especially in elderly patients, traumatic lesions of the elbow.

The biceps, triceps, supinator, and antebrachial extensor muscles must perform isotonic and isometric exercises.

Primary treatment is mainly based on physical therapy planned in phases ranging from isotonic exercises of the elbow muscles to active movement within a limited range to full active movement to the assumption of

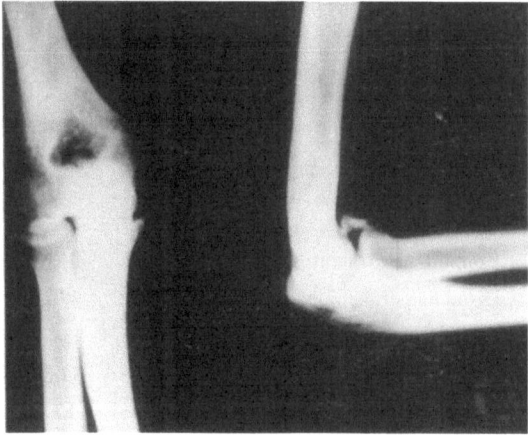

Fig. 1. - Radial head fracture.

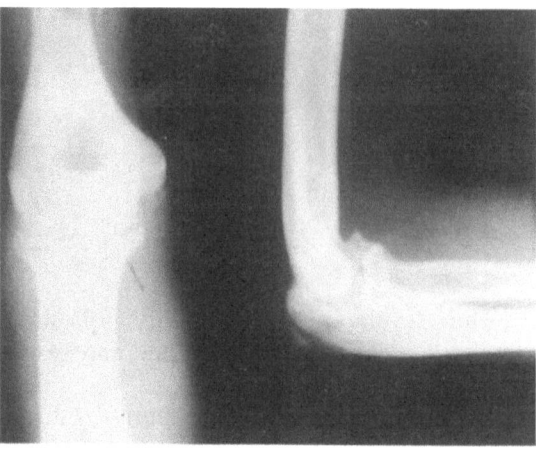

Fig. 2. - Same case as Fig. 1 with severe, rapidly evolving stiffness.

specific positions against the force of gravity for progressively longer periods.

The final treatment usually begins when fracture healing is already under way or, in cases of pure dislocation, when the capsuloligamentous lesions have healed (usually 30-40 days).

The first step in this phase is the goniometric measurement of the residual range of flexion-extension and pronation-supination in order to obtain reliable data for monitoring the process of functional recovery.

The next step is to carefully examine the tone and trophism of the biceps and triceps. As in the knee, decreased muscle tone and trophism prevent full recovery of joint function.

EMG allows precise quantitative evaluation and is very widely used in these cases.

Comparison with the contralateral elbow indicates a significant muscular deficit in the affected elbow that must be treated promptly if satisfactory functional recovery is to be attained.

This goal is usually achieved in the third and final phase of the rehabilitation program, with the use of electrical stimulation and selected resistive exercises.

Thorough application of the physical therapy techniques described above is usually enough to prevent the onset of stiffness. This complication does also depend upon the complexity of the trauma, but is too often brought on by inadequate rehabilitation.

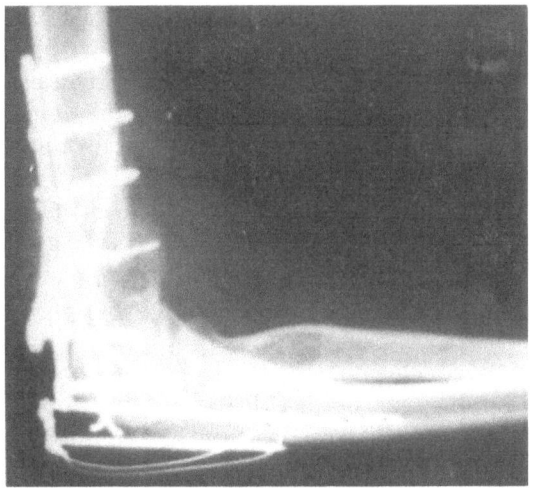

Fig. 3. - Severely comminuted fracture treated with multiple internal fixation devices.

A careful analysis of our patients' medical histories revealed that the stiffness was a result of the above iatrogenic factor in over 65% of the cases.

In this study, severe stiffness occurred in cases of either pure dislocation or complex fracture. A shoulder-hand syndrome was present in 6 cases.

The treatment program used in this study consists of the following phases:

1) Standard radiographic examination to reveal possible anatomical changes and check the calcic tone. In cases of osteoporosis (algo-neurodystrophic syndrome) the treatment varies, as will be described later.

2) Registration EMG of the biceps, triceps, supinator, and antebrachial flexor and extensor muscles to check for possible neuromuscular lesions. Once this possibility is excluded, an EMG with spectral analysis of the biceps and triceps should be taken to calculate the quantitative differences in the affected elbow compared to the contralateral elbow.

3) Electrical stimulation of the biceps and triceps. The same therapy may be used for the antebrachial extensors. Periodic exams using spectral analysis to check biceps tone and trophism.

4) If necessary, application of orthosis in order to guarantee that the degree of range of motion attained during the therapy session is maintained throughout the rest period.

5) Passive motion exercises using the hold-relax technique.

6) Hot packs to prepare for the physical therapy sessions should be applied with careful attention to the risks.

In cases complicated by a shoulder-hand syndrome, the treatment is not only longer but also intended primarily to counteract the manifestations of the syndrome (local edema and osteoporosis), in the knowledge that once these problems are overcome, the range of motion deficit would be more easily corrected. It is a well-known fact that the use of pulsed electromagnetic fields together with electrical stimulation yields satisfactory results in these cases.

EVALUATION OF THE RESULTS

Whether the patient is able to overcome the stiffness and recover a larger range of joint motion depends essentially upon two

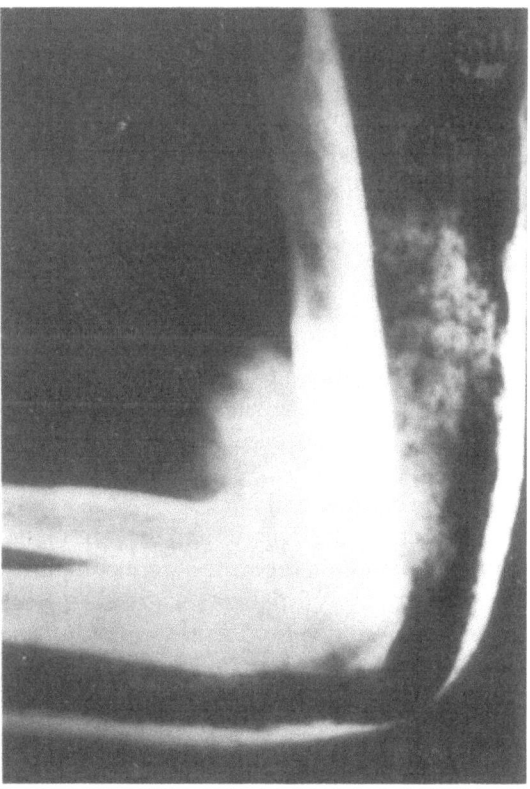

Fig. 4. - After removal of the fixation devices, the good anatomical reconstruction contrasts with the development of both extensive calcifications and severe stiffness.

factors. The first is how much time has passed since the onset of the limitation and the second is how severe the deficit is.

Good results are possible if the stiffness is treated within one year from its onset. Naturally, the greatest recoveries are achieved in the cases with the most severe limitations.

In light of these two elements, the patients of this study are divided as follows:

Table 4

Severe or very severe stiffness	Slight or moderate stiffness
26 (63.3%)	15 (37.7%)
12 onset more than 1 year before treatment	5 onset more than 1 year before treatment

In evaluating the results, it is necessary to keep in mind some basic considerations. As in other joints, it is necessary to evaluate the so-called *useful sector*, a section of the range of motion that, if functional, allows the execution of most movements.

In the elbow this sector is located between 90 and 160 degrees.

The recovery of range of motion on either side of this sector should always be sought, but coming up short of complete recovery should not be considered failure, since several authors (Meziaire *et al.*) refer to these extreme degrees of range of motion as the *luxury sector*.

On the other hand, an evaluation based solely on the amount of range of motion recovered can be deceiving, because even if a large range is recovered (which usually happens in the most severe cases), it might not include the entire *useful* range.

Therefore, the degrees and the percentage of range of motion recovered were compared.

None of the 26 patients with severe stiffness had motion in the *useful sector*. Of these, 14 had slight mobility. In 13 cases the stiffness lasted for 10-14 months.

The average recovery of range of motion was 60 degrees (40%). In 4 cases the recovery

was insignificant and arthrolysis was prescribed.

Overall, of the 22 cases of successful use of physical therapy, 18 regained the *useful sector* of motion. The average period of ambulatory physical therapy was 7 weeks.

The 15 patients with moderate or slight stiffness had motion in the *useful sector*. Seven patients even regained the *luxury sector*, and 8 patients increased their range of motion by 22%.

In conclusion, elbow stiffness is highly undesirable, can be disabling, and may appear even after correct conservative and surgical treatment.

Unsatisfactory results are often due to failure to do physical therapy as part of the prophylaxis, the primary treatment, and the final treatment, resulting in the complication of lesions whose functional recovery should be certain.

As proof of this are the cases in which the anatomical reconstruction of the elbow was imperfect, yet the functional result was quite good.

Furthermore, in terms of functional recovery, radiographic study has an entirely relative value. Elbows that radiographically show anatomical changes may have negligible functional limitation and vice versa − elbows with normal radiographs may develop severe stiffness.

This observation forces us to shift our attention to other well-known factors, such as capsuloligamentous trophism and elasticity, both of which should respond to a well-executed physical therapy program.

Less well-known perhaps is the importance of the muscle factor, primarily that of the biceps. A spectral analysis of the elbow muscles supports this observation, confirming that the best functional results are achieved in cases where physical therapy is aimed toward recovery of muscle tone and trophism. As a matter of fact, excellent recovery coincided with the moment in which the spectral analysis of the biceps of the affected elbow matched that of the healthy contralateral one.

REFERENCES

1) BRODEUR A.E., SILBERSTEIN M.J., GRAVISS E.R., LUISIRI A.: The basic tenets for appropriate evaluation of the elbow in pediatrics. *Curr. Proble. Diag., Radiol.* Sept.-Oct. 1983; **12**: 1-29.

2) COTHAY D.M.: Injury to the lower medial epiphysis of the humerus bofore development of the ossific centre. Report of a case. *J. Bone Jt Surg.* 1967; **49-B** (4): 766-767.

3) DELEE J.C., WILKINS K.E., ROCKOOD C.A.: Fracture separation of distal humeral epiphysis. *J. Bone Jt Surg.* 1980; **62-A**: 46-51.

4) DIXON R.A.: Reversed dynamic slings. A new concept in the treatment of post-traumatic elbow flexion contractures. *Injury* 1976; **8**; 35-38.

5) GREEN D.P., MC COY H.: Turnbuckle orthotic correction of elbow flexion contractures after acute injuries. *J. Bone Jt Surg.* 1979; **61-A**: 1092-1095.

6) HANSEN P.E., BARNES D.A., TULLOS H.S.: Case report of arthrographic diagnosis of an injury pattern in the distal humerus of an infant. *J. Pediat. Orthop.* 1982; **2**: 569-572.

7) HOLDA M.E., MANOLI A., II, LA MONT R.L.: Ephiphyseal separation of the distal end of the humerus with medial displacement. *J. Bone Jt Surg.* 1980; **62-A**: 52-57.

8) PIZZETTI M., CARUSO I.: *Medicina fisica e riabilitazione..* Ed. Lombardo, Roma, 1987.

9) ROBACK D.L.: Elbow arthrography: brief technical considerations. *Clin. Radiol.* 1979; **30**: 311-312.

10) KNAPP M.E.: Physical therapy in fractures about elbow joint (read at the annual session at Cleveland, Ohio — Sept. 3 1940) *Arch. Phys. Ther.* 1940; **21**: 709-715.

11) WILSON P.D.: Capsulectomy for relief of flexion contractures of the elbow following fracture. *J. Bone Jt Surg.* 1944; **26**: 71-86.

Conclusions

L. Perugia

The elbow is among the orthopedist's most "difficult" joints for many reasons. It is a relatively small joint, in reality made up of three separate joints that are structurally different from one another: the humeroulnar is a hinge joint, the humeroradial a gliding joint, and the proximal radioulnar a pivot joint. Furthermore, the most important of the three, the humeroulnar joint, has a peculiar anatomical configuration that makes it anatomically complex and functionally simple only in appearance, while the humeroradial joint has a functional role not only in flexion and extension, but especially in the sophisticated movements of forearm pronation and supination. It must also be kept in mind that important vascular and neural structures run through the elbow area, making it very susceptible to neurovascular complications accompanying or following elbow fractures.

Despite its anatomical and functional complexity, the elbow was relatively neglected by orthopedists for quite a long time. This neglect was probably due to the fact that complete functional recovery of a joint in the upper limb does not possess the urgency of complete functional recovery of a weight-bearing joint. In the last decade, however, the proliferation and diversification of scientific interests together with a greater demand for physical well-being, which can be considered a reflection of growing social and economic affluence, has brought increased attention even to the least vital sectors of the medical field. The result for the field of orthopedics and traumatology was a rigorous reevaluation of the upper limb, initially involving the shoulder and increasingly incorporating the elbow. This volume is a result of this growing interest.

This text, which begins with the structural and functional anatomy of the elbow, analyzes the various aspects of traumatic lesions of this joint, including diseases of the soft tissue and the rare lesions of the musculocutaneous nerve. The most attention, however, is justly given to fractures, which are evaluated in both the short and long term. Traumatic lesions of the elbow pose many problems, all of which deserve close attention. Some aspects, however, demand particular consideration because of the long-term residual effects, the complexity and difficulty of treatment, the old or new problems they present, or the interest that the recent therapeutical progress stimulates. These are the themes that I intend to probe in order to emphasize the most modern and interesting aspects.

In children, supracondylar fractures are the most common traumatic injuries. These fractures do not usually pose particular problems as far as therapeutic indication, since conservative treatment is always preferred for slightly displaced or reducible fractures, while fractures that are irreducible and/or accompanied by neurovascular lesions usually require surgical treatment. Such fractures, however, can severely damage the growth cartilage, pathologically altering bone growth and thereby causing varying degrees of axial deviation of the elbow. Thanks to recent studies, those of our institution included, it has been shown that there is no connection between degree of fracture displacement or accuracy of reduction and extent of possible axial deviation of the distal humerus. In other words, any supracondylar fracture can cause axial deviation severe enough to require osteotomy. Yet not only for this reason is the elbow of the child one of the most difficult areas for the orthopedist. In infants, an accurate evaluation of the traumatic lesions and the shifting of the growth plates may be very difficult, especially when these are entirely or almost entirely composed of cartilaginous tissue. On the other hand, traumatic lesions of these plates during any stage of growth can cause severe and possibly irreparable growth disturbances in the elbow. These facts should convince orthopedists to conduct very careful evaluations of injured elbows in children, so as to prevent diagnostic errors that can cause irreparable lesions.

In recent years motor vehicle accidents have become a common cause of severe trauma, responsible for fractures that are at times very complex. The elbow, and particularly the distal humerus, is among the areas most susceptible to multiple, severely displaced fractures that require the orthopedist's maximum effort to achieve a satisfactory functional result. This is only possible through anatomical reconstruction of the articular surfaces as well as stable internal fixation that allows very early joint mobilization. This text contains two very interesting articles dealing with such fractures. Both emphasize the need for a posterior approach, a solid fixation using epiphyseal screws and either tubular or T-shaped dia-epiphyseal plates, and the avoidance of temporary fixation devices, such as Kirschner wires, that can put off functional rehabilitation. Adhering to these guidelines is the only way to achieve a satisfactory result, even if it is not as good as the effort required by this surgery deserves.

Radial head fractures are among the most common fractures in the elbow region. Undisplaced fractures do not usually create therapeutical problems, while displaced and/or comminuted fractures usually require surgical treatment, that in adults may consist of either simple resection or prosthetic replacement of the radial head. This is a classic dilemma of elbow surgery. Prosthetic replacement restores the normal length of the bone and thus prevents instability of the proximal radioulnar joint as well as proximal subluxation of the radius at the distal radioulnar joint, both consequences of radial head resection. This text contains two chapters that contribute significantly to the resolution of this dilemma. The prosthesis guarantees good clinical results at least over the short and middle term. Over the long-term, however, degeneration of the prosthesis is frequently observed in the

form of crepitation and fragmentation or detachment of the stem, this in addition to degenerative phenomena of the capitulum humeri. Even though radial head resection often causes distal radioulnar subluxation, it for the most part yields satisfactory clinical results that appear stable over time. These findings clearly indicate radial head resection as the treatment of choice, since prosthetic replacement exposes the elbow to inconveniences as well as the risk of reoperation to remove the prosthesis; these negative aspects of prosthetic replacement are not balanced by the advantages, which are more theoretical than practical.

Pure dislocation is another common traumatic syndrome of the elbow, which unlike other lesions has not received the attention it deserves until recently. Dislocation is considered a minor problem, yet it often results in reduced elbow mobility and/or periarticular calcifications, joint instability, and long-term degenerative arthritis, found to varying extents in almost half of the patients with elbow dislocation. In recent years several studies, including the one by Patella et al., have reported a direct correlation between duration of immobilization and extent of residual articular deficit. This finding should lead to a reduction of the classic period of immobilization from 20 days to 10-12 days, also considering the fact that prolonged immobilization does not guarantee stability. Rapid mobilization, on the other hand, even has a positive effect on the calcifications, which in our experience and that of other authors seem to develop in fewer cases when the period of immobilization is less than two weeks.

In the elbow, loss of mobility is almost inevitable in injuries whose treatment has yielded unsatisfactory results; most unsatisfactory results are regarded as such exclusively due to the loss of mobility. In other words, while therapeutical failure for most joints consists of the persistence of pain, for the elbow, stiffness is the element that most often causes the unsatisfactory rating. This is the reason why arthrolysis plays such an important role in the treatment of elbow lesions. The advent of arthroscopic surgery has certainly opened up new possibilities in this area of joint disease. In the elbow, however, arthroscopic arthrolysis does not seem to guarantee the same satisfactory results obtained in other joints such as the shoulder and the knee. Therefore, arthroscopic arthrolysis should be reserved for selected cases and substituted with open management when the stiffness is severe and persistent. This procedure, however, is also susceptible to complete or partial failure. From this point of view, the operation proposed by Kenya Tsuge is very interesting, but there is not yet enough data to support its validity. In my opinion, this is one of the areas of elbow disease that most needs research, so that orthopedists will be able to prescribe either arthroscopic or open management that is less vulnerable to failure.

The same considerations apply for total elbow arthroplasty, which has not yet reached that high degree of reliability that has been achieved in other joints. There are two reasons for this: the first is the field of bioengineering's relative lack of attention for elbow prostheses because of their infrequent use; the second is the anatomical complexity of the elbow along with the structural features of the distal humerus, which, because of the reduced thickness and the essentially cortical structure of the bone, make implantation difficult and stability of both cemented and cementless prostheses problematic. However, in the last decade qualitative progress has been made in the field of elbow replacement-thanks to the invention of unconstrained prostheses, which in most cases have replaced the old hinged prostheses which were almost guaranteed to loosen shortly after implantation. The most recently conceived prostheses can be implanted with fewer unknowns regarding long-term results, and thus are highly indicated for use in traumatic syndromes of the elbow, that is, in patients who are often quite young. As stressed by Souter, however, the indications in this area are relatively limited and, most importantly, the prosthetic implantation must be planned and executed very carefully by a surgeon with experience in this procedure on elbows with rheumatoid arthritis.